MINDFUL HEROES

STORIES OF JOURNEYS THAT CHANGED LIVES

EDITED BY

Terry Barrett,
Vin Harris and
Graeme Nixon

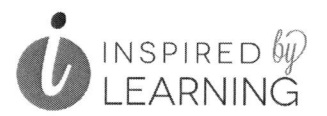

INSPIRED by LEARNING

MINDFUL HEROES:
STORIES OF JOURNEYS THAT CHANGED LIVES

Edited by Terry Barrett, Vin Harris and Graeme Nixon

Published by Inspired By Learning, Aberdeen, Scotland, UK

© Terry Barrett, Vin Harris and Graeme Nixon
Attribution-NonCommercial-NoDerivatives 4.0 International (CC BY-NC-ND 4.0)

This is a human-readable summary of (and not a substitute for) the license. Disclaimer.

You are free to:

- **Share** – copy and redistribute the material in any medium or format
- The licensor cannot revoke these freedoms as long as you follow the license terms.

Under the following terms:

- **Attribution** – You must give appropriate credit, provide a link to the license, and indicate if changes were made. You may do so in any reasonable manner, but not in any way that suggests the licensor endorses you or your use.
- **NonCommercial** – You may not use the material for commercial purposes.
- **NoDerivatives** – If you remix, transform, or build upon the material, you may not distribute the modified material.
- **No additional restrictions** – You may not apply legal terms or technological measures that legally restrict others from doing anything the license permits.

Notices:

- You do not have to comply with the license for elements of the material in the public domain or where your use is permitted by an applicable exception or limitation.
- No warranties are given. The license may not give you all of the permissions necessary for your intended use. For example, other rights such as publicity, privacy, or moral rights may limit how you use the material.

How to cite this book:
Barrett, T., Harris, V., Nixon, G. (Editors) (2019) Mindful Heroes: Stories of Journeys that Changed Lives. Aberdeen, Scotland: Inspired By Learning.

Find us on the web and order eBook or paperback at www.inspiredbylearning.eu
Paperback also available from Samye Ling Bookshop https://www.samyelingshop.com/
Cover and Text Design, Graphics and Formatting by Maja Petrović, Zagreb, Croatia
Cover artwork by Colin Curbishley contact through http://www.shallal.org.uk/
Design consultancy and support by Jacky Seery
Printed by Book Printing UK, Remus House, Coltsfoot Drive, Woodston, Peterborough PE2 9BF

ISBN (Paperback): 978-1-909876-11-8

ACKNOWLEDGEMENTS

We would like to thank the mindful heroes for sharing their stories of developing their mindfulness practice together with developing mindfulness and compassion initiatives in professional and community settings. We are grateful to the Mindfulness Association for their encouragement and support in producing this book. We appreciate the professional guidance, commitment and attention to detail of David McMurtry from Inspired by Learning. Maja Petrović has done a wonderful job of the design, formatting and graphics that really present these stories in an appealing and engaging manner. The front cover artwork by Colin Curbishley is very inspiring. Thank you to Jacky Seery for design consultancy and support.

DEDICATION

We dedicate this book that it may inspire individuals and groups to develop their mindfulness and compassion. The royalties of this book are going to the Everyone Project which supports groups who may not otherwise have the opportunity to participate in mindfulness courses.
www.everyoneproject.org

Terry Barrett, Vin Harris and Graeme Nixon (Editors).

TABLE OF CONTENTS

Section 1 Mindful Heroes
1. Mindful Heroes Stories: An Introduction - Terry Barrett and Donald Gordon — 1
2. The Journey of Mindful Heroes - Vin Harris — 9
3. Masters in Mindfulness: Compassion and Insight Applied to Multiple Lives and Professions - Graeme Nixon — 25

Section 2 Stories of Mindful Heroes in Educational Settings
4. Introduction to Stories of Mindful Heroes in Educational Settings - Terry Hyland — 37
5. As the Stars Align: Effects of Mindfulness on Children with Autism Spectrum Disorder (ASC) - Donald Gordon — 41
6. Dragons and Weebles: Mindfulness with Adolescents - Heather Grace Bond — 59
7. Combining Poetry and Mindfulness: Stories of Creating New Spaces in Higher Education -Terry Barrett, Naomi McAreavey and Larry McNutt — 73

Section 3 Stories of Mindful Heroes in Health Settings
8. Introduction to Stories of Mindful Heroes in Health Settings - Paul D'Alton — 91
9. The Road Taken: Exploring lived experiences of mindfulness in people on substance recovery journey - Jana Neumannova — 93
10. Finding my Bliss: Top tips for introducing mindfulness to healthcare staff - Ian Rigg — 107
11. Doing what needs to be done: mindful compassion training for nurses - Gavin Cullen — 121

Section 4 Stories of Mindful Heroes in Business Settings
12. Introduction to Stories of Mindful Heroes in Business Settings - Joanne O' Malley — 139
13. Is there Time for Mindfulness in Business? Making the case for a healthier approach to time management - Susan Grandfield — 143
14. Lost in Work: My Story of Recovery - Tarja Gordienko — 157

Section 5 Stories of Mindful Heroes in Sport Settings
15. Introduction to Stories of Mindful Heroes in Sports Settings - Karl Morris — 171
16. Mindful Learning and Coaching in Alpine Skiing - John Arnold — 175
17. Its Golf....but not as we know it: Golf as a mindfulness practice and a metaphor for life - Vin Harris — 189
18. The Mindful Curling Olympic Team - Misha Botting — 203

Section 6 Stories of Mindful Heroes in Creative Arts Settings
19. Introduction to Stories of Mindful Heroes in Creative Arts Settings - Sarah Moore (Fitzgerald) — 217
20. Dare to Create! Meditation, Insight and Creative Processes in Music - Susanne Olbrich — 219
21. Heroes of the Stage: Connecting with the Joy of Performing - David Waring — 235

Section 7 Stories of Mindful Heroes in Community Settings
22. Introduction to Stories of Mindful Heroes in Community Settings - Jane Negrych — 251
23. The Autobiography of a Mindfulness Community in Eight Short Chapters - John Darwin — 255
24. Turning Empathic Distress into Compassion – A Hero's Journey for Family Carers - Jacky Seery — 271
25. The Mindfulness for Everyone Project - Vin Harris, Alan Hughes and Julie McColl. — 287

CHAPTER 1

MINDFUL HEROES STORIES: AN INTRODUCTION

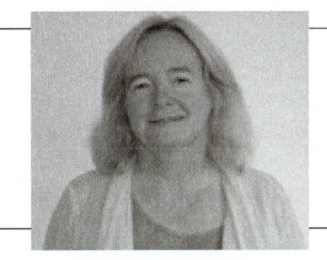

Terry Barrett

terry.barrett@ucd.ie
terrybarrett500@hotmail.com

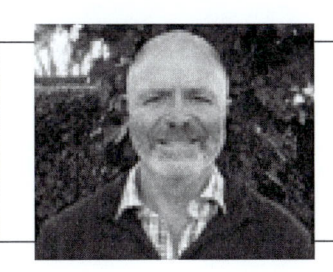

Donald Gordon

dm.gordon@btinternet.com

WHAT IS THIS BOOK ABOUT?

STORIES OF MINDFUL HEROES

Everyone loves stories. This book tells the stories of a constellation of mindful heroes. This book is about mindful heroes: ordinary people, like you and me, who followed the path of mindfulness and went on a hero's journey. These mindful heroes developed their own personal mindfulness practice together with studying mindfulness. They benefited from their growth in mindful awareness, compassion for self and others and insight. Then they wanted to share this and provide others with the opportunity to develop their potential in their own ways. On their journeys they changed their own and sometimes others' lives. They share their stories of their personal and professional journeys with you.

> Human beings need stories. From our very earliest years, it's how we make sense of the world. These days, given that we're bombarded with fragments of information from everywhere, it seems to me that we need complete, complex stories more than we ever have before (Moore Fitzgerald 2014a).

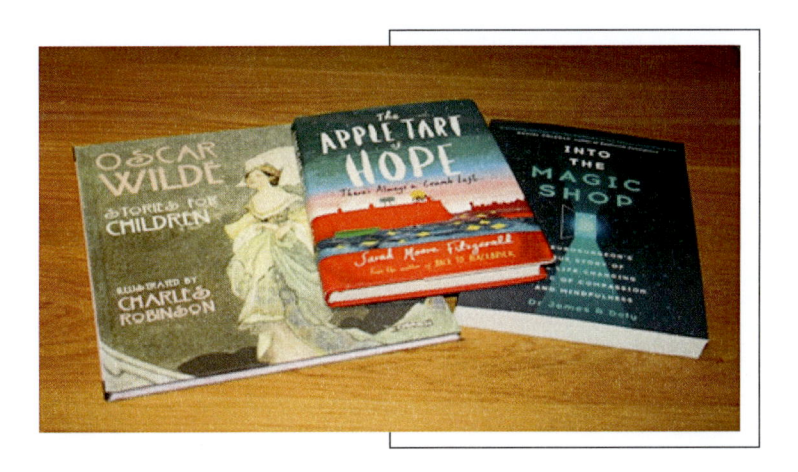

Figure 1: Storybooks for people of all ages (Wilde, 2015; Moore Fitzgerald, 2014b; Doty, 2016). Photo: © Terry Barrett 2018

WHAT IS MINDFULNESS?

John Kabat-Zinn's (1994) classical definition of mindfulness is "paying attention in a particular way; on purpose, in the present moment, and non-judgmentally" (p.4). It combines the intention to be attentive with an attitude of self-compassion. There are both formal and informal mindfulness practices. Formal mindfulness is meditation practices like mindfulness of breath where we give attention to our breath going in and out of our bodies, and bodyscan where we give attention to the sensations in each part of our body in turn starting with our toes and ending with the tops of our heads. Informal mindfulness practice is giving non-judgemental attention to the activities of daily life: having a shower, drinking a cup of tea, going for a walk or reading a chapter of a book. The five facets of mindfulness are observing, describing, acting with awareness, non-judging of inner experience (our thoughts and emotions), and non-reactivity to inner experience, (Baer et al., 2006). The idea of mindfulness is explored further in Chapters 2 and 3.

WHY READ THIS BOOK?

THE HERO'S JOURNEY

This is the first book on mindfulness to adopt a Hero's Journey approach. The reason why we chose this theme is that the Hero's Journey helps us to make sense of and give meaning to the challenges and opportunities, the dragons and the angels, the quests and adventures we experience in our lives. This archetype story resonates with the inner hero in many women and men. This book is inspired by Joseph Campbell's Hero's Journey (1949). At the start of the Hero's Journey, the hero has a crisis, a challenge or a feeling that all is not right or a call to adventure. The hero goes to a new world where challenges are faced with the help of new resources, people and learning. When the hero returns to the old world there is a natural wish to share the treasures found in the new world with others. The hero returns to the world of the familiar with a motivation of applying the insights, skills and actions to making the world a better place. Batman, Luke Skywalker in Return of the Jedi, Neo in The Matrix and Elizabeth Gilbert in Eat, Pray, Love are all archetypal heroes who spring to mind. Religious traditions also have their own real-life heroes who made this journey: Mohammad, Jesus, Mary (Our Lady), the Buddha and Kisa Gotami all left the world of the familiar, journeyed into unfamiliar territory and eventually returned to be of service in improving the human condition. Mindfulness practitioners and writers have shared the fruits of their journey with us including Sharon Salzberg, Pema Chodron, Tara Brach, Ruby Wax, John Kabat-Zinn and Jack Kornfield. Many poets in their poems distil the wisdom from their heroic travels including Mary Oliver's The Journey and Seamus Heaney's Digging. Hero stories are not primarily about the person in the story but more about re-invigorating the heroic response in readers. The mindful heroes in this book engaged in an ongoing process of developing a personal mindfulness practice, learning about the human condition, along with developing the courage and commitment needed in moving towards authentic expressions of mindfulness. For example, Susanne Olbrich in Chapter 20 discusses:

> how long-term mindfulness practice has played an important part in liberating my creative energy as a musician. Additionally, mindfulness has found its way into my work in many ways big and small. When I do my accounts or book concerts, when I perform, prepare a workshop or speak with piano pupils' parents, when I work on a new piece of music or rehearse with other musicians, my intention and practice is to do so with presence and heart: to care, to notice, and to be fully alive in the process.

EXPRESSIONS OF MINDFULNESS IN PROFESSIONAL AND COMMUNITY SETTINGS

The authentic expressions of mindfulness presented by authors of the chapters from 10 different countries in this book, are about how they creatively applied mindfulness together with other approaches to a variety of settings across Education, Health, Business, Sport, Creative Arts and Community Work. The emphasis in these stories is on developing potential as well as working with pathology. The purpose of the book is to inspire and engage others in: exploring mindfulness, developing their personal mindfulness practice, applying mindfulness, compassion and insight to different professional and community settings and learning from recent research. The authors (or lead authors) of these chapters were postgraduate students, well established in their professional careers, who chose to study on a MSc Programme in Studies in Mindfulness. The University of Aberdeen in partnership with the Mindfulness Association provides an MSc Studies in Mindfulness Programme. This programme combines the development of personal mindfulness practice with the design and facilitation of mindfulness initiatives in professional and community settings together with reviewing and contributing to current research in this field. The authors draw on their work-based projects or professional enquiries completed as part of this programme to share with you what they have learnt. In Chapter 24 Jacky Seery who was a family carer herself talks about the course she gave to a group of family carers that combined mindfulness, compassion and Qigong movement:

> The greatest – and totally unexpected - gift I received on this exceptionally rewarding journey came about when I began to share the juicy, sweet fruits of my training in mindfulness and compassion with a small group of highly stressed family carers. The very act of opening my heart to these unsung caring heroines and then extending heartfelt compassion to them contributed so much to my own long-term healing and overall sense of wellbeing and fulfilment in life.

Some chapters in this book are about teaching the Mindfulness Based Living Course (MBLC) designed by the Mindfulness Association e.g. Chapter 25 The Mindfulness for Everyomne Project. A larger number of chapters are about adapting the MBLC course and creatively combining it with other approaches to meet the needs of particular groups. Two examples of chapters of this type are Chapter 6 Dragons and Weebles: Mindfulness with Adolescents and Chapter 24 Turning Empathic Distress into Compassion: A Hero's Journey for Family Carers. The largest number of chapters are not about teaching mindfulness but about sensitively and confidently adapting mindfulness, compassion and insight approaches in integrated ways in professional and community settings. Two examples of these types of chapters are Chapter 7 Combining Poetry and Mindfulness: Stories of Creating New Spaces in Higher Education and Chapter 14 Lost in Work: My Story of Recovery.

HOW THE BOOK BEGAN AND HOW WE WROTE IT?

Terry finished her Postgraduate Diploma in Studies in Mindfulness. Later she spent a summer weeklong retreat on Holy Isle, a small island in Scotland. And that is when the book began…….

Touch of spray of wave on my face
Steady myself on the small rubber boat.
Feel the magic of the tiny island of Holy Isle
A calm so deep after a week retreat.
Heather asks: "Will you edit a book for us?"
I respond: "Yes."

See the large island of Arran from the big boat
As we voyage towards the mainland.
Have an insight to ask Vin and Graeme to be co-editors.
See the gap between what I do and who I am
Get smaller and smaller.

The book comes alive at the writers' retreat.
Clink of glasses to toast its head and heart.
The buzz of peer review
The laughter of camaraderie.
The silence of meditation
And of mindful walking snake-like
in the Eskdalemuir countryside.

Feel the heartfulness of the heroes' stories.
Sense the growth from personal practice
To creation of places and spaces
for others to develop in their own ways.
Bear witness to the tapestry
and textures of emotions,
research and actions.
Tired but happy as I edit another chapter
in Neidin, my little nest.

Touch of spray of wave on my face
Steady myself on the small rubber boat.
With Holy Isle behind us now again
In my mind's eye I see people reading,
Glimpsing a common humanity.
Noticing flashes of inspiration.
Spotting their own possibilities
For voyages of adventure and discovery.

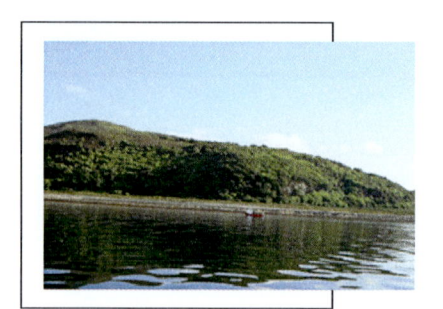

Figure 2: The Mindful Heroes Book by Terry Barrett
Photo Holy Isle from the water © Terry Barrett 2018

We saw writing this book as a practice of mindfulness, compassion and insight. As editors we meditated together in silence at the start of our initial meetings about the vision, purpose and theme of the book and at the start of all subsequent meetings. We worked together to facilitate a writers' retreat for book chapter authors in a community centre in the countryside in Scotland. This combined discussing the mindful hero theme of the book, peer-reviewing the first draft of our chapters in groups, blocks of writing time, doing mindfulness practices, enjoying good company and the Scottish countryside and celebrating the start of our book.

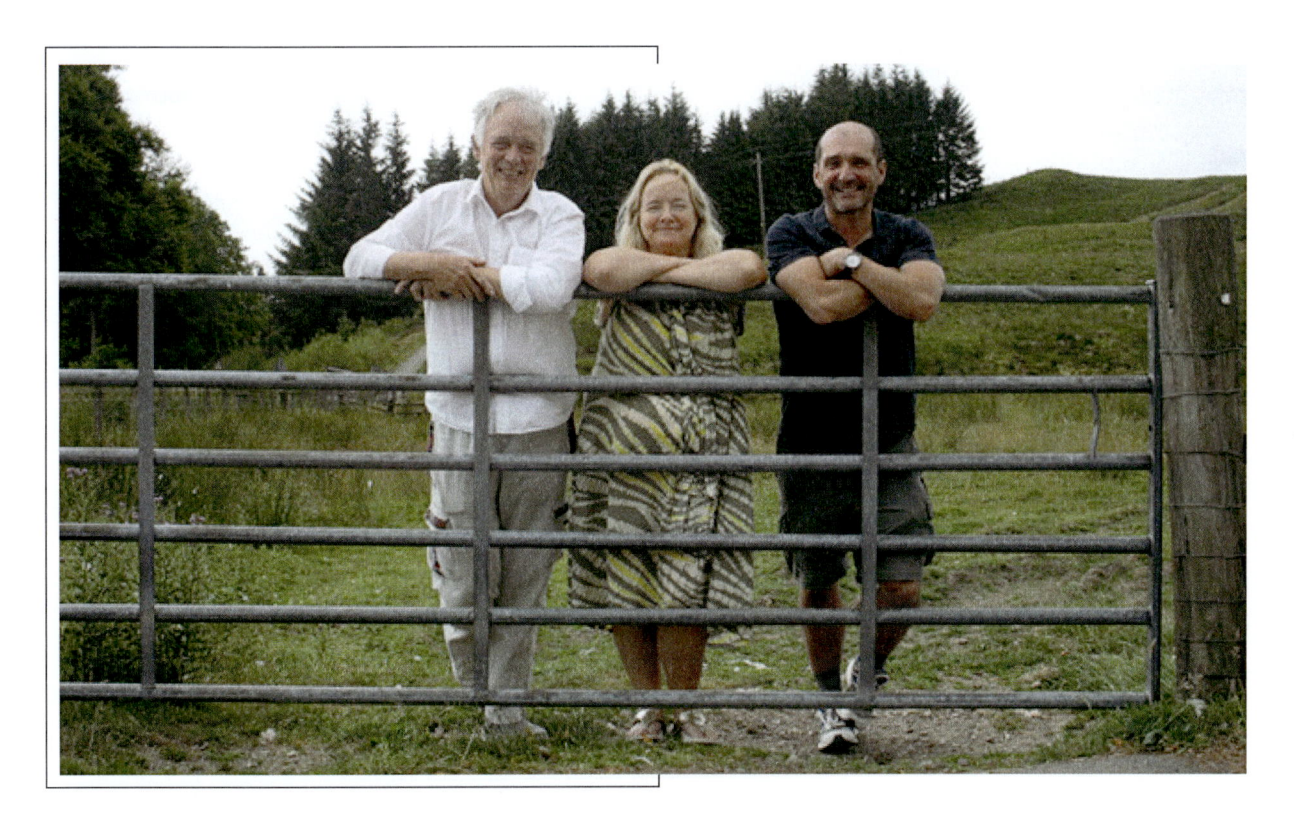

Figure 3: The Editors Vin Harris, Terry Barrett and Graeme Nixon at the writers' retreat in Scotland Photo © Terry Barrett 2018

In this retreat authors got insights for their chapters from: discussing them with peers, silent writing and mindfulness practices. We tried to be self-compassionate as we were kind to ourselves in realising that a first draft was just that, and the nature of writing is re-writing and with time, feedback and hard work we would arrive at a chapter we would be happy to share with the public.

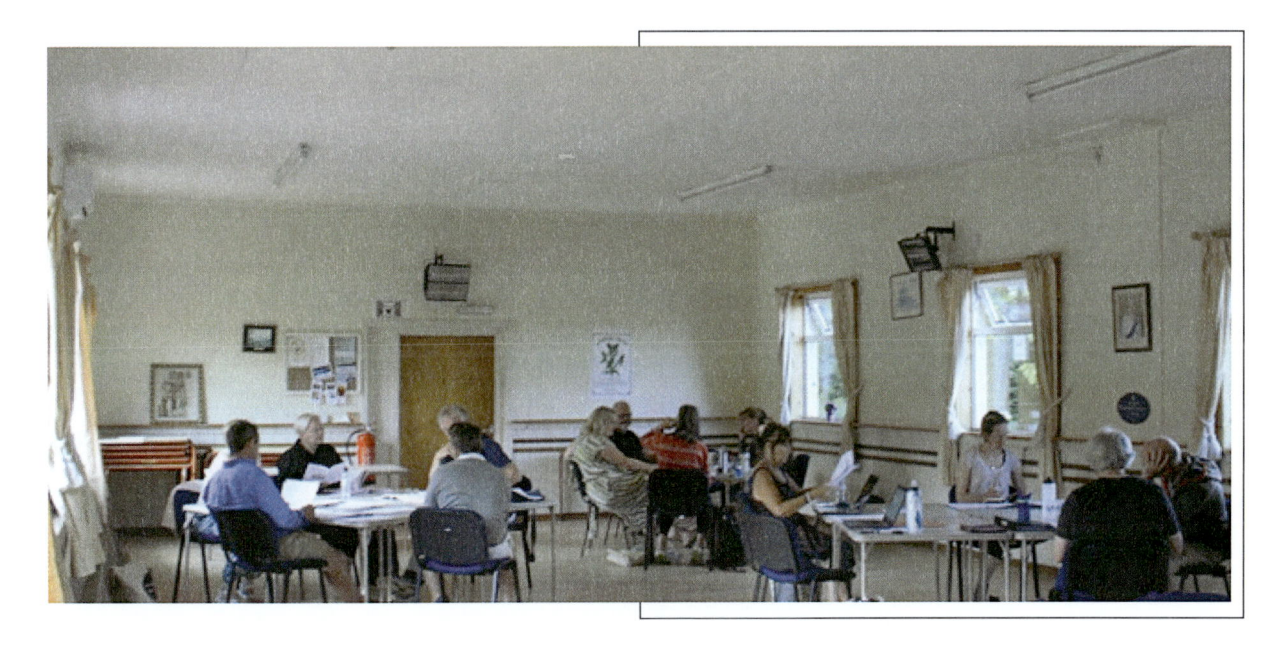

Figure 4: Three groups peer reviewing first drafts of chapters at the writers' retreat Photo: © Terry Barrett 2018

We also tried to be compassionate to you the reader, writing in accessible ways and finding ways to engage you with the chapters that value your experiences and your stories. This book is very much a collective enterprise as together we helped it to take shape. Conversations in groups and pairs helped us to tell our stories.

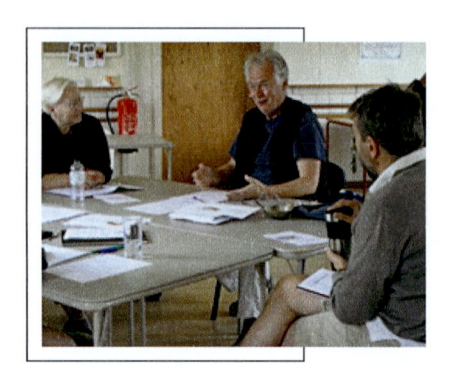

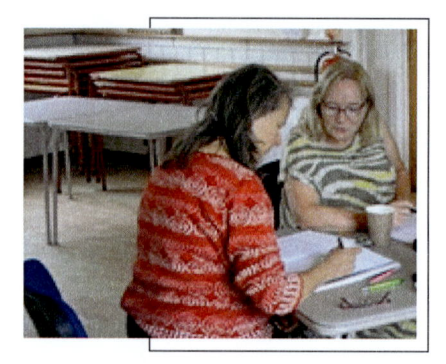

Figure 5: Book conversations at the writers' retreat Photos: © Terry Barrett 2018

By the end of the retreat we had a real sense of writing "our" book together. We look forward to it being read worldwide, and we have given you our e-mail addresses so the conversations can continue. And now that we have finished the book, we look forward to book launches, reunions, conferences and workshops in different countries.

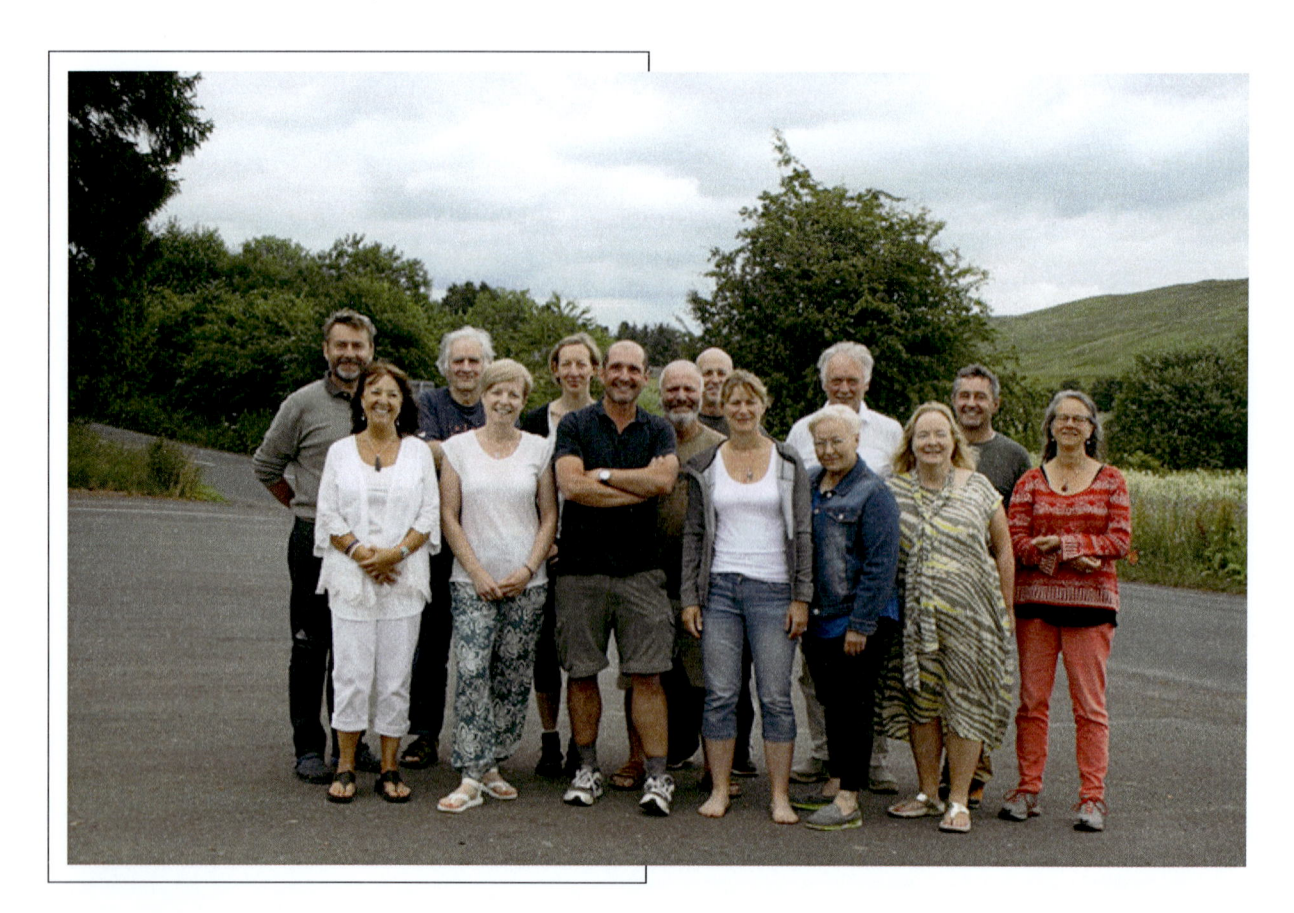

Figure 6: The authors at the writers' retreat Photo © Terry Barrett 2018

HOW TO READ THIS BOOK?

Having read this introduction we strongly recommend that you read the next two chapters (Chapter 2 The Journey of Mindful Heroes and Chapter 3 Masters in Mindfulness: Compassion and Insight Applied to Multiple Lives and Professions) first. These two chapters set the scene for the rest of the book. In Chapter 2, much like the archetypal hero, Vin Harris contends that all Mindful Heroes, in one way or another, go through four recognisable stages, namely Departure, Descent, Initiation and finally the Return where the mindful hero shares the gifts learned in helping others to live in mindful and meaningful ways. He discusses how the journey from doing to being, in becoming more mindful, actually comprises journeys within journeys or circles within circles in returning time and again to relating to our experiences with mindful awareness. In Chapter 3, Graeme Nixon explores the blend of experiential and academic learning in this MSc Studies in Mindfulness programme. The MSc represents a graduated approach covering interlinked practices in mindfulness, compassion and insight that allow participants to see, hold and relate to the workings of their inner environment with spaciousness, warmth and perspective. Graeme provides a thoughtful consideration of the causes and conditions that have given rise to the growth of secular mindfulness in modern society, touching on the imperatives of becoming more aware, more compassionate, and the need to find meaning and fulfilment in life.

Having read the three introductory chapters, then choose whichever of the stories of the Mindful Heroes that you are most drawn to reading first. Pick the section which interests you the most: Education, Health, Business, Sport, Creative Arts or Community Work. In reading these chapters, you are invited to reflect on two interlinked aspects of the hero's journey, namely, the process involved in personal transformation in following the path of mindfulness, and how the journey translates into expressions in everyday life and work. In many ways, these expressions mark the Return in the journey. The first chapter in each of these sections is an introductory chapter. In this chapter a specialist in the particular field responds to the chapters in the section and makes links between these chapters and their own practice, research and writing together with current issues in the field.

In each chapter there are invitations for you to Pause and engage personally with the ideas and stories of the chapter. As a reader you are invited to engage in a variety of formal mindfulness meditation practices as part of your engagement with the chapters in this book, and you will see these Pause and Practice opportunities. There are opportunities to: Pause and Reflect on questions on how this chapter relates to you and your stories, Pause and Watch video clips and Pause and Listen to audio clips. You can choose to take up these invitations to stop, slow down and connect your experiences to the experiences in these chapters or read the chapter straight through and return to these reflective opportunities later. At the end of each chapter there is a Further Resources section which provides you with links to various resources to explore the topic further.

The book itself may also be seen as a Return and it is hoped that readers find some benefit in making their own lives and those with whom they come into contact that little bit happier, and be inspired and helped in leading meaningful, free lives. The royalties from the book will go towards supporting the work of The Everyone Project. This project supports the teaching of mindfulness courses to groups of people who may not otherwise have access to these opportunities. These groups include carers, those recovering from addiction, asylum seekers and young people, adults and elderly people on low incomes. You can read more about the Everyone Project in Chapter 25.

May this book contribute to you reducing suffering and the causes of suffering and increasing happiness and the causes of happiness. May you experience true joy!

FURTHER RESOURCES

Holy Isle
Centre for World Peace and Health
(Retreats and Courses).
http://www.holyisle.org
Joseph Campbell Foundation
https://www.jcf.org/
The Mindfulness Association
http://www.mindfulnessassociation.net/
The MSc Studies in Mindfulness, University of Aberdeen
https://www.abdn.ac.uk/study/postgraduate-taught/degree-programmes/946/studies-in-mindfulness/

REFERENCES

BAER, R. A., SMITH, G.T., HOPKINS, J., KRITEMEYER, J. and TONEY, L. (2006). Using Self-Report Assessment Methods to Explore Facets of Mindfulness. Assessment 13 (1), pp. 27-45
CAMPBELL, J. (1949). The Hero with a Thousand Faces (1st ed.). Princeton, NJ: Princeton University Press. (2nd ed. 1968, 3rd ed. 2008).
DOTY, J.R., (2016) Into the Magic Shop. London: Yellow Kite
KABAT-ZINN, J. (1994). Wherever you go, there you are. New York, NY: Hyperion Books.
MOORE FITZGERALD, S. (2014a) Interview with Martin Doyle 19th November 'Human beings need stories. It's how we make sense of the world ' Irish Times
https://www.irishtimes.com/culture/books/sarah-moore-fitzgerald-human-beings-need-stories-it-s-how-we-make-sense-of-the-world-1.2004263
MOORE FITZGERALD, S. (2014b) The Apple Tart of Hope. London: Orion Children's Books
WILDE, O.(2015) Stories for Children Illustrated by Charles Robinson. Dublin: The O'Brien Press.

CHAPTER 2
THE JOURNEY OF MINDFUL HEROES

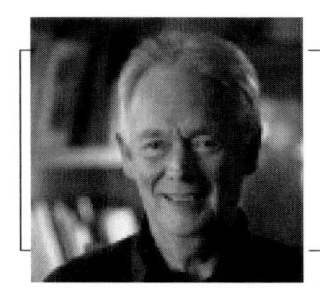

Vin Harris

vinharris.hkt@gmail.com

THE PATH OF MINDFULNESS?

MINDFULNESS – THE STORY SO FAR

Have you noticed that the world we live in never stops changing? This was always so but changes happen faster than ever before and it has become impossible to predict what surprises tomorrow will bring. Today our body, mind and spirit are challenged in ways that our ancestors could never have imagined. An ever increasing number of people now practice mindfulness in order to survive and thrive during these confusing times. Much has been written about the theory and practice of mindfulness. If asked to sum up what it is and why it works, I would say: "mindfulness is a way of allowing things to get better by not making them worse".

Training in mindfulness involves paying attention to a support such as breath, sound or bodily sensations. There is no need to adopt a particular world view; we relate to experience without philosophy, as it is rather than as it is supposed to be. What could be more natural than that? Maybe the simplicity of mindfulness practice is exactly what is needed when everything feels too complicated.

When introduced to mindfulness, people become aware of an autonomous tendency of mind to move away from the chosen mindfulness support towards distraction. Mindfulness training rests on the premise that practitioners can notice when attention is no longer with the chosen support and so return to a state of presence. Noticing distraction and coming back to being with the support is the essence of practice. It may well be that practice does not make perfect, but it does strengthen the innate capacity to be awake where we are rather than dreaming of another time and place.

So what is the value of learning to live in the here and now? When thinking about the dramas from the past or anticipating preferred futures, it is very easy to get lost in excessive involvement with hopes and fears. The repetition of our habitual tales, that may or may not be true, defines who we believe we are and the world we think we inhabit. Meditation is not a technique to prevent the arising of thoughts. Through the intention to become familiar with what is happening, as stories come and go they are simply witnessed; they lose their power to disturb and deceive. The mind remembers how to rest.

Resting cannot be brought about by force: the teaching of mindfulness offers an invitation to stay where we are and let go of the stories we tell ourselves. Just noticing habitual patterns as they arise establishes the conditions for them to subside naturally. There is no doubt this method settles the agitated mind, providing relief in troubled waters. However, we humans love stories and we are fascinated by travel: we may want a peaceful predictable life but we yearn for inspiration and adventure. Mindfulness enables practitioners to be more at ease with life and of course the importance of this benefit is appreciated. Nevertheless, if the injunction to "be here now" becomes a mindless mantra that is revered as the entire purpose of meditation, at some point it will conflict with a deeper imperative; the quest for meaning and purpose.

Mindfulness is a way of learning to deal directly with life. During most mindfulness courses as well as instruction on formal meditation practices there will also be training in paying attention to what is happening during everyday activities. Meditation in this new reincarnation has already helped many people to cope with the pressures of present day society. Having made significant steps towards establishing its place in the world, mindfulness is now in a position to help bring about positive change. Originally secular mindfulness was conceived as an intervention to alleviate physical and mental suffering. More recently it has found employment in the enhancement of personal well-being and professional effectiveness. In other words, not only is mindfulness proving beneficial in clinical settings for the relief of human problems, it also has a role to play in the pursuit of human potential. This is what inspires our current adventure. "On such a full sea are we now afloat. And we must take the current when it serves, or lose our ventures" (Shakespeare, 1599, Julius Caesar, 4.iii).

Later in this chapter I will describe some key elements of the Mindfulness Association's approach to training in Mindfulness-Compassion-Insight-Wisdom. We will explore in some detail the affinity it has with Joseph Campbell's understanding of the Hero's Journey and the wisdom it awakens in anyone who is ready to bring the universal imagery back to life. Before looking to where mindfulness might go next, it may be useful to reflect on how we came to be where we are now.

DOING (ALMOST) NOTHING

Perhaps because mindfulness has been presented as philosophically neutral, there has been little resistance to its pervasive influence. Jon Kabat-Zinn describes mindfulness as "paying attention in a particular way; on purpose, in the present moment, and non-judgmentally" Kabat-Zinn, 1994, p.4). The biggest obstacle to implementing this radical alternative to constant striving is not that it is difficult to do; if anything it is too simple. It feels counterintuitive to believe that resting will be helpful in dealing with the relentless demands of the 21st century and the complexity of our human condition. Baer (2003) and Shapiro et al. (2006) refer to an ever increasing body of research which affirms the life-changing impact of mindfulness. It seems that remarkable results are achieved when we allow things to be as they are. So is it even possible to do nothing; can we learn to rest without initiating yet more doing?

I particularly like this explanation of meditation:

> Meditation is not a matter of trying to achieve ecstasy, spiritual bliss or tranquillity, nor is it attempting to be a better person. It is simply the creation of a space in which we are able to expose and undo our neurotic games, our self-deceptions, our hidden fears and hopes. We provide space through the simple discipline of doing nothing. Actually, doing nothing is very difficult. At first, we must begin by approximating doing nothing, and gradually our practice will develop. So meditation is a way of churning out the neuroses of mind and using them as part of our practice. Like manure we do not throw our neuroses away, but we spread them on our garden; they become part of our richness (Trungpa, 1976, p.2).

This was written by the influential Tibetan Buddhist teacher, Chogyam Trungpa. I was fortunate to be part of a generation of spiritual seekers whose lives were touched by the migration of Tibetan Buddhism to the West. We were inspired, but we certainly found it difficult to believe that meditation is not something special to be assimilated. I still find it amazing that advice coming from such charismatic teachers, representing an uncompromised lineage from an ancient culture, could be so pragmatic yet so appropriate for our well-intentioned if somewhat eccentric generation.

I feel deeply grateful that my life has been blessed through a connection with Tibetan Buddhism but I also appreciate the way in which secular mindfulness has helped me to hear what my Buddhist teachers were trying to tell me all along. This has been my path: your path may be different. However, as you turn your attention to the world within, you set out on a journey that is likely to have deeper implications. My wish is that mindfulness can become a guesthouse for travellers whatever their quest may be; a safe resting place open to any pilgrim who seeks shelter from the storm.

MYTHOLOGY AND POETRY

If anyone in distress finds some benefit from a brief introduction to mindfulness, then surely no one could dispute that this has been worthwhile: but hopefully many of us will continue to practice with the aspiration to enrich our own lives and the lives of others. Could viewing this human life as a mythological journey prepare us to embrace the inevitable challenges that will be encountered on the way? What would it be like to regard our mindfulness practice as a lifelong quest?

In the Power of Myth, Joseph Campbell reflects on our need for myths and stories:

> Mythology is not a lie, mythology is poetry, it is metaphorical. It has been well said that mythology is the penultimate truth - penultimate because the ultimate cannot be put into words. It is beyond words. Beyond images, beyond that bounding rim of the Buddhist Wheel of Becoming. Mythology pitches the mind beyond that rim, to what can be known but not told (Campbell and Moyes, 1991, p.206).

We are invited to engage with mythology, poetry and metaphor as expressions of penultimate truth. Knowing about mindfulness is never enough and might sometimes be an obstacle; science can provide confidence in the purpose and benefits of practicing mindfulness yet the essence of meditation in all its many forms always has been and still remains the art of a beginner's mind.

The well recognised connection between mindfulness and poetry is explored further in chapter six of this book. Poetry conveys subtle meaning in the teaching and practice of mindfulness: it touches the parts that concepts cannot reach. Similarly mythology can make a vital contribution as the emphasis of practice shifts beyond attending to immediate suffering with mindfulness and compassion towards exposing the underlying causes of suffering through insight on the quest for inner freedom. Without interference from an excess of thinking, stories are able to transmit wisdom and inspiration directly to the heart that understands the meaning beyond the sum of the words.

Pause and Reflect

Heroes and Villains:
Take a few moments to bring to mind some of the characters in your favourite books and films. Allow them to be alive in your inner world.
What do you admire about your heroes? What qualities and values do they represent that you may have or aspire to develop?
What do you dislike about the villains? What faults and mistakes do they embody that you wish to be free from?
How is the experience of reflecting on Heroes and Villains different from telling yourself how you should and should not act?

A PATH FOR OUR MINDFULNESS JOURNEY

My own meditation practice has been supported and guided for many years by the Buddhist view of the world. There is some debate as to whether Buddhism is a religion or merely a philosophy of mind. At this point I am more interested in the fact that the Buddha suggested there is a reliable path leading from confusion to clarity. It could be argued that ultimately the very notion of following a path is an illusion and perhaps a hindrance. However, in my experience, living within the metaphor of being on a journey has been extremely helpful. William Blake said: "If the fool would persist in his folly he would become wise" (Blake, 1976, p.45). Like the archetypal fool, when I set out on my search for wisdom it was not clear where I was going or how I might get there. The path of Buddhism has helped me commit to pursuing my folly when I might otherwise have completely lost my way or given up altogether.

Mindfulness is learning to discover where you are rather than worrying about where you have come from or where you are going. Yet in conversations between fellow practitioners and tutors, we often refer to being on a mindfulness journey. The metaphor resonates and so this question arises: is it possible to practice and teach mindfulness in a way which honours the present moment, provides a sense of direction to sustain the long term journey and still allows freedom for the immediacy of personal exploration? It occurs to me that we don't need to invent such a path when one already exists. The Hero's Journey is a universal narrative that transcends cultural norms and religious beliefs. Might this perspective on the human condition inform the search for purpose and meaning? Can it guide and support mindfulness practitioners on a path that continues beyond pathology towards potential?

THE HERO'S JOURNEY

TREASURE MAP

The Hero with a Thousand Faces (Campbell, 2008) gathers together numerous tales of an adventure or quest that appears in myths, legends, parables, folklore and literature from countries all over the world and throughout the ages. In more recent times film makers have been influenced by Campbell's work: the ancient principle of a Hero's Journey continues to weave its magic and awaken our imagination. This story has no end.

Campbell (2008) and others such as Vogler (2007) developed models of varying complexity to chart the territory that a hero passes through on his/her journey. There are many variations but the basic plot is quite simple:

> A hero ventures forth from the world of common day into a region of supernatural wonder: fabulous forces are there encountered and a decisive victory is won: the hero comes back from this mysterious adventure with the power to bestow boons on his fellow man (Campbell, 2003, p.xxiv).

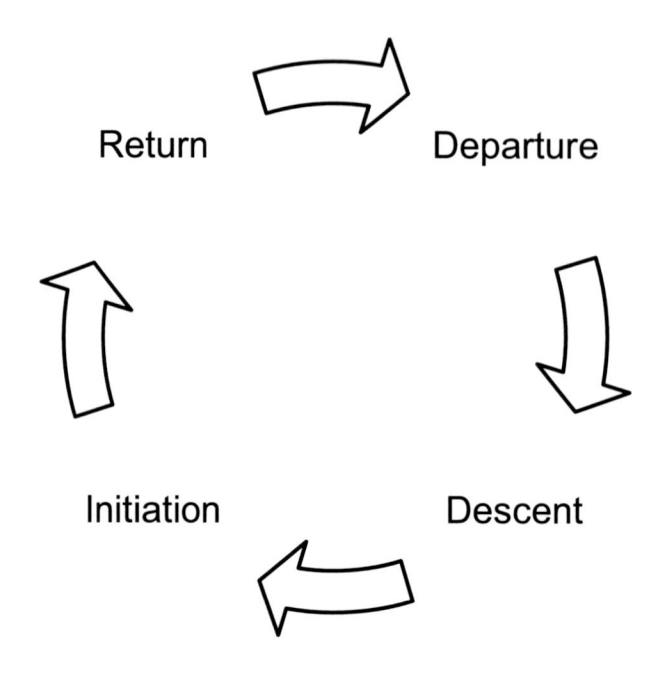

Figure 1: Key Stages of the Hero's Journey

1. Departure: leaving the normal world and entering strange new territory.
2. Descent: encountering obstacles and receiving help.
3. Initiation: facing challenges and finding freedom.
4. Return: coming home and being able to help others.

Can we also understand this archetypal story of the Hero's Journey as a guidebook, a treasure map for our own mission to discover human potential?

THE STONE IN MY SHOE

Albert Einstein reflects on the driving force behind human aspirations:

> Everything that the human race has done and thought is concerned with the satisfaction of deeply felt needs and the assuagement of pain. One has to keep this constantly in mind if one wishes to understand spiritual movements and their development (Einstein, 2006, p.26).

The pursuit of happiness is normal and of course we all do our level best to avoid suffering. The tragedy is that we often pursue these objectives in ways that ironically deliver the opposite of what was intended. As Bob Dylan sings: "You can't live by bread alone, you won't be satisfied. You can't roll away the stone if your hands are tied" (Dylan, 1994, p.693). There is no sustainable happiness in the mundane world and, although it may not have been apparent when setting out, the quest reveals a spiritual dimension.

An underlying feeling of unease creates momentum. The contemporary Tibetan meditation master, Mingyur Rinpoche suggests: "the yearning for a state of complete, uninterrupted happiness pulls at us. In a sense, we're homesick for our true nature" (Mingyur, 2007, p.55). The path that leads to freedom from suffering is not always easy but in my experience the diversions end up being more painful. I may ignore the stone in my shoe for a while, but it is always there unless I am fulfilling my potential. Once started the Hero's Journey is almost inevitable.

THE JOURNEY OF MY LIFE

As I describe a few pivotal moments from the story of my life, in the hope that it will inspire you to see the Hero's Journey reflected in your life, I can still hear the reassuring voice on the radio from story time at primary school: "Are you sitting comfortably?...then I'll begin".

DEPARTURE

For no apparent reason I have always been practical and love making things. From an early age I wanted to be a joiner and work with wood, which did happen eventually, but before that I went to Warwick University to study literature. It was as if the world had woken up. Outrageous sounds of Hendrix, Grateful Dead and Captain Beefheart; songs brought back from the edge of space by Dylan, Cohen and Joni Mitchell; introduction to a world in and out of time by the genius of Shakespeare, Blake and Eliot; art forms that spoke to and for a crazy generation, optimistic sincere seekers of delight and truth. With perfect timing people, music and books came into our lives with messages from beyond. I always assumed that my journey would take me to India but somehow I ended up in Scotland.

Surprising as it may now seem, the world managed to function without Internet, email or Facebook. A friend of mine had been told (by none other than David Bowie) that in a place called Samye Ling in Scotland, there were: "some far out Tibetan dudes who really know where it's at". Following the call to adventure we headed North. He was right.

DESCENT

When I first moved into Samye Ling in the early 1970s, it was a small community very different from the large institution it is now. Akong Rinpoche, a Tibetan Lama who had escaped from Tibet, was the head of the community and under his guidance we were introduced to Buddhism and hard physical work. Community members were given jobs that matched their personal needs as well as serving the greater purpose. I certainly needed bringing down to earth after the heady days of university and one of my early jobs was looking after a small herd of dairy cows; feeding, milking, cleaning up a lot of shit.

One day I was talking with Akong Rinpoche about his big dream to build the Samye Project and his aspiration that we would do the work ourselves. I had pretty much forgotten my childhood wish to be a woodworker but in that very moment I remembered it and said: "I always wanted to be a woodworker.... I'll go away and learn joinery skills and then come back to help build the temple". Along with my friends who had also gone off to learn various building skills, I returned to Samye Ling ready for the adventure ahead of us. Over a ten-year period we built the main temple. It was a huge endeavour and we encountered many personal and practical challenges. We had spiritual guidance plus hands-on help from Akong Rinpoche, this remarkable Tibetan Lama, who was ready to do whatever was needed to help us wake up.

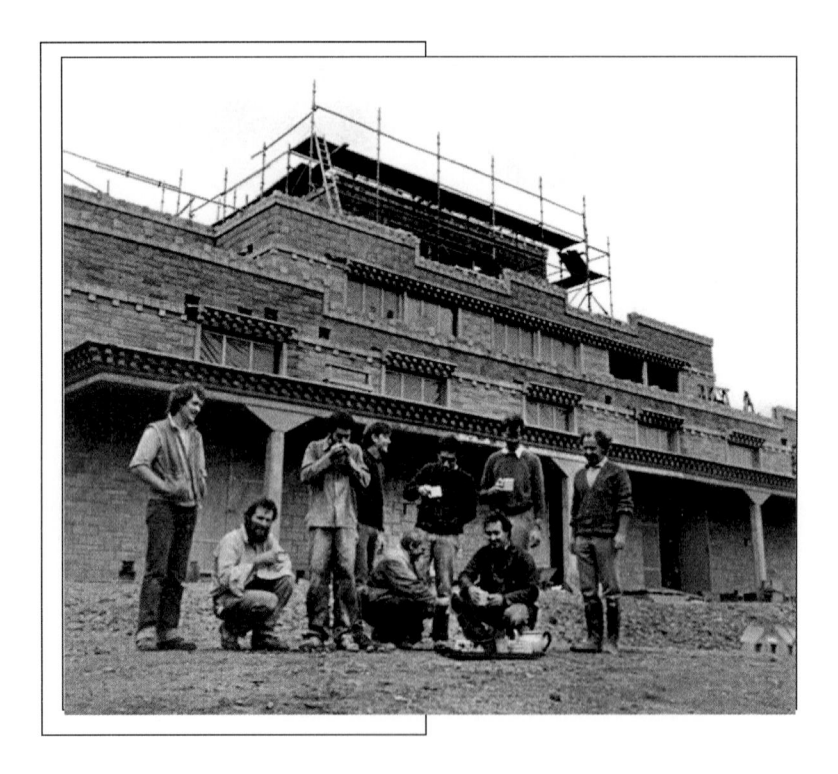

Figure 2: Samye Ling Temple during construction 1980's. Photo © Samye Ling Archive

INITIATION

The most memorable explanation of initiation that I have heard didn't come from my Buddhist teachers but from a woodwork guru. It was my first day at the training centre and one of the tutors, Reg Brown came over to my work bench. I remember his exact words: "You need to understand that learning a craft is like receiving an initiation. You can't get it from a book, you can't figure it out for yourself, you must receive it from someone else". Having just left Samye Ling I was surprised to be hearing about this topic in a joinery workshop! Reg Brown continued: "Once you've received the initiation you know you are going to die, so you need to do two things with what you've been given. You need to add to the tradition and you need to pass it on to others". This captures the essence of the initiation process; an introduction to an unfamiliar world by someone who can show us the ways of the new territory in which we find ourselves.

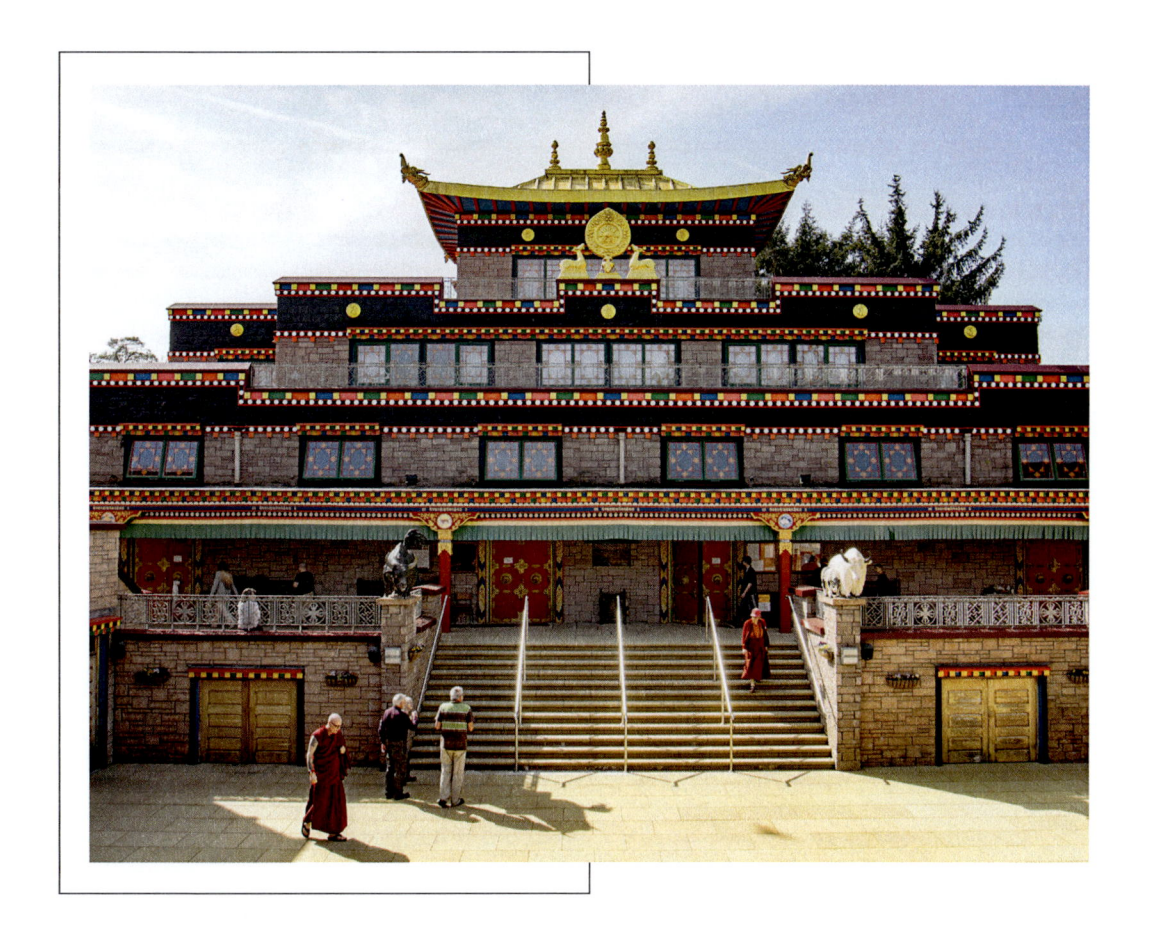

Figure 3: Samye Ling Temple as it is now. Photo © Samye Ling 2019

RETURN

During a period of semi-retirement from my business, I was fortunate to be able to help bring the final stage of Samye Project to completion. Before he died in 2013, Akong Rinpoche finally saw the realisation of his dream that started to come alive in the 1970s. Rather than rushing into another big project I decided to pause. I spent three months in retreat on Holy Isle. There was no particular agenda other than to take some time and space to connect with the Buddhist practices I had received. However, during that retreat, I began to reflect on how much meditation had helped throughout my life. It was time to pass on what I had understood.

Mindfulness is a very accessible way to make the benefits of meditation available, particularly when many people may have neither the time to engage in extensive study nor the inclination to adopt a religious view of life. I had already studied and practiced with Rob Nairn and helped to establish the Mindfulness Association, it seemed obvious that I was now in a good position to help others to bring meditation into their daily life through teaching mindfulness.

When teaching mindfulness I am happy if anyone experiences respite from suffering and perhaps glimpses of happiness that can be found by simply being present. I also see a need to offer support to practitioners who are ready to leave behind the secure prison of their own limitations. I hope that seeing mindfulness practice in the context of the Hero's Journey will guide our search for freedom without prescribing what we may discover.

MINDFULNESS FOR LIFE

A VISION FOR MINDFUL LIVING

Rob Nairn envisaged an approach to training in mindfulness that integrates Mindfulness-Compassion-Insight-Wisdom (for more information see link to Mindfulness Association website in Further Resources at the end of this chapter). This idea was developed and became an experiential training programme for the MSc Studies in Mindfulness Studies at the University of Aberdeen. The same training materials are presented in Mindfulness Association courses at weekends and week-long retreats to groups throughout the UK and Europe. Shaped by the experience of tutors and participants, the training modules have evolved into their present form over a period of ten years. The emerging Mindfulness for Life initiative brings together practitioners who want to continue their mindfulness journey and find new ways to express their inner freedom through compassion in action.

I find it helpful to summarise the training pathways as follows:

- Mindfulness – Knowing what is happening when it is happening.
- Compassion – Accepting what is happening when it is happening.
- Insight – Recognising what is happening when it is happening.
- Wisdom – Understanding what is happening when it is happening.

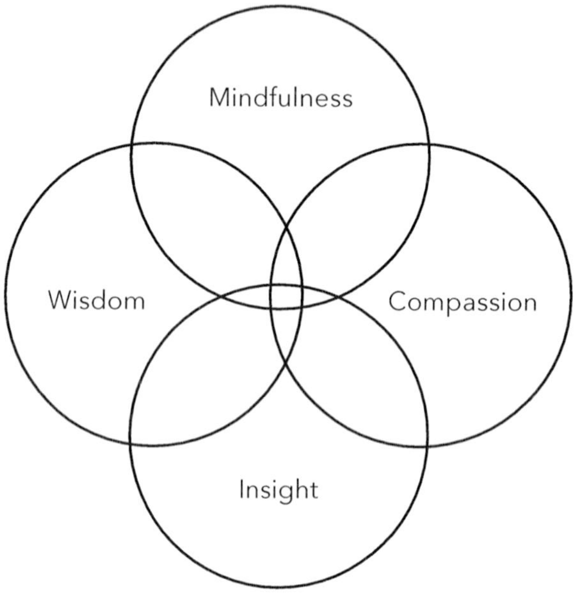

Figure 4: Key Elements of the Mindfulness Association's Training

A WAY OF LIFE

It may be convenient to deliver mindfulness training as a standardised menu of products. However, I am concerned that the transformative power of meditation will be forgotten if short term "mindfulness based interventions" become the only option that is available. Everyone needs a break from a stressful life but package holidays are no substitute for a lifelong adventure accompanied by experienced fellow explorers. More than a New Year's resolution – mindfulness is for life.

Later in this book you will read the stories of some Mindful Heroes who brought what they had discovered into a wide range of social and professional contexts. It is important to keep in mind that their primary ambition was not to find the shortest route to qualifying as a mindfulness teacher. With genuine commitment to study and practice, they first set out on a life-changing personal journey. Their experiences gave them the confidence, flexibility and creativity to find a way to use what they had learnt to help others. It seems to me that the path they walked has a significant connection with the Hero's Journey and I want to share my personal reflections on this Journey of Mindful Heroes.

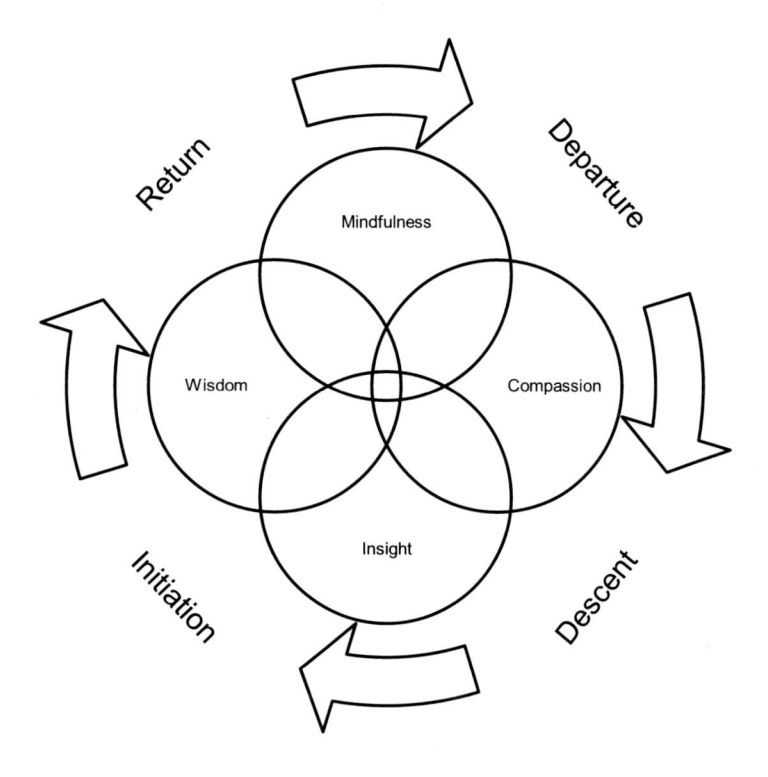

Figure 5: The Journey of Mindful Heroes

THE JOURNEY OF MINDFUL HEROES

STAGE1 - MINDFUL DEPARTURE

> What you know you can't explain, but you feel it. You've felt it your entire life, that there's something wrong with the world. You don't know what it is, but it's there, like a splinter in your mind, driving you mad (The Matrix, 1991).

Joseph Campbell remarked, "We must be willing to get rid of the life we've planned, so as to have the life that is waiting for us. The old skin has to be shed before the new one can come." (Osbon, 1991, p.18). In the "Departure" stage of the story, the hero lives in an ordinary world and receives some kind of call to embark on an adventure. The Hero's Journey may begin with a crisis which disrupts the comfortable routines of life: or perhaps there is a yearning for a voyage of discovery born of dissatisfaction with the predictable everyday world. But the prospect of leaving home is still frightening and it may be tempting to play it safe and live with what we know rather than making a bold leap into the unknown.

Similarly, an interest in mindfulness may be precipitated by grief, concerns for the health of a loved one, personal illness, a dramatic shift in circumstances, a feeling of relentless pressure at work. Alternatively, when everything is going reasonably well, there may be an underlying feeling that something is wrong and there must surely be more to life than this. The characters in your favourite movies or storybooks needed guides and mentors to encourage them to heed the call to adventure and face the challenges that lie ahead. How can we expect our exploration of the world within to be any different?

You probably already suspect that the truth is not "out there" and that problems cannot be resolved by attempting to manipulate the circumstances of your life to align with your preferences. However, it is still not easy to remember that the causes of happiness and suffering are to be found within; particularly in days like these when there is an onslaught of media messages assaulting your senses, persuading you to chase after the dazzling displays of useless information, products and services on offer.

Unlike the mythical heroes of a less materialistic age, we may not have access to mysterious helpers with the wisdom to point us in the right direction. Therefore, I feel it is especially important that we do what we can to look after one another as we step out from the everyday world of mindless doing and place our trust in an alternative way of being.

Sometimes you may feel that the practice is not working, that your mind is more chaotic than you realised. Is mindfulness after all not the anaesthetic you had hoped for? On the Journey of Mindful Heroes we are not going shopping for the secret formula that is guaranteed to make our problems go away. We already have what we need but, as my granny used to say, "We can't see for looking". Are you ready to leave behind the weight of expectations? Rather than accumulating a new bag of tricks with which to play the same old game, when you cross the threshold into a new world, this call to adventure asks if you are willing to enter into a fresh new relationship with whatever may happen. "For we are a travelling light and we spark in the moment we're in" (Greig, 2006, p.46).

Pause and Reflect

The Call to Adventure:
Why not give yourself some time to take a break. Sit still for a while and let the story of your life play out in your mind's eye.
Can you remember how and why you started to take an interest in learning about mindfulness?
What inspiration and assistance did you receive from friends, mentors, books, videos or unforeseen circumstances that appeared in your life?
How does it feel as you appreciate how events that you could never have imagined were able to unfold?

STAGE 2 - COMPASSIONATE DESCENT

> When you put your hope in gods, your fear of demons worsens. Once you know the sacred nature of the world and beings, demons and gods have one taste (Patrul, 2017, p.85).

The "Descent" stage of the journey begins as the hero enters a world where different rules apply. In this fluid and ambiguous place it is hard to know who to trust; enemies may be helpers in disguise and friends may inadvertently divert you off course. The hero may well feel disorientated, insecure and probably inadequate for the trials ahead.

A disorderly confusing world may be revealed when you practice mindfulness and start to notice what is going on in your inner world. To witness chaos in the space created through the simple discipline of doing almost nothing can be a salutary and humbling experience. Sleeping demons of anxiety, guilt, shame and insecurity may be awakened. Your inner critic may offer plenty of unwelcome advice. Without self-compassion, inner conflict will always prevail and it will be more or less impossible to continue your journey. Acceptance is the key that opens the door to compassion.

If you accept whatever arises, your mindfulness practice can bring a sense of ease and genuine growth. Perhaps fear of demons is a tendency to suppress what feels unacceptable and hope in gods may be an impulse to fabricate preferred alternatives. Serving either of these insatiable tyrants is exhausting. Witnessing this endless struggle, how could anyone not be moved to compassion for our human condition? When I have compassion for myself then compassion for others flows without hesitation. Although I may not yet realise the sacred nature of the world and beings, through cultivating kindness and acceptance it is at least possible to find a less complicated way to meditate and live.

In many stories, the hero learns to face seemingly insurmountable obstacles. Each test is daunting but it develops courage and confidence in preparation for greater challenges. Your instincts tell you to avoid uncomfortable situations, to run away from problems. It feels scary to hold your ground. If you apply the practice of compassion to smaller issues first, your trust in the power of acceptance to generate change will grow stronger.

Friends may offer you a way back to the comfort zone you left behind but are they really being compassionate? Could it be more beneficial when people you don't like to be with show the path you need by directing attention towards your own limitations? How do you know who to trust? When you learn to take responsibility for your own journey, preference and aversion no longer rule your life. Compassionate connection becomes a reality: "Whatever obstacles arise, if you deal with them through kindness without trying to escape then you have real freedom" (Akong, undated).

Pause and Reflect

Facing the Situation:
Now may be a good time to rest, taking time out to be with the sensations in your body as breath comes and goes.
Are there any difficult situations in your life these days? I would be surprised if there are none! Instead of trying to avoid or fix the problems, what would it be like for even a short time to allow everything to be just as it is?
If you could see yourself through the eyes of a kind and wise friend, how would you deal with these present obstacles?

STAGE 3 – INITIATION THROUGH INSIGHT

> In our being there is a primordial yes that is not our own; it is not at our own disposal; it is not accessible to our inspection and understanding…..Basically, however, my being is not an affirmation of a limited self, but the "yes" of Being itself, irrespective of my own choices (Merton, 2015, p.15-16).

The "Initiation" phase of the journey delivers the ultimate challenge. This is the big one: the innermost cave, the most intimidating enemy, the fiercest monster, the impossible feat of strength, skill and courage. The life of the hero and the fate of everything he or she holds dear is at stake. Failure is not an option, victory seems impossible. All that has been learnt until now with help from mentors and allies has prepared the hero for this. The final test must be faced alone. In order to accomplish what appears impossible you let go of everything you think you know. What you think you know defines who you think you are; who you think you are limits the possibility of what you think you can and cannot achieve:

> And what you do not know is the only thing you know
> And what you own is what you do not own
> And where you are is where you are not (Eliot, 2001, p.18).

The battle seems to be with external forces, but an inner victory is achieved which can only be won by surrendering to a greater reality. Through initiation, the hero connects with the divine, experiencing a profound transformation. The reward turns out to be less than was anticipated yet more than could have been imagined. Eventually we all become ready to deal with what we fear most. There is no longer any need to avoid what might be lurking in the shadows and anything is now possible: "what looks large from a distance, close up ain't never that big" (Dylan, 1994, p.680).

If you are like me, the last thing you want to do is confront your hidden hopes and fears. When you do, you realise you are tired of carrying them, there is a palpable sense of relief when you finally set them free. Insight is that "Aha!" moment which cannot be planned.

> Once the mind sees clearly that it is creating suffering, its inherent wisdom lets go of the processing that creates it, just as we let go of a very hot object as soon as we register the pain it is causing (Teasdale, J.D. and Chaskalson, M., 2013, p.120).

You might have expected that following a moment of insight, you see what is going on and then you have to decide what to do. But it is not quite like that. When you recognise what is going on change follows naturally. Without deference to external authority or reference to philosophy, simply witnessing the complex self-perpetuating activity of mind provides conditions where insight reveals itself.

In daily life and during meditation, are you sometimes aware of a sense of being on duty? A restless insecurity telling you it is not ok to let go, an insidious anxiety reminding you that the world will cease to function properly unless you maintain control. Off duty, at rest but still knowing, the mind is aware of its own superficial thinking as well as subtle attitudes and habitual patterns below the surface. Normal logic would suggest that letting go of striving might lead to stagnation and the hero might become ineffective. However, through initiation the hero gets out of his or her own way and steps into a greater way of being; extraordinary feats are accomplished with ease. When the tedious background noise of hopes and fears subsides we are already in tune with the primordial yes.

Pause and Reflect

Letting Go:
Take a few moments to be comfortable, turning your attention inwards, allowing yourself to reflect on what you have been reading.
Can you bring to mind times in your own life when faced with big challenges you have found a strength you didn't know you had?
Have you ever discovered a solution to a problem or had a creative idea that as soon as it appeared seemed completely obvious?
What happens when you stop being who you think you are supposed to be?

STAGE 4 - RETURN WITH WISDOM

> The person who has found the way can pass on the gracious teachings to others;
> Thus he aids himself and helps the others, too. To give is then the only thought remaining in his heart (Milarepa, 1999, p.79).

The hero who set out left behind the ordinary world, answering the call, looking beyond the boundaries of known experience for solutions to everyday problems. The territory was strange and the laws were often contrary to normal logic. Nevertheless, what the hero discovers will be of great value if it can be carried back into the world where the journey began. It may be fascinating to stay in that special world but the quest would be incomplete. The hero honours the initial inspiration for setting out on the journey; indeed as understanding increases the commitment to help others grows stronger. Sometimes at the end of the story the hero returns to share a treasure that will benefit everyone: often the true reward is simply that the mundane world now appears transformed.

Through training in insight you become aware of limiting habitual patterns which invariably reinforce feelings of isolation. When you expose these agendas and see how you have been arranging your life around unacknowledged insecurity, you will also recognise the alternative; living in connection with the world. Einstein expresses the possibility and value of seeing through the illusion of separation:

> A human being is a part of the whole called by us universe, a part limited in time and space. He experiences himself, his thoughts and feeling as something separated from the rest, a kind of optical delusion of his consciousness. This delusion is a kind of prison for us, restricting us to our personal desires and to affection for a few persons nearest to us. Our task must be to free ourselves from this prison by widening our circle of compassion to embrace all living creatures and the whole of nature in its beauty. (Einstein, 2005, p.206).

As wisdom shows you limitless potential, compassion motivates you to do whatever you can to free yourself and others from suffering and the causes of suffering. It is as if the energy that was trapped in exclusively serving one self is now set free. You return from your journey wiser, more compassionate, ready to engage in meaningful activity. Not dreaming of escape, awake in the world. But old habits look for a new way to survive. It is easy to be drawn into playing the same game wearing different clothes. After a while you may find yourself settling into an amended version of the world you thought you had left behind for good. As TS Eliot reminds us: "the only wisdom we can hope to acquire is the wisdom of humility: humility is endless" (Eliot, 2001, p.16). The journey still continues. Circles within circles, slowly learning not to make a crisis out of a drama, growing in confidence that somehow the fool will always find the way home. From time to time, if we are fortunate, there will be that precious opportunity to help our fellow travellers. And remember, it doesn't have to be perfect: "If we waited till our dance was pure, who would get off their arse?" (Greig, 2006, p.125).

CIRCLES WITHIN CIRCLES

Stories have a coherent structure whereas there is always some mystery in the play of life. As the history of each individual unfolds, it is as if there are several interwoven narratives from which intricate patterns emerge, perhaps not recognisable except in moments of freedom from expectations. The perennial challenge is to somehow find the courage to accept myself as I am.

The cyclical form of the Hero's Journey is perfectly conveyed by TS Eliot: "We shall not cease from exploration and the end of all our exploring will be to arrive where we started and know the place for the first time" (Eliot, 2001, p.43). Interconnected journeys without beginning are endless circles; the play of years, weeks, days or timeless moments. One act approaches resolution, another one unfolds. New characters enter the stage, their voices echoes of an earlier scene. So it seems the play goes on until I am ready to sit so still that I can see what is really happening and I am silent enough to hear what I most need to learn. And so the story continues…

Pause and Reflect

Sharing Your Treasure:
It is easy to dwell on our faults and weaknesses so let's do something different.
Why not acknowledge your unique talents and strengths? What treasures have you discovered that could help others?
How can you translate what you have learnt into a language that can be heard and understood in the everyday world?
How will you be able to manifest your inner values as effective activity?
Don't worry if you think you don't know the right answer. Be willing to hear whatever response may arise in your heart.

FOLLOW YOUR BLISS

IMPLICATIONS FOR STUDY, PRACTICE AND TEACHING

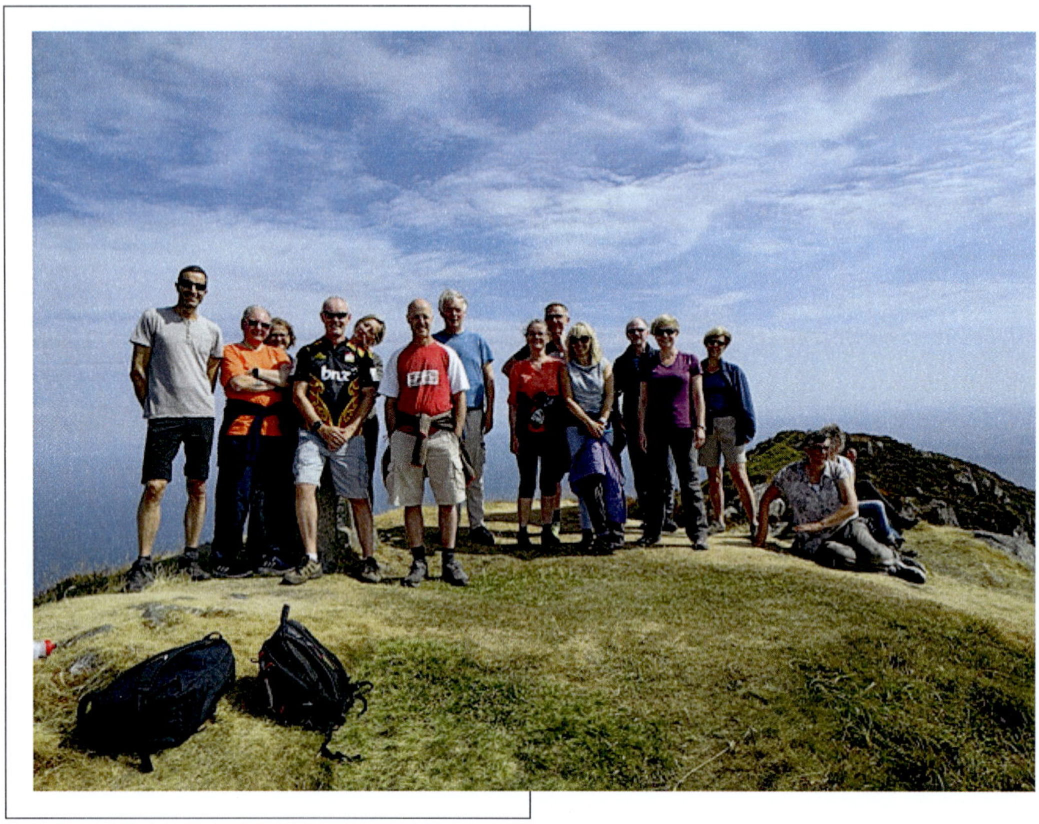

Figure 6: Mindfulness for Life group on top of Holy Island. Photo © Michael McTernan 2018

In the next chapter, Graeme Nixon will tell you about how an unexpected partnership between meditation practice and academic study has flourished. Indeed the initial idea of linking Mindfulness-Compassion-Insight to the Hero's Journey first came about when I was teaching with Graeme at Samye Ling on the MSc Studies in Mindfulness Studies at the University of Aberdeen. Some students had struggled to find secular sources to refer to in their insight assignments. We presented the Hero's Journey to illustrate how once insight has been found within then it appears everywhere.

"There's a divinity that shapes our ends, rough-hew them how we will". (Shakespeare, 1609, Hamlet, 5.ii). We plant seeds but we cannot know how they will grow. The case studies in the following sections of this book are examples of the activity that flourished as Mindful Heroes made the journey their own. Their stories affirm the life changing impact of mindfulness practice. When set free the human spirit is generous; we naturally want to share the benefits we have discovered with others. However, there is a danger that after a brief excursion, you might consider that mindfulness training is completed when in reality the adventure has only just begun. If this happens you may return with some interesting souvenirs from an entertaining holiday. That is not enough: you and others deserve more.

I hope you will choose to be a Mindful Hero: regarding your mindfulness practice as a lifelong series of courageous journeys into the unknown, may you reveal the ever present treasure that eliminates inner poverty.

ENTERING THE FIELD OF BLISS

Do you know that special feeling when out of nowhere a wonderful opportunity presents itself to you? When this happens my head may try to find excuses but my heart knows there is no choice. There is a sense of freedom as I let go of what I thought I wanted and act in alignment with my deeper purpose. There is a feeling of greatness and at the same time I am in awe of the mysterious interconnected forces at play. Probably this is what Joseph Campbell means by the directive to follow your bliss and the promise that:

> If you do follow your bliss you put yourself on a kind of track that has been there all the while waiting for you, and the life you ought to be living is the one you are living. When you can see that, you begin to meet people who are in the field of your bliss, and they open doors to you. I say follow your bliss and don't be afraid, and doors will open where you didn't know they were going to be (Campbell and Moyes, 1991, p.120).

In writing this book with my fellow travellers, it feels like we have set out on an inspiring adventure that had been searching for us. The power of auspicious coincidence is showing itself to be alive and well in the 21st century as this project brings to life the Journey of Mindful Heroes. Universal patterns affirm individual aspirations: in the mirror of myth we recognise our own true face.

I trust these stories we share will serve as a reminder of what you have always known and that you will choose to follow your bliss: now more than ever, our world needs mindful heroes.

Pause and Reflect

Your mission, should you choose to accept it.....
This chapter comes to an end but before you move on it might be worthwhile to pause for a minute or two. Allow yourself some space and see clearly where you are now.
Do you perhaps have a sense of the next episode of your story being whispered in your ear?
Maybe it is more like a loud banging at your door that is calling you to action?
This journey is endless: are you ready?

FURTHER RESOURCES

AKONG: A REMARKABLE LIFE. Film. Directed by Chico Dall'Inha. UK: AMP & HKT, 2017. A film about the life of Akong Rinpoche, founder of Samye Ling.
He was my hero: a friend, mentor and teacher for more than 40 years.
FINDING JOE. Film. Directed by Patrick Takaya Solomon. USA, 2011. A truly inspirational film, Finding Joe is a great introduction to the work of Joseph Campbell.
THE MINDFULNESS ASSOCIATION.
Website http://www.mindfulnessassociation.net/ Information about the founder Rob Nairn and his publications plus current training programmes.
VIN HARRIS. LinkedIn page https://www.linkedin.com/in/vin-harris-806aa912/
My contact details, information about my current projects, some guided practices, links to my podcasts and other interesting and inspirational content.

REFERENCES

AKONG, R., (undated). Quotes. Available: http://www.samyeling.org/quotes/
BAER, R. A., (2003). Mindfulness Training as a Clinical Intervention: A Conceptual and Empirical Review. Clinical Psychology: Science and Practice, 10, pp. 125-143.
BLAKE, W., (1976). Poems and Prophesies. London: Dent.
CAMPBELL, C. and MOYES, B., (1991). The Power of Myth. New York: Anchor Books.
CAMPBELL, J., (2003). The Hero's Journey, Joseph Campbell on His Life and Work. Novato, California: New World Library.
CAMPBELL, J., (2008). The Hero with a Thousand Faces. Novato, California: New World Library
DYLAN, B., (1994). Bob Dylan Lyrics 1962-1985. London: Harper Collins.
EINSTEIN A., (2005), The New Quotable Einstein (collected and edited by Alice Calaprice). Princeton, New Jersey: Princetown University Press.
EINSTEIN, A., (2006). The World As I See It. New York: Citadel Press.
ELIOT, T.S., (2001). Four Quartets. London: Faber & Faber.
GREIG, A., (2006). This Life, This Life. New and Selected Poems 1970-2006. Northumberland: Bloodaxe.
KABAT-ZINN, J., (1994). Wherever You Go There You Are. Mindfulness Meditation for Everyday Life. Great Britain: Piatkus Books.
McTERNAN, M., (2018). Holy Island photo taken by Michael McTernan.
MERTON, T., (2005). The Pocket Thomas Merton. (edited by M. Inchausti). Boston and London: New Seeds.
MILAREPA, (1999). The Hundred Thousand Songs of Milarepa. (translated by G.C.C Chang). Boston and London: Shambhala.
MINGYUR, Y., (2007). The Joy of Living, Unlocking the Secret & Science of Happiness. New York: Harmony Books.
OSBON, D.K., (1991). Reflections on the Art of Living, A Joseph Campbell Companion. New York: Harper Collins.
PATRUL, R., (2017). Enlightened Vagabond, The life and Teachings of Patrul Rinpoche. (Collected and translated by M. Ricard). Boulder: Shambhala.
SAMYE LING,. (undated) Photo by kind permission of Samye Ling Archive.
SHAKESPEARE, W., (1599). Cited from (1980). The Complete Works of Shakespeare, The Alexander Text. London and Glasgow: Collins
SHAKESPEARE, W., (1609). Cited from (1980). The Complete Works of Shakespeare, The Alexander Text. London and Glasgow: Collins
SHAPIRO, S. L., CARLSON, L. E., ASTIN, J. A. and FREEDMAN, D., (2006). Mechanisms of Mindfulness. Journal of Clinical Psychology, 62 (3), pp. 373-386.
TEASDALE, J.D. and CHASKALSON, M., (2013). How does mindfulness transform suffering? II: the transformation of Dukkha. Mindfulness, Diverse Perspectives on its Meaning, Origins and Applications. (edited by Williams, J.M.G. and Kabat-Zinn, J.). London and New York: Routledge.
THE MATRIX. Film. Directed by The Wachowskis. USA: Warner Brothers, 1999.
TRUNGPA, C., (1976). The Myth of Freedom and the Way of Meditation. Boston, Massachusetts: Shambhala.
VOGLER, C., (2007). The Writer's Journey: Mythic Structure for Writers, Third Edition. California: Michael Wiese Productions.

CHAPTER 3

MASTERS IN MINDFULNESS: COMPASSION AND INSIGHT APPLIED TO MULTIPLE LIVES AND PROFESSIONS

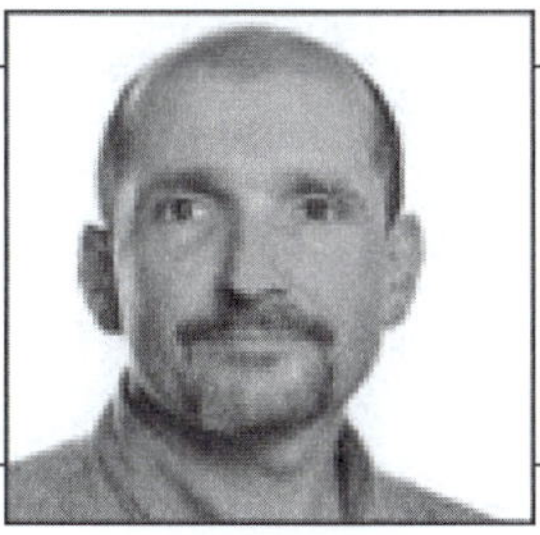

Graeme Nixon

g.nixon@abdn.ac.uk

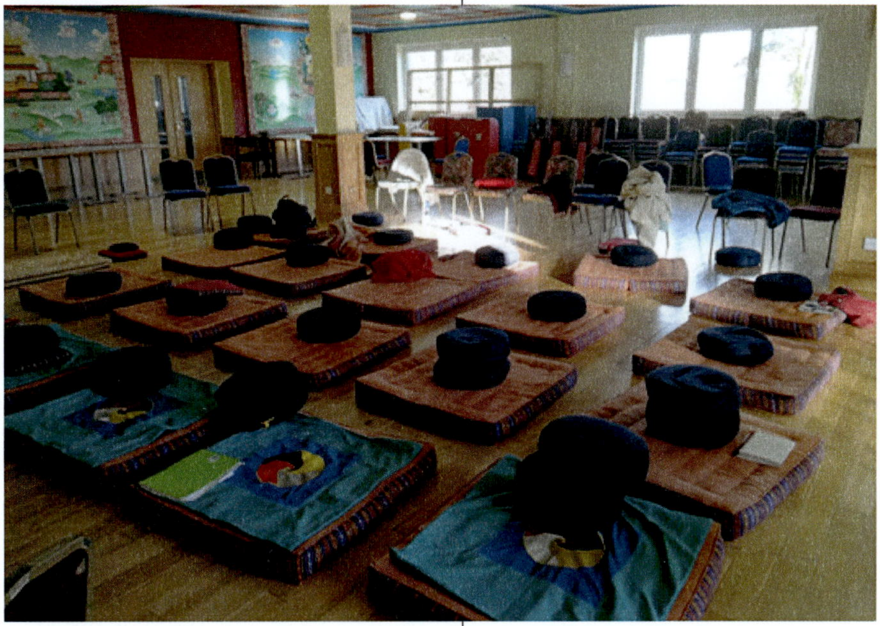

Figure 1: Samye Ling MSc classroom (empty) Photo © Graeme Nixon 2018

THE PATH OF MINDFULNESS?

We are amidst a mindful revolution. This is evident in column inches in newspapers; entire shelves in book shops; colouring books; political pronouncements; medical referrals; tailored package holidays, as well as in welcome criticality and satire. Since Jon Kabat-Zinn, in the late 1970's, began his work to bring a secular meditation approach to stress reduction, mindfulness has been the object of research and application, initially within clinical or health contexts but increasingly in diverse settings. Mindfulness meditation is a treatment for pathology, disease or dysfunction, but is increasingly being used as a way of developing human potential in diverse fields such as such as learning, communication, relationality, leadership, performativity, spirituality, and meaning making (to name but a few).

It is this view of mindfulness as developing human potential rather than treating pathology that underpins the MSc Studies in Mindfulness programme at the University of Aberdeen, Scotland, UK, (where I work as a lecturer). Since 2010 we have offered an MSc Studies in Mindfulness degree programme within the School of Education. This postgraduate programme has attracted over three hundred students from multiple professional contexts from all over the world. Students have included nurses, doctors, psychotherapists, psychologists, business managers and coaches, teachers, social workers, prison officers, yoga teachers, chaplains, athletes, sports coaches, actors, musicians, dancers, academics, software engineers, environmental consultants, naturalists and mindfulness teachers. Indeed, this book is a testament to the breadth of applications that the Studies in Mindfulness programme has facilitated and to the appeal of a study of mindfulness approach that provides a staged experiential training in Mindfulness, Compassion and Insight alongside an opportunity to reflect on practices and examine how these practices could be of impact in diverse settings. This book offers a sample of the experiences of students on the programme who have applied and researched mindfulness, compassion and insight in the worlds of Education, Health, Business, Sport, Creativity and Community work.

It may be helpful before discussing the content of the MSc to outline its genesis. Before working as an academic I was a secondary school teacher in Scotland specialising in Religious, Moral and Philosophical Studies. This was born of a lifetime's interest in how humans try to address the great existential questions (something, as a hopeful agnostic, that I remain interested in!). Having dabbled in meditation in my teens and introducing it (via the study of Buddhism) to my school pupils, I used to take school groups to the Samye Ling Tibetan Buddhist Centre and Monastery, which is nestled in the Scottish borders, for study weekends.

When, in 2005, having secured a lectureship at the University of Aberdeen in the School of Education, I continued to take student teachers to the monastery. It was there, along with my colleague and friend Dr David McMurtry, as well as Samye Ling monk and long-time meditator Choden, that I began discussing the need to explore the benefits of a secularised form of meditation (mindfulness) and the possibility of developing a Master's degree. At the same time published writer on meditation Rob Nairn and others affiliated with Samye Ling were keen to explore how mindfulness could be studied in a western institution in ways where it would be not just about human pathology but potential.

These discussions evolved over the next few years. For me it was an interesting experience petitioning an ancient University (Aberdeen was founded in 1495) to develop a Master's degree in mindfulness but this process was invaluable in sharpening our thinking about the need for the programme to not only be about and in mindfulness, but also embody a mindful, objective and secular approach to such study (the consonance of mindfulness and secularity is something I will explore further below). The other elements we thought indispensable to the experiential and academic training we were offering were compassion for self and others, and the cultivation not only of mindful but insightful awareness. These would be (and I hate the term) our 'unique selling points'! We wanted our mindfulness programme to be more than a teacher training programme for any specific mindfulness-based intervention. Instead, our programme would be a profound and critical immersion in mindfulness practice, its theoretical underpinnings, and an examination of its potential applications for multiple professions.

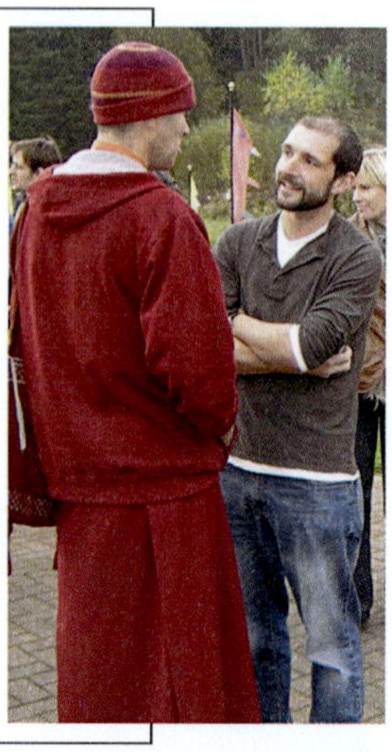

Figure 2: The Author in discussion with Choden (in robes), Samye Ling Photo © Graeme Nixon (2008)

THE GROWTH, NATURE AND APPLICATIONS OF MINDFULNESS

Universities in the UK and elsewhere are introducing an ever-increasing number of people to mindfulness. The programme we developed at Aberdeen in partnership with the Mindfulness Association, based in the School of Education, perhaps represents a move towards more holistic, pastoral and multi-professional applications of mindfulness. This contrasts with the dominant clinical settings for mindfulness to date.

Mindfulness is the awareness that emerges through paying attention purposefully to present experiences without judgement or preference. It is attention regulated to rest upon immediate experience, leading to a greater recognition of mental events. Mindfulness is an orientation to experience in which one engages with an attitude of kindness and curiosity. Rob Nairn, who taught on our programme, defines it as observing thoughts, without preference, no matter what they are. Mindfulness as practiced and taught in UK Universities, is secular and does not involve or require involvement in any religion or commitment to any particular belief system. That said, secular mindfulness is a form of meditation, and can draw upon Buddhist practices and psychological theory. Mindfulness has recently emerged, however, as a secular approach to meditative practice, with no reference to metaphysical, enchanted or supernatural beliefs. Given the (often unreflective) antipathy to 'religion' in increasingly secular developed countries, this is perhaps worth emphasising.

Interestingly, such antipathy is often not directed towards Buddhism, as shown by the range of Buddhist images in places as diverse as garden centres and restaurants. Interestingly the interest in Buddhism (Christopher Hitchens thought Buddhism is regarded with "thoughtless exceptionalism" (cited in Harris 2015, p29)) is not reflected in adherence or commitment. For example, only 0.4% Scots at the 2011 census self-identified as Buddhist, though I suspect a much greater percentage have Buddhist iconography around their homes! Steve Bruce (2017) contends that the appeal of Buddhism and nature of western borrowings from Buddhism is thrown into relief by the relatively little borrowing that has taken place from Islam (which he calls the 'unpillaged Eastern religion').

Reasons for this apparent immunity to antireligious sentiment may lie in Buddhism's apparently philosophically pragmatic, non-theistic approach, and in its appeal to individual experience rather than any institutional or theistic rule. Having said that, mindfulness simply involves paying attention to our experiences without judgement, and this is something that happens to be found in a range of spiritual, mystical traditions and philosophical traditions.

> **Pause and Reflect**
>
> Do you think there is a tendency to sanitise or psychologise Buddhism in the west, ignoring that Buddhism, like other traditions, has its Gods, enchantment, and sinners as well as saints?

Such secular mindfulness-based approaches and interventions are burgeoning. This has happened primarily within mental health and medical settings. Two approaches to health care in which mindfulness is a core aspect can be broadly delineated: mindfulness-based stress reduction (MBSR) and mindfulness-based cognitive therapy (MBCT). These forms of mindfulness intervention are used to treat an increasing range of psychological disorders such as depressive relapse, sleep and eating disorders, psychosis and borderline personality disorder. It should also be mentioned that mindfulness approaches can also be discerned within dialectical behaviour therapy and acceptance and commitment therapy. Both latter approaches place emphasis on the development of acceptance and present moment awareness as core to a range of therapeutic conditions.

Within these approaches to mindfulness there is a combination of formal, informal, short and more extended mindfulness practices, all of which are designed to develop awareness of attention, observation without reaction and categorisation of the activities of the mind and body. These approaches maintain many of the same practices and tend to favour an eight-week structure, and also can includes cognitive therapeutic inputs aimed at allowing participants to develop awareness that thoughts are not facts and recognition of automatic thoughts, thereby allowing practitioners to come to a degree of understanding about, and control over, their thought processes.

The growth of these mindful-based interventions since Kabat-Zinn first introduced mindfulness into the health context in 1979, is impressive. Kabat-Zinn's hope that mindfulness 'be developed and tailored in the future to specific classes of individuals and diagnoses' (Kabat-Zinn 2002) seems to becoming a reality. Mindfulness based approaches have also been applied to other, non-medical contexts such as sport, business and education. In these areas the ability to observe experience non-judgementally has been explored as a means to not only enhance well-being and communication, but also performance. In other words mindfulness is increasingly being seen as a way of enhancing professional efficacy in multiple contexts. This multiplicity of contexts and applications has been, since 2010, the broad scope of the MSc programme at Aberdeen, and this book is a celebration of this diversity.

THE ABERDEEN MSC:
A BLEND OF EXPERIENTIAL AND ACADEMIC LEARNING

The Aberdeen MSc in Mindfulness is a blended distance learning part-time programme which typically takes four years. All our students are professionals balancing the demands of study with their work. The face to face teaching elements take place on the university campus (real and virtual) and also at Samye Ling and the Holy Island (a retreat centre affiliated to Samye Ling). Our course tries to balance a stepped experiential training with academic rigour and criticality. This can, to be honest, be one of the most challenging and enriching aspects of being involved in the programme.

The experiential modules (Mindfulness, Compassion and Insight) lead to an opportunity for the students to develop skills in research into their professional context, culminating in a work-based project or dissertation. Most of the chapters by our graduates in this book represent abridged versions of these projects. These modules introduce students to theoretical positions and practices relating to Mindfulness, Compassion and Insight. Students are led through each practice by a tutor who then guides an enquiry into their experiences. Another common approach is that students discuss the practice experience with each other in small groups (see figure 5). For each of these modules students have to write an assignment that evidences reflection on personal mindfulness practice; understanding of relevant theory and explores the possible (or actual) applications of each of these themes and concepts within their professional context.

The structure of the MSc allows students to cultivate the ability to pay attention to present moment awareness (mindfulness); interact with experience acknowledging the tendency to judge (acceptance); relate to the experience and self with good will (compassion) and begin to grasp the nature of both experiencer and experience (insight). These stages are interlinked and sequential. Paul Gilbert and Choden describe this trajectory thus:

> mindfulness and compassion work together but from different positions. Compassion helps us to reorganise our minds by generating particular motives and feelings, while mindfulness helps us to step back and disengage from emotional thinking loops that suck us in, thereby providing the stability and perspective which is the basis for insight (Gilbert & Choden, 2013, p49).

This sequence recognises that as students develop skills in mindfulness there is a degree of settled awareness and less stormy relationality with thoughts and feelings. This in turn can lead to the surfacing of hitherto suppressed psychological conditions. This can lead to painful reactions. Our course is based on the view that an explicit compassion training is necessary for practitioners to be able to relate to and accept these negative states. Once practitioners have developed the capacity and compassionate resources to be present with these inner challenges, this then creates conditions whereby they can begin to discern the origins and nature of that which causes psychological distress (insight). This awareness in turn diminishes the power these conditioned habits of mind exerts over us. This experiential trajectory maps onto a Buddhist progression from single pointed mindfulness to insight meditation, suffused with compassionate awareness. However, though the shape of the training parallels the journey taken by some Buddhists, there is no requirement whatsoever that our students subscribe to any aspects of Buddhism.

Half way though Year 2 of the MSc students are introduced to approaches to research, which they can then put into practice, initially in a small-scale way, in their professional context. They are taken through a staged introduction to research frameworks or paradigms, methodologies, ethical considerations and data handling and analysis. The small-scale project they develop can be seen as a means by which they can develop skills for reflective and reflexive professionalism and demonstrate a degree of understanding of the research process. Students have, for example, based this on a series of post mindfulness intervention interviews with three colleagues in the health service, a focus group with class of secondary pupils in a school or a pre and post intervention survey with colleagues in a business organisation. It should be stressed that during the 'research phase' of the MSc and in prior modules, that mindfulness and academic thinking/awareness are explored as closely linked. Indeed, we argue that the intelligence of meditation (sometimes called "discriminating awareness") and academic criticality overlap; that our students can engage in mindful research. Perhaps this contrasts with populist misunderstanding of meditation as being "inner peace"?

This small-scale project hopefully demonstrates a degree of mastery of process which our students then take forward into the last stage of the MSc in which they design, implement and write up a work-based project or dissertation. These tend to be larger in terms of ambition and participants. In each of the sections of this book that follow you can look at abridged accounts of our students' dissertations or research projects, as well as the story of their journey to, during and since the MSc.

MINDFULNESS IN CONTEXTS

The experiential modules are accompanied by a series of inputs and themes which aim to provide several contexts in which mindfulness has emerged, been articulated or explored (such as evolutionary psychology, neuroscience and social theory). This allows students to gain a robust criticality about mindfulness, its appeal and to interact with research into mindfulness in a discerning and scholarly way.

We think there is a need to locate mindfulness in scientific, social, philosophical and ideological context. This is an interesting aspiration given much of our teaching takes place at a Buddhist monastery! In a series of lectures, we aim to offer these contexts, thereby hopefully navigating the temptation to fall into easy binaries around the secular or spiritual origins and nature of mindfulness practice, or to avoid any accusations that our MSc is a form of Buddhist seminary (as one tabloid newspaper would have it when we first launched the degree!).

In these contextual lectures we explore the emergence of mindfulness set against social change which has, according to Alain De Botton (2013) seen a clumsy secularisation in western or Euro-American culture. The unarguable decline in the influence of, and attendance or adherence to, the churches as traditional arbiters of knowledge has had consequences. In an increasingly postmodern context the traditional 'stories' and rituals of our tribes are not working as they once did. Where once, religious institutions choreographed the social and psychological lives of people, there is now a confusing array of representation; a crisis of legitimation which is given greater impetus by the panoptical powers of technology.

Figure 3 (below) may capture the movement from a time where enchanted explanations were offered for areas of life out with our knowledge, to a situation where our psychological equilibrium is disturbed by a glut of information with no concomitant increase in the scope of our agency (our capacity of to act independently and to make own free choices). There is therefore a deficit between the information we are exposed to, and our perceived capacity to act skilfully. There is therefore an appetite for a 'thinking skills' technique which allows us to navigate this confusing time more skilfully; immunising us from the urge to catastrophise: making us aware of what we can and cannot effect (what the Stoic philosophers described as the 'dichotomy of control'), and offering a form of voluntary community.

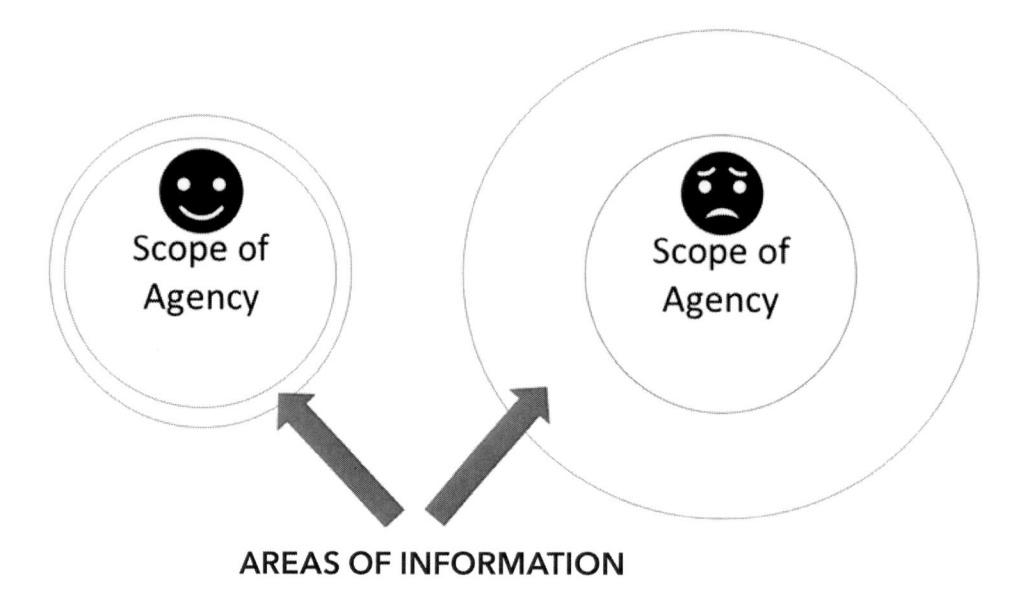

Figure 3: The Action-Information Deficit

> **Pause and Reflect**
>
> Does the Action-Information Deficit model resonate with you? Do you think technology has been a factor impacting psychological wellbeing? What practical steps can you take to have a skilful relationship with technology and the information it presents?

What we have therefore is a democratisation of consciousness. As the meta-narratives or big stories are treated with increasingly incredulity, the micro-narratives of individuals come to the fore. In the postmodern belief supermarket, the personal or individual quest for knowledge, truth, contentment and happiness becomes normative, with no one tradition holding power.

As I write these words in March 2019, I reflect that 502 years ago Martin Luther, with his protest over the perceived abuses of the Church, may have ushered in modern western democratic consciousness; his rallying call a demonstration of the power of individual conscience over institutional control, and a model for individual autonomy ever since:

> Unless I'm convinced by proofs from Scriptures or by plain and clear reasons and arguments. I can and will not retreat, for it is neither safe nor wise to do anything against conscience. Here I stand. I can do no other. God help me! (Luther 1521 cited in Ganns 1914).

Interestingly not only was Luther's protest made possible by political support, but by the newly discovered technology of the printing press. The emergence of the internet in the late twentieth century has perhaps lent new impetus to this democratisation of consciousness, though perhaps not without an impact on our equanimity! The irony of Luther's attempt to reform his Church is not only the resultant schism, but a demonstration that the institution itself could be defied or ignored. The Reformation therefore may have been instrumental in the decline of Christianity as more and more people followed Luther's modelling!

According to De Botton (2013), the result of abandoning traditional ways of organising our minds and orientating to the cosmos has been to ignore what these traditional ways gave us. The babies thrown out the bath water, for him, include:

- Rituals as ways of organising our experience around the rhythm of life
- Forgiveness as a means to resolve psychological blocks
- Being held as a sense of surrender to something out with ourselves
- Community as a way of orientating with others and experiencing common humanity
- A pessimistic (or realistic) view of the human condition as a means of dealing with the reality of suffering
- A view of education and art as about fulfilment and exploration of the good life
- Pilgrimage as a formalisation of our ambitions, goals and journeys
- Mental exercises as a way of relating to our own thinking
- Role Models as guides on how to live our lives
- Modesty about fulfilment rather than some sense of entitlement to be happy
- Myths as great stories we deliberately tell ourselves with perennial metaphorical significance

In reflecting on these perhaps we can see the opportunity costs of secularising so clumsily and the appetite for something to fill what Victor Frankl (2004) described as the existential vacuum (a time when many feel a loss of meaning in their lives)? Secular mindfulness may allow us to fulfil many of these needs, maintaining our modern individual integrity but without subscribing to some metaphysical tradition. The emergence of secular mindfulness may therefore by symptomatic of a time when people want absolution (acceptance), ritual, community, coherence and the guidance of a more experienced other, but without having to buy into a particular set of supernatural beliefs. Richard Holloway perhaps describes the process by which we have replaced religion (in this case the ritual of confession) with psychology:

> The ecclesiastical monopoly of the process has been over for a long time, and the practice of it has been largely secularised by the psycho-therapeutic professions which have taken over as the main ports at which the cargoes of human despair are now unloaded (Holloway 2013, p70).

Pause and Reflect

Do you agree with the idea that society has secularised clumsily, with little thought to replace the ways that religion choreographed our public and private lives?

MINDFULNESS AND THE ELEPHANT IS THE ROOM!

As previously mentioned much of the teaching in the Aberdeen MSc takes place at a Tibetan Buddhist monastery. It is rather interesting to think that, while we extol the potential of secular mindfulness in the quiet of a temple space, around us the prayer wheels and flags turn and flutter; monks and nuns chant petitions to Bodhisattvas, and images of Tara, Chenrezig and Shakyamuni Buddha are sentinel around every corner.

One of the first things we offer our students is a tour of the monastery and its precincts, followed by an input on the possibility and purposes of secular mindfulness. In a way, then, we surface that the elephant is the room and hopefully address any worries that we are proselytising into a religious tradition. Students are encouraged to reflect on the fact that, during the process of secularisation and democratisation of consciousness there was also an increasing awareness of other traditions (including the wisdom or dharma traditions of the east). I have already outlined some of the reasons why Buddhism may appeal to the western mindset in terms of apparent agnosticism and lack of hierarchy. Add to this an apparent lack of supernaturalism and perceived compatibility with the scientific approach; the espousal of a non-material route to contentment, and view that all phenomena is ephemeral and changing. We can therefore see that aspects of Buddhism, in many ways, have a great deal of appeal for the western mind which has largely rejected the authority of traditional institutions; adopted the scientific temper (albeit selectively in many cases), and is increasingly finding the conditions of late capitalism too fast, stressful and empty of lasting contentment!

This is, of course, why places like Samye Ling and the Holy Island, and to an extent, mindfulness have flourished. The seeds of Buddhist teachings brought to the west, particularly in the late 1960's, fell on fertile ground in that zeitgeist, the inscrutable lamas quickly were pedestalled and cushioned above contradiction; their religion shaped to fit the existential vacuum of their adopted country, stripped of deities, karmic agency and samsaric realms. Alternatively, these aspects of the religion were quickly psychologised by western devotees.

This cherry-picking from the dharma traditions is something that certain critics of secular mindfulness focus on, adding to concerns about lack of grounding in lineage the criticism that there is also a loss of ethical compass when we attempt to secularise mindfulness. One of my former colleagues at the university who was a Tibetanist scholar (and Buddhist) claims that secularity in the context of mindfulness, acts like a form of ideological prophylactic! For him describing mindfulness as secular prevents the possibility of insemination by religious ideas, but also blocks us from the benefit of its birth tradition!

SECULAR MINDFULNESS AND THE PAX ROMANA!

Criticisms of secular mindfulness like the one above are considered as part of our MSc programme, as well as other criticisms relating, for example, to the quality of research; uncertainty about the active ingredient; subjectification or personalising of injustice and suffering; unacknowledged group effect; passivity or lack of translation to social activism; lack of diversity and inclusion within mindfulness practitioners, and the perceived instrumentalisation of mindfulness and applications in what are perceived to be unethical corporate or military settings (the so-called McMindfulness phenomenon).

The response to many of these criticisms or concerns can often be that these caveats are not to do with mindfulness per se but how it is perceived, taught and applied in certain contexts. That said, it would be literally mindless of us as academics and teachers not to explore these criticisms and attempt to address them, especially as some are under-researched or have a certain amount of evidential weight. For example, I have written elsewhere (Nixon et al. 2016) about the demographics of mindfulness and this was evident in the research we conducted with our MSc cohorts 2010-13.

Our degree programme aims to be inclusive, deliberately exploring the consonance of secular awareness with mindfulness, but also allowing our students to maintain the integrity of their own ideological position (religious or otherwise). Though 'sacred awe', mindfulness and mysticism are ubiquitous to religion, they are perhaps more fundamentally hardwired within sentience or self-awareness. It could even be argued that allying them to any one tradition is to weld them to the metaphysical and moral superstructure of institutions which inevitably serve themselves more than their followers. Such institutions, in seeking to preserve themselves, blunt any radical moral, political or spiritual consciousness and use their eschatology (belief in an afterlife) as a means by which to defer action and encourage people to accept their (often unfair) situation. Indeed, the criticism often levelled at secular mindfulness from certain religious groups that it can be used as a tool for controlling or training employees/populations in acceptance of unfair situations could equally be levelled at religious traditions themselves. That is, it could be argued that religions in some forms are just that, a systematic way of encouraging people to accept the unfairness of the human condition, an organised way of deferring contentment and action until some presumed hereafter!

Not only does no tradition have a monopoly over mindfulness but these traditions sometimes domesticate it to serve their own interests and seek to sever it from moral action in society. Appeals to enchantment and flawed human nature can erode our individual conviction and autonomy, making it ok to be a flawed moral character. Repentance or the quest for merits may reinforce this and strengthen institutional control. Criticism from certain traditions that secular mindfulness is without moral compass does seem a little patronising, born of a flawed assumption that religion and ethical awareness are conflated. Our students come from incredibly diverse contexts, and in each of these professional settings there are codes of ethics which seek to enshrine and enact pro-social behaviour.

Moreover, as Sam Harris (2014) has argued, when positing the need for a 'contemplative science' mindfulness, if practiced correctly has, at its heart an ethical valency which is evident in the attitude of kindness, curiosity and compassion that one should adopt when investigating our thought-scapes. As Rob Nairn (1999) has observed 'right' mindfulness has two components; technique (the ability to settle the mind), and attitude (the quality of awareness with which we observe our thoughts). Many of the criticism of secular mindfulness are based on the idea that when it is stripped of its religious 'lineage' mindfulness is some kind of amoral psychological technique. Arguably to try to practice without an attitude of kind, compassionate curiosity is not be mindful at all.

Our programme therefore allows people of all faiths and none to develop mindful awareness. We have had Christian chaplains and Muslim imams who have sought to develop skills in mindfulness to enhance their pastoral role and devotional practice. We also argue that to be secular is to be in and of the world, which is not far removed from definitions of mindful awareness. It is important, at the outset of the programme, to differentiate secular (of the world, as opposed to religion) from secularism (the opposition to religion).

Though we don't go as far as Harris (2015) who argues that religious stylisation around mindfulness should be removed and can be a barrier to accessing any benefits of practice, we argue that people of all faiths and none can benefit, and do not have to take refuge in any tradition. The analogy I have come to use to explain this is based on my own undergraduate study of the last pagan Roman emperor Julian. Julian was emperor for a few short years in the late 4th century CE and he wanted to restore the old faiths and turn back the clock in the face of increasingly Christian homogeneity. He therefore sent architects and builders to restore sites such as the Temple in Jerusalem, the Agora in Athens, the Great Pyramids and the Delphic Oracle. His aim was to restore the market place of beliefs that had existed prior to Constantine's 312 CE conversion to Christianity; to make the empire a place where people could access and explore spirituality in their own ways. Julian died in battle after three short years as emperor, his dream unfulfilled and his reign the target of ridicule by subsequent Christian polemic.

However perhaps Julian's vision is the rather grandiose metaphor for the MSc Studies in Mindfulness at the University of Aberdeen! We preside over a 'pax romana' for our students who come to and journey within mindfulness in their own ways, exploring consonance with their own experiences and beliefs, the idea that we can, through observing our thoughts with an attitude of kindness, live with greater equanimity, realising that other centres of experience (humans) are equally subject to swirls of anxiety and rumination.

In line with Julian's vision our students explore commonalities within spiritual and philosophical traditions. After all, the post Edenic fall of humanity posited by the Abrahamic traditions; the view that we obscure reality with illusions in the Dharma traditions, and Plato's parable of the cave whereby we confuse projected shadows for the real, are all really at heart saying that to be human is to be a creative, autonomous, freethinking being. However, to be made thus is also to be capable of anxiety, misperception, rumination and shame. Arguably therefore these great traditions have, at their very foundation, the idea that a great deal of human suffering is the result of our own thought processes as thinking beings, William Blake's 'mind-forged manacles' perhaps? Interestingly the secular, naturalistic narrative that evolutionary psychology offers, as espoused by Paul Gilbert (2013), parallels this account, offering a form of absolution by evolution for our condition.

The Mindfulness MSc programme at the University of Aberdeen is therefore (dare I say it) a very broad church indeed! We also discuss the opportunity cost of the 'eastward glance' the danger that we ignore the fact that mindful resources and traditions are pre-existent in indigenous traditions within the West. It has been interesting to observe these being increasingly surfaced and growing in confidence in response to the emergence of mindfulness couched in terms of Buddhist frameworks. Christian mindfulness has become more prominent and those of a more secular persuasion such as the philosopher Massimo Pigliucci (2017) have been keen to point out that ancient Stoic philosophy anticipates much that secular (or Buddhist) mindfulness espouses.

Furthermore, as our student embark on their own research projects we introduce the idea that mindful awareness and the 'scientific temper' are closely aligned. In other words, to be mindful is to have a curious beginner's mind, an openness and an awareness of our own preferences (hypotheses) about phenomena. Mindful research is therefore arguably consonant with good science! Francis Bacon, the philosopher who formalised the scientific method in the 16th century argued that, in order to understand phenomena in themselves we must be wary of various 'idols' that lead us astray. He described these as idols of the market place; the tribe; the theatre, and the cave. These can be interpreted to mean that the good scientist should be wary of the demands of economics (market place), pre-existing stories of our society (tribe), the urge for entertainment (theatre), and habits of the mind (cave). Personally, I think such wariness or awareness of these engines of preference is not only characteristic of good science but mindfulness!

Similarly, the contemporary psychologist Ellen Langer (2009) has written a great deal about mindfulness and learning. Her thinking is captured in Figure 4 below:

MINDFUL	MINDLESS
Actively engaged in present	Automatons
Aware of context and multiple perspectives	Stuck in a rigid perspective
Drawing new distinctions	Rely on distinctions made in the past.
Guided by rules and routines	Governed by rules and routines.

Figure 4: Mindful v. Mindless learning, adapted from Langer (2009)

Langer's summary again places mindfulness and scientific awareness similarly. It also suggests that to cling to established orthodoxies, to offer undeserved deference to various authorities, either of secular or religious origin, is be mindless.

Hopefully I have demonstrated in this discussion that mindfulness, as taught in the Aberdeen University programme aims to explore the potential benefits of mindfulness in many areas of life, amongst diverse groups of professionals. To an extent therefore, in presenting an approach to mindfulness that is not exclusive to any philosophical or religious tradition we are also aiming to develop ideological mobility; a grasp of how wisdom traditions have framed the ubiquity of human suffering and tried to address it.

> **Pause and Reflect**
>
> Do you think Bacon's idols (Cave, Tribe, Marketplace and Theatre) and how we relate to them, may be at the heart of a lot of unhappiness?

CONCLUSIONS

In October 2015 the United Kingdom government launched the Mindful nation report. This report, written by a cross party parliamentary group, suggested that mindfulness should be explored within Health Care, Education, Criminal Justice and Business:

> What is already clear is that it [mindfulness] is an important innovation in mental health which warrants serious attention from politicians, policymakers, public services in health, education and criminal justice as well as employers, professional bodies, and the researchers, universities and donor foundations who can develop the evidence base further (The Mindfulness Initiative 2015, p.6).

The University of Aberdeen's Studies in Mindfulness programme has, as this book demonstrates, been meeting the aspirations of the Mindful Nation report for some time. Our degree is continuing to recruit large numbers of students from a broad range of professions. As its programme director I consider myself in a very privileged position. As you may have read above, one of the casualties of clumsy secularisation, and perhaps the neo-liberalisation of schooling, may have been a view of education that centres on addressing questions about what it is to lead a good life and how to find happiness or contentment. In working on the Studies in Mindfulness programme I consider this a central concern and think myself fortunate to work alongside an inspiring range of people who are also seeking to answer these questions and investigate the role of how relationality to our thinking may play a part in the potential for personal and professional contentment. These people are the heroes of this book.

I hope you, the reader will experience some of this in the chapters that follow as a selection of graduates and students outline their journey to the MSc, research within it, and ongoing impact on their lives. In this book you will look at, for example, how Don used mindfulness to work with autistic children; how Ian's colleagues responded to a mindfulness intervention in the health service; how Susan examined the potential of mindfulness for dealing with the stress of the 'always on' culture within business; how John explored mindfulness in ski coaching as a more embodied approach; how Susanne researched the potential of mindfulness for the creative process, and how John has developed a mindfulness intervention for elderly people. These are just a sample of this books chapters but perhaps give a flavour of the richness and range of how mindfulness can be explored. I hope this book gives you even a little of the pleasure and satisfaction reading it, as I have had working with its contributors.

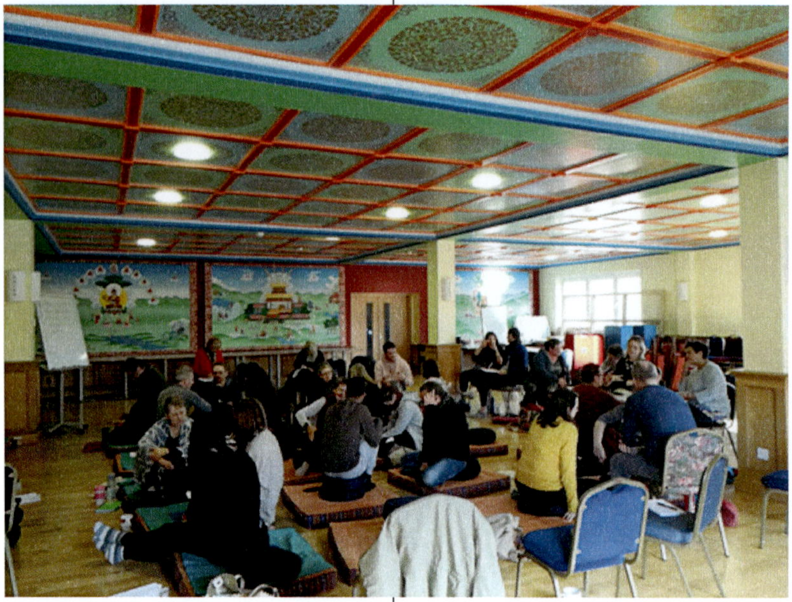

Figure 5: MSc students discussing practice experience Photo © Graeme Nixon (2018)

FURTHER RESOURCES

Sam Harris' Blog on Consciousness, Meditation and Secularism
https://samharris.org/podcast/
Published Journal Article on the MSc Studies at mindfulness at the University of Aberdeen
https://www.tandfonline.com/doi/full/10.1080/02643944.2015.1127990
University of Aberdeen MSc Studies in Mindfulness programme information
https://www.abdn.ac.uk/study/postgraduate-taught/degree-programmes/946/studies-in-mindfulness/

REFERENCES

BRUCE, S. (2018) Secular Beats Spiritual: The Westernization of the Easternization of the West, London: Oxford University Press
DE BOTTON, A. (2013) Religion for Atheists: A non-believer's guide to the uses of religion. London: Penguin
FRANKL, V. (2004). Man's search for meaning. Reading: Random House
GANNS, H. G. (1914) Luther, Martin, The Catholic Encyclopedia. New York: Robert Appleton
GILBERT, P., & CHODEN. (2013). Mindful compassion. London: Constable-Robinson.
HARRIS, S. (2015) Waking Up, Searching for Spirituality without Religion. London: Penguin
HOLLOWAY, R. (2013) Leaving Alexandria: A Memoir of Faith and Doubt. Edinburgh: Canongate
KABAT-ZINN, J. (2002). Commentary on Majumdar et al.; Mindfulness meditation for health. The Journal of Alternative and Complementary Medicine, 8, 731–735.
LANGER, E. (2000) Mindful Learning. Article in Current Directions in Psychological Science, Volime 9, pp220-223LUTHER, M. (1521) Luther's Response to the Inquisition at the Diet of Worms https://www.britannica.com/event/Diet-of-Worms-Germany-1521 (accessed 15th November 2017)
THE MINDFULNESS INITIATIVE (2015) Mindful Nation UK, Report by the Mindfulness All-Party Parliamentary Group (MAPPG) http://themindfulnessinitiative.org.uk/images/reports/Mindfulness-APPG-Report_Mindful-Nation-UK_Oct2015.pdf (accessed 15th November 2017)
NAIRN. R. (1999) Diamond Mind, a Psychology of Meditation. Massachusetts: Shambhala
NIXON ET AL. (2016) Studies in mindfulness: widening the field for all involved in pastoral care Pastoral Care in Education Vol. 34
PIGLIUCCI, M. (2017 How to Be a Stoic: Using Ancient Philosophy to Live a Modern Life. London: Rider Books
SEGAL, Z., WILLIAMS, J., & TEASDALE, J. (2012). Mindfulness-based cognitive therapy for depression: A new approach to preventing relapse. New York, NY: Guilford Press

CHAPTER 4

INTRODUCTION TO STORIES OF MINDFUL HEROES IN EDUCATIONAL SETTINGS

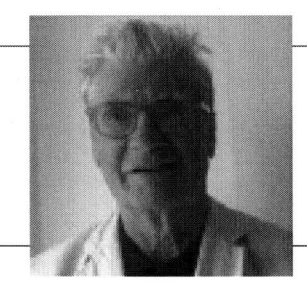

Terry Hyland

hylandterry@ymail.com

THE PATH OF MINDFULNESS?

I have taught in schools, colleges and universities throughout the UK and retired as Professor of Education at the University of Bolton in 2009. I am currently a Director and Trustee at the Free University of Ireland in Dublin where I teach philosophy and mindfulness to 'second chance' mature students. Mindfulness has become something of a boom industry over the last few decades thanks largely to the work of Kabat-Zinn (1990) who developed a Mindfulness-Based Stress Reduction (MBSR) programme in his work at the Massachusetts Medical School in 1979. Since then the work of Kabat-Zinn and associates (Williams & Kabat-Zinn, 2013) has been responsible for a massive global expansion of interest in mindfulness-based interventions in a diverse range of domains including work in schools, prisons, workplaces and hospitals, in addition to wide applications in psychology, psychotherapy, education and medicine (Purser, Fordbes & Burke, 2016).

Siegel (2007) has suggested that "at the heart of mindfulness is the teachable capacity for reflection" and that this "'earnable skill is just a breath away from being readily available as the fourth "R" of basic education" (pp.259-260). Siegel's work has shown that "resilience can be learned through experience" (p.215), and he picks out the key features of mindfulness strategies - approaching rather than avoiding difficult states, replacing rumination with observation based on curiosity and kindness, and the reflection on thoughts and feelings using notation and labelling (pp.216-225) - as ways of establishing calm and stability by integrating left and right hemispheres of the brain.

The "present-moment reality" developed through mindfulness is widely acknowledged in educational psychology as not just "more effective, but also more enjoyable'" (Langer, 2003, p.43) in many spheres of learning, and there is now a wealth of evidence aggregated through the Mindfulness in Education Network (http://www.mindfuled.org) about the general educational benefits of the approach. On the basis of work done in American schools, Schoeberlein and Sheth (2009) list a wide range of benefits of mindfulness for both teachers - improving focus and awareness, increasing responsiveness to student needs, enhancing classroom climate - and students in supporting readiness to learn, strengthening attention and concentration, reducing anxiety and enhancing social and emotional learning . As they put it:

> Mindfulness and education are beautifully interwoven. Mindfulness is about being present with and to your inner experience as well as your outer environment, including other people. When teachers are fully present, they teach better. When students are fully present, the quality of their learning is better (p.xi).

Such claims about the close interrelationships of mindfulness and educational processes and practices are fully reflected in the present book through the accounts of teachers working in a diverse range of contexts and making use of a wide variety of mindfulness strategies.

WORKING WITH CHILDREN WITH AUTISTIC SPECTRUM CONDITION

The close links between mindfulness, education and therapy – all aimed at enhancing mind/body wellbeing through cultivating present moment awareness and emotional resilience (Hyland, 2018a) – are exemplified in Donald Gordon's work (Chapter 5) with children identified with Autistic Spectrum Condition (ASC). Grounded in recent research in the field, Gordon's work with such children is supported by a sound philosophical principle of seeking to align the life we ought to be living with the one we actually live. This provides a solid ethical foundation for mindfulness work with ASC children aimed at helping them to achieve their full human potential in all aspects of life and learning.

It is heartening to note Gordon's insistence on grounding all teaching/learning in this sphere within what he described as the "compass of bliss" which incorporates the values of loving-kindness and compassion drawn from the spiritual traditions (essentially Buddhist roots) which provide mindfulness practice with its deep and powerful meaning and significance. Gordon's concern with the problems of assessment and measurement in education are also to be welcomed since such questions have been at the heart of the commodification and commercialisation of practice popularly labelled 'McMindfulness' (Purser & Loy, 2013; Hyland, 2017, 2018b) in recent years. Although it is not clear that the modified assessment scheme used here managed to avoid all the dangers of tick box educational measurement, the content of the programme making use of nature walks and environmental interventions was enough to ensure positive outcomes for the ASC children.

MINDFULNESS WITH ADOLESCENTS

Heather Grace Bond's imaginative work with young students (Chapter 6) is firmly rooted in philosophical questions about the meaning and purpose of education. This is to be applauded since aspects of the contemporary mindfulness in schools movement often neglect such questions in favour of concerns with enhancing traditional academic goals (Hyland, 2015; O'Donnell, 2015). Bond's recommendations for practice – informed by progressive educators such as Rousseau and Freire – is fully aligned with the mindfulness practices grounded in the Buddhist traditions alluded to in her account of working with adolescents.

References to the importance of Aristotelian ethics in this context were apt since Aristotle's "middle way'" philosophy concerned with the cultivation of virtue is on all fours with the fostering of the brahma-viharas (virtues and meditation practices to cultivate them). These are loving-kindness, compassion, sympathetic joy and equanimity – in Buddhist mindfulness practice. Bond provides a comprehensive survey of the empirical research on young people's development in these emotionally volatile years, and utilises this to good effect in her programme informed by the compassion/self-compassion work by Kristin Neff and Paul Gilbert. The mythical metaphors foregrounded in Bond's description of both her personal mindfulness journey and her learning/teaching strategies were well chosen and added imaginative depth to the recommendations for practice.

MINDFULNESS AND POETRY

The creative use of poetry in mindfulness theory and practice is well-established (Santorelli & Kabat-Zinn, 2001). Many of Thich Nhat Hanh's poems, for example, can be said to encapsulate the core aims and values of mindfulness practice (Hanh, 1999). This rich tradition is exemplified to great effect by Terry Barrett, Naomi McAreavey and Larry McNutt (Chapter 7) in their account of the use of a broad and diverse range of poetry with higher education students and staff. With the aim of creating mindful spaces for reflection and personal transformation, poems by, for instance, Philip Sydney and Robert Hayden are linked with appropriate images to foster the appropriate environmental spaciousness. Reading, writing and listening are imaginatively inter-connected in the learning/teaching sessions to create an authentic climate of contemplative pedagogy. Moreover, such work helps to shift educational processes away from their obsession with cognitive aims towards the affective and psychomotor domains of education which are crucial to the cultivation of mindful awareness (Weare, 2004; Hyland, 2011).

MINDFULNESS, SPIRITUALITY, ETHICS AND EDUCATION

Recent negative developments resulting in the commodification of mindfulness practice were alluded to earlier. These were serious enough to cause Kabat-Zinn (2015) to express:

> concerns that a sort of superficial "McMindfulness" is taking over which ignores the ethical foundations of the meditative practices and traditions from which mindfulness has emerged, and divorces it from its profoundly transformative potential (p.1).

Mindfulness, we are reminded, can "never be a quick fix," and there are grave dangers in ignoring "the ethical foundations of the meditative practices and traditions from which mindfulness has emerged" (p.1.).

There can be little doubt that all of the educational applications of mindfulness described in the chapters in this section of the book manage to avoid the pitfalls noted by Kabat-Zinn. The foundational principles and values undergirding mindfulness spiritual traditions are fully reflected in all the accounts, and it was refreshing to note the foregrounding of Buddhist ethical precepts – what Kabat-Zinn rightly refers to as the 'universal dharma' (2015, p.1) – in the statements of inspirational sources and operational approaches.

REFERENCES

KABAT-ZINN, J.(1990). Full Catastrophe Living (London: Piatkus)
KABAT-ZINN, J.(2015). Mindfulness has huge health potential – but McMindfulness is no panacea; The Guardian, 20.10.15;
http://www.theguardian.com/commentisfree/2015/oct/20/mindfulness-mental-health-potential-benefits-uk , accessed 3.11.17
HANH, Thich Nhat (1999). Call Me By My True Names (Berkeley, CA: Parallax Press)
HYLAND, T.(2011) Mindfulness and Learning: Celebrating the Affective Dimension of Education. (Dordrecht, The Netherlands: Springer Press)
HYLAND, T. (2015). On the Contemporary Applications of Mindfulness: Some Implications for Education; Journal of Philosophy of Education, 49 (2),170-186
HYLAND, T. (2017). McDonaldizing Spirituality: Mindfulness, Education and Consumerism; Journal of Transformative Education , 17 (4),334-356
HYLAND, T. (2018a). Philosophy, Science and Mindfulness (Mauritius: Scholars' Press)
HYLAND, T. (2018b). The Degeneration of Contemporary Mindfulness: re-asserting the ethical and educational foundations of practice in mindfulness-based interventions; in Brewer, L.(ed)(2018) Meditation: Practices, Techniques and Health Benefits (New York: Nova Science Publishers)
LANGER, E. (2003). A Mindful Education. Educational Psychologist, 28 (1), 43-50
O'DONNELL, A.(2015). Contemplative Pedagogy and Mindfulness: Developing Creative Attention in an Age of Distraction; Journal of Philosophy of Education, 49 (2), pp.187-202
PURSER, R. & LOY, D. (2013). Beyond McMindfulness; Huffington Post, 1/7/13, http://www.huffingtonpost.com/ron-purser/beyond-mcmindfulness_b_3519289.html;accessed 14/7/17
PURSER, R.E., FORBES, D. & BURKE, A. (2016) (eds) Handbook of Mindfulness: Culture, Context and Social Engagement (Switzerland: Springer International Publishing)
SANTORELLI, S. & KABAT-ZINN, J. (2001). Poetry for Mindfulness Based Stress Reduction in Mind-Body Medicine (University of Massachusetts Medical School : Centre for Mindfulness in Medicine, Health Care and Society)
SCHOEBERLEIN, D. & SHETH, S.(2009). Mindful Teaching and Teaching Mindfulness. (Boston: Wisdom Publications)
SIEGEL, D.J. (2007). The Mindful Brain. (New York: W.W. Norton & Co).
WEARE, K. (2004) Developing the Emotionally Literate School (London: Paul Chapman)
WILLIAMS, J.M.G. & KABAT-ZINN, J. (eds) (2013). Mindfulness: Diverse Perspectives on its Meaning, Origins and Applications (Abingdon: Routledge)

CHAPTER 5

AS THE STARS ALIGN: EFFECTS OF MINDFULNESS ON CHILDREN WITH AUTISTIC SPECTRUM CONDITION (ASC)

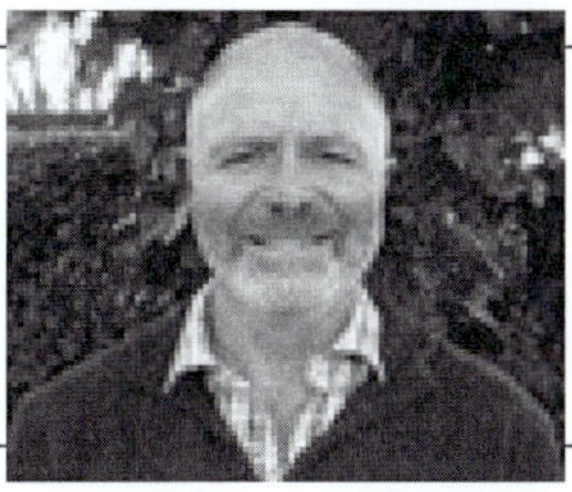

Donald Gordon

dm.gordon@btinternet.com

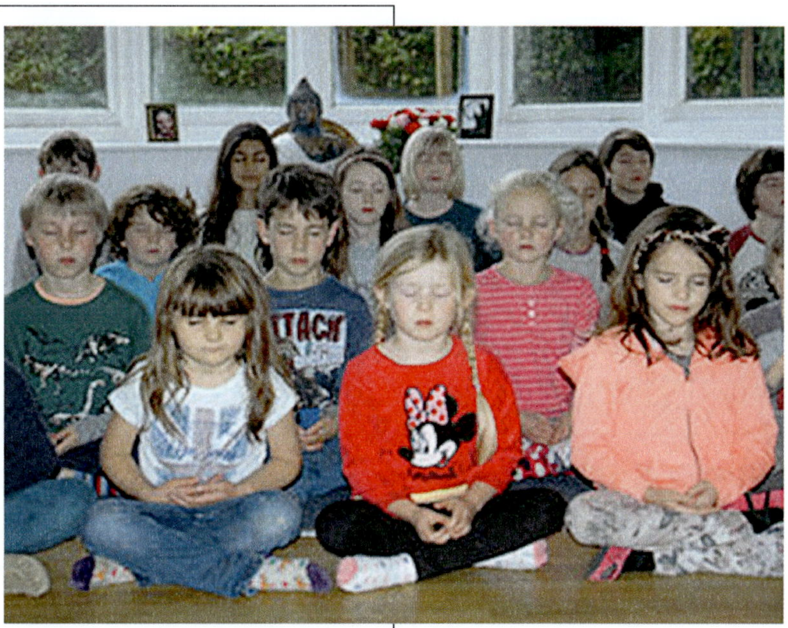

Figure 1: Children Meditating Photo by DharmaBN1

INTRODUCTION

ALIGNMENT OF STARS

As the stars aligned, so too did my journey into mindfulness and working with children with Autistic Spectrum Condition (ASC). The seeds for training in mindfulness were planted a long time ago: an inclination towards matters both spiritual and scientific from a very early age; studying ecology while taking optional courses in world religions and bioethics at university; to a career spanning work in education and environmental conservation, including time spent in Southeast Asia. It is perhaps not surprising that the combination of mindfulness and time spent in nature has represented an evolving theme to my journey, discussed more at the end of the chapter.

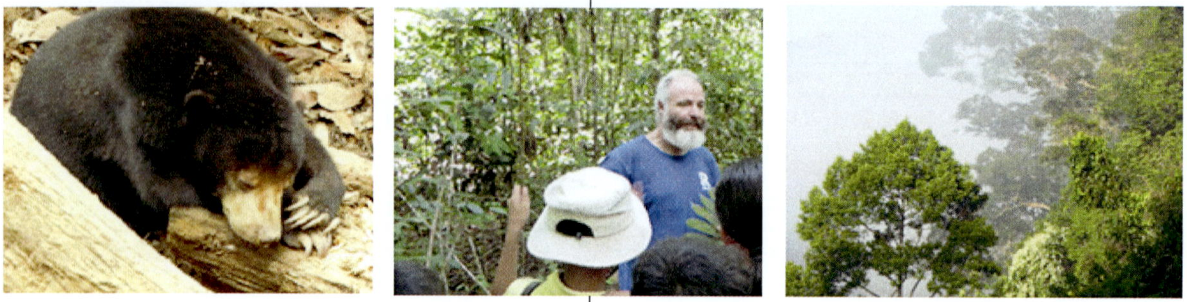

Figure 2: Conservation and Environmental Education in Malaysia Photos © Donald Gordon 2014

Rather unexpectedly, early formative experiences came together about fifteen years ago when my eldest son was invited to visit Samye Ling Monastery, Scotland as part of a school trip. When asked about his experience, he remarked, something to the effect, that "spending an hour meditating was a complete waste of time, particularly when it could be used to play football!" Intended or not, his reverse psychology worked, and my curiosity was piqued. It wasn't long afterwards that I started attending courses in various aspects of meditation, leading into forming the first, and by all accounts, rather challenging cohort of students who participated in the MSc Studies in Mindfulness programme which started in 2010.

Coinciding with my growing interest in mindfulness, I was appointed to teach science at a Special Needs School in the U.K. that works with students with learning and communication difficulties from five to nineteen years of age. Around seventy percent of those students had a diagnosis of Autistic Spectrum Condition (ASC). Teaching special needs was new territory - indeed, my first day jitters were not helped much by being confronted by a very tall and direct student on the school yard, who looked me up and down and, after considerable inspection, stated within earshot of all willing to listen "you've got to be kidding!" It proved an important lesson in maintaining equanimity and a sense of humour – we became friends and I taught at the school for ten years.

With a commitment to enabling students to reach both academic and personal potential, the school became increasingly interested in the contribution mindfulness could make to student wellbeing, along with the development of life, academic and communication skills. A couple of trial interventions in offering mindfulness to students yielded encouraging results. In one such study I conducted in 2010, a seven-week course of mindfulness was offered to fifteen students, comprising one class in each of key stages three (eleven to fourteen years of age), four (fourteen to sixteen years) and five (sixteen plus). Results from the study showed that students perceived the most positive effects of mindfulness to be on concentration (forty percent of students felt their attention had improved) and mood (over thirty percent felt that they had become happier), while more than twenty-five percent of students felt they had become less calm; the latter result often referred to as the waterfall experience where the mind appears to be more agitated when first engaging with mindfulness practices.

The momentum and results gained on the back of these trials ended up convincing senior management to offer instruction in self-awareness to all students as part of the school curriculum. The development of the Self- Awareness Programme, so-called to allay fears that we were offering any sort of religious indoctrination, commenced at the beginning of the 2010 academic year. The school also provided financial support for me to participate in the MSc Studies in Mindfulness programme in order to further mindfulness at the school and to begin building a more robust evidence base as to the benefits or otherwise of offering instruction in this area to students with ASC. The stars continued to align…

FOLLOWING MY BLISS

As outlined by Vin Harris in Chapter 2, Joseph Campbell (1949) alluded to the need to apply insight and courage in returning time and again to aligning the life you ought to be living to the one you are living. He continued by stating that this journey is often not linear (circles within circles) but necessary in enabling individuals to achieve full potential.

In developing this analogy a bit further, my own journey into teaching children with special needs may be framed using a compass where the arrow pointing North (N) represents a state of being in flow with life. As illustrated in Figure 3, this arrow firmly points to expressions in education, the natural world, poetry, youth development and human psychology. Mindfulness has not only been part of this journey in terms of expression but also in helping me to approach life in ways which are authentic given my personality and life experiences.

> **Pause and Reflect**
> **Insight Practice – Reflective Questions**
>
> Allow the mind to gently settle on the breath and then gradually ask yourself each question three times, allowing pauses to write down anything that emerges:
>
> What are my strengths?
> What are my values?
> What would I like to do in life?

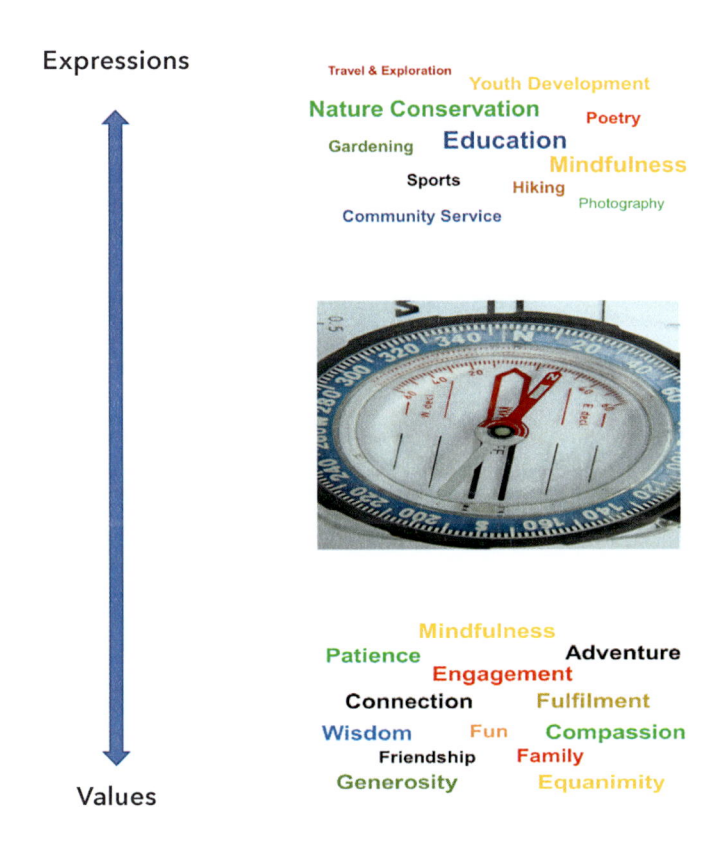

Figure 3: Compass of Bliss

The expressions in Figure 3 are also informed and coloured by values at the heart of mindfulness and more formal spiritual traditions: being aware of what is happening while it is happening without preference (mindfulness); responding in ways that are helpful to both myself and others (compassion); and in the analogy of the Return in the Hero's Journey by Joseph Campbell (1949), having the opportunity to connect with and support fellow travellers. Not surprisingly, mindfulness, self-kindness and connection with common humanity are also the three inter-related components of self-compassion identified by Neff (2011) and outlined in the self-compassion break.

Pause and Reflect
Self-Compassion Break

Bring to mind a slightly uncomfortable situation. Then, with hands on heart, repeat the following to yourself three times:

- This is a moment of difficulty (mindfulness)
- Difficulty is part of life (common humanity)
- May I be kind to myself (self-kindness)

In the analogy of the compass, it is perhaps not surprising that the arrow is not pointing due north. In my own experience, when this arrow has deviated from my bliss either in terms of core values or expression, there is a certain unease that sets in – the greater the drift, the greater the unease! The sense that something isn't quite right also promotes an increasing fascination with the existential vacuum mentioned by Graeme Nixon in Chapter 3 in the writing of Frankl (2004). The compass also underscores the deeper imperative of meaning and purpose as mindfulness is considered in its wider context of awakening full human potential.

Against this personal and professional background, the time was ripe to explore the effects of mindfulness on children with Autistic Spectrum Condition (ASC). More specifically, I was intrigued to see how my personal journey in mindfulness could be applied and adapted in contributing to the development and wellbeing of students at the school. The journey began with an exploration of the evidence base in the application of mindfulness with children, with particular reference to those with ASC. A full reference to the MSc thesis on which the following is based is provided at the end of the chapter (Gordon, 2014).

THE EVIDENCE BASE – GROWING

MINDFULNESS AND YOUNG PEOPLE

Coyne et al (2008) assert that the state of literature regarding assessment of acceptance and mindfulness in children and adolescents is much like the population it is trying to assess, namely, young and developing. Despite this, there is growing evidence as to the impacts and effects of mindfulness on young people in the context of such programmes as Mindfulness-based Cognitive Therapy for Children (MBCT-C), Mindfulness-based Stress Reduction (MBSR) for Children, Dialectic Behaviour Therapy for Adolescents (DBT-A) and the Mindfulness in Schools Project (.b curriculum). For further details of these programmes, please see Further Resources at the end of the chapter.
Much of the literature associated with these programmes points in the direction of improved wellbeing and attention, reduced worry, anxiety and reactivity, and greater calmness, self-regulation and awareness (Weare, 2013). A meta-analysis carried out by Zoogman et al (2015) found mindfulness interventions to be helpful overall and a promising intervention for young people. Using the .b curriculum, the Welcome Trust is currently funding the My Resilience in Adolescence Project (MYRIAD), aimed at assessing the effectiveness of mindfulness training in young adolescents and whether this training is effective and cost-effective in schools (MYRIAD, 2018). Not surprisingly, when it comes to children with special needs, research and evaluation of the potential effects of mindfulness are even more limited but emerging.

MEASURING THE EFFECTS OF MINDFULNESS

A further difficulty in measuring the effects of mindfulness on children and adolescents, particularly those with special needs, is in the use of standardised research instruments (e.g. questionnaires) able to validate emerging claims. Research that I conducted as part of Professional Enquiry in the MSc Studies in Mindfulness programme identified four main research instruments that had been developed for children in assessing the effects of mindfulness. Unfortunately, none had been developed for use with children having special needs (Gordon, 2012).

Following careful scrutiny of these four instruments, it was decided to trial the Child and Adolescent Mindfulness Measure (CAMM) with our students, given the following:

- CAMM was designed for children between the ages of nine and eighteen; other measures were not designed for children as young as nine.
- CAMM is based on a limited number of questions (ten), whereas other measures include up to thirty-two questions.
- CAMM is a single variable measure of mindfulness, able to show changes from pre to post intervention with respect to acting with awareness and being able to accept internal experience without judgement.

In trialling CAMM, it was found that many of our students found the original research instrument difficult to understand in terms of language used as well as understanding the meaning to some of the questions being asked. A link to the original CAMM questionnaire may be found in the Further Resources section at the end of this chapter. Subsequently, a much more user-friendly version of CAMM was prepared (Appendix 1) through the input of eight students and working in conjunction with the Speech and Language Therapy (SALT) Department at the school. Modifications included simplifying the language to questions being asked and accompanying these questions with visual symbols. Visual symbols are used extensively at the school given that many students with ASC have a visual style of learning.

AUTISTIC SPECTRUM CONDITION (ASC)

Autistic Spectrum Condition (ASC) is considered a spectrum condition as it manifests itself differently in each individual (Siegel, 2003). Characteristics of ASC include varying degrees of difficulty in the areas of social interaction, verbal and nonverbal communication, and repetitive behaviours. Asperger's Syndrome is part of that spectrum.

---

1. Attention shifting, where attention may be hard to get, hard to shift or both.
2. Lack of curiosity and preference for the familiar, particularly where novelty may be perceived as unsettling or threatening.
3. Reinforcer saliency or finding rewards (things of interest) that work.
4. Arousal regulation - may involve hyper or hypo-sensitivities to stimuli and what these individuals tend to seek out or avoid colours the way they see the world.
5. Perseveration or tireless engagement in repetitive behaviours.
6. Perceptual inconstancy - experiencing sensory input (e.g. visual, auditory) in ways that are different to others. There is evidence that children with ASC are more orientated to senses that are proximal (e.g. close and include senses associated with touch, smell and body movement) rather than distal (e.g. far and include senses such as sight and hearing).
7. Processing speed - auditory processing is a common problem in people with ASC, many of which have a visual style of learning.
8. Affiliative orientation – represented by a lack of desire to be with or like others. This results in a desire to be alone, and there is a strong motivation to please oneself rather than others. Students with ASC tend not to respond well to social praise, encouragement or peer pressure.
9. Theory of Mind - the ability to put oneself in another person's shoes. This development need makes it difficult for people with ASC to understand and respond to others in ways that are age-appropriate and naturally empathetic. Related to difficulties with both verbal (receiving, processing and responding) and non-verbal communication (recognising and responding appropriately to social cues).

Figure 4: Development Needs in Students with ASC Adapted from Siegel (2003).

Siegel (2003) outlines nine primary deficits or development needs in individuals with ASC. These are outlined in Figure 4 and are instructive in considering the contribution that mindfulness may make to the development and learning of students with ASC.

Consequently, typical strengths with an autistic learning style include:

- Preference for visual and logically ordered information
- Learning through cognition rather than through social routes.
- Comfortable with habitual forms of learning in preference to problem solving approaches.
- Preference for routine, predictability and structure.
- High motivation with special interests
- Attention to repetition, precision, and consistent accuracy, with a highly attention specific style of thinking (Jordan (2004), Singhania (2005) and Siegel (2003).

In contrast to the deficit model presented in Figure 4, evidence is beginning to point towards a unique learning style on the part of individuals with ASC. Proponents of SAACA (Single Attention and Associated Cognition in Autism) argue that the learning style of individuals with ASC is based on single interest attention, often using one sensory mode at a time. Further, there is a close connection between sensory-motor systems, the interest system and that of attention in a sensory-motor interest loop (Lawson, 2011).

Manifestations of ASC typically include low self-esteem, depression, issues with anger management, impulsivity in the face of emotions such as anger, and poor attentional skills due to a range of external (social alienation/bullying) and internal (blame, self-criticism, lack of interest) factors. Restoratives to emotional balance include retreat to places of solitude, constructively channelling excessive energy into physical activities, repetitive actions (routine) such as rocking or manipulating an object such as a stress ball, diverting attention to another task, helping others (being needed), discussing a problem from different perspectives, cue-controlled relaxation (e.g. a card/object that takes you to a place of safeness) and engagement in special interests, away from environments that lead to an overstimulation of the senses (Atwood, 2007).

RATIONALE FOR THE STUDY

In reviewing the literature, it became apparent that there was great potential for training in mindfulness to tap into and support the unique learning style of students with ASC, particularly given the use of single-focus sensory supports (e.g. breath, sound, tactile objects) in settling the mind and developing faculties such as attention. Evidence was also suggesting that training in mindfulness resonates well with emotional restoratives and addresses a number of manifestations (anxiety, depression, anger) that are prevalent in individuals with ASC. Further, training in mindfulness provides an alternative way of learning about and relating to patterns of thought and emotion in ways that are spacious, responsive and skilful. Against this background and the fact that little research had been done in this area, a study on the effects of mindfulness on an ability to act with awareness and accept internal experience without judgement was warranted.

RESEARCH QUESTION AND OBJECTIVES

Question: Does training in mindfulness enhance the ability of students to (a) act with awareness and (b) accept internal experiences without judgement?

Objectives:
1. To conduct an evaluation of student's perceptions to (a) act with awareness and (b) accept internal experiences without judgement before and after a mindfulness intervention.
2. To map key aspects of the mindfulness intervention against development needs and learning on the part of students with ASC.

STUDY APPROACH, RESULTS & EVALUATION

EVALUATION OF STUDENT PERCEPTIONS

As Self-Awareness was a curriculum subject at the school, all classes, along with their form tutors, received one forty-five minute lesson in mindfulness per week with an opportunity to practice materials learned during morning form times (registration periods). Form tutors were also encouraged to set aside about five minutes during at least two registration periods per week in order for students to consolidate practices learned. For the purposes of the study, the structured mindfulness intervention spanned thirty-one weeks (Figure 5), was offered to classes from key stages two through five and included use of a pre and post CAMM research instrument to evaluate student perceptions as to the effectiveness of mindfulness in allowing them to act with awareness and accept internal experiences without judgement. The intervention shown in Figure 5 was based on the practices learned on the MSc Studies in Mindfulness Programme and subsequently adapted for use with students at the school.

Term	Weeks	Major theme	Main Activities
Autumn I	7	Recognising the Unsettled Mind	- Mindful walking/movement - Recognising the Unsettled Mind - Settling the Mind
Autumn II	7	Settling the Mind	- Settling, grounding, resting (SGR) and using supports (sound, breath, stones, candles) - Three Minute Breathing Space - Compassionate Body Scan
Spring I	6	Kindness Practices	- SGR & use of Supports - Place of Safeness Practice - Kindness Practice Oneself & Others - Self Compassion Break
Spring II	5	Kindness & Self compassion	- Soles of the Feet Practice - Compassionate Walking - Kindness and Self Compassion Practices
Summer I	6	Compassion for Self and Others	- SGR & use of Supports - Soften, Soothe, Allow Practice - Tonglen (taking and sending) - Role Play & Three Minute Breathing Space

Figure 5: Overview of the Mindfulness Intervention

In total, results from thirty-nine students were used to assess change resulting from the mindfulness intervention. The results (Figure 6) are presented in terms of scores increasing, decreasing or staying the same in going from pre to post intervention. Overall, it was found that twenty of thirty-nine students (fifty-one percent) showed an increase in the overall CAMM score, eighteen of thirty-nine students (forty-six percent) showed a decrease, while one student recorded the same score. The most pronounced change was in Key Stage Three (eleven to fourteen years of age), where the number of students showing an increase in score was almost twice those showing a decrease.

Number of Students

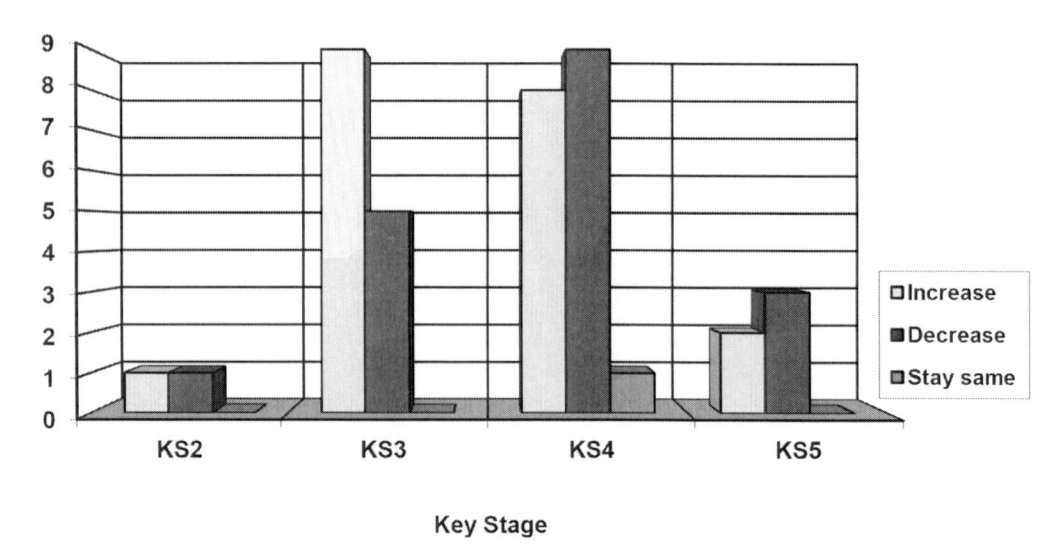

Figure 6: Change in CAMM Score by Key Stage

At first glance, these results may be reflective of younger children being more open and receptive to new experiences, including engagement with mindfulness practice – that is, before the trials, tribulations and scepticisms of the teenage years set in (Bernay, 2009). For schools looking to introduce mindfulness programmes, the implication is that access to and acceptability of mindfulness may be enhanced by introducing interventions such as this at relatively early key stage years.

Of perhaps more interest, however, were the results shown with the Key Stage Four students (fourteen to sixteen years of age). To that end, four semi-structured interviews were conducted – two with students showing an increase in CAMM score and two showing a decrease to gain insight into what might be accounting for these results. The first line of enquiry was to ask students if they understood the questions being asked, fully expecting this not to be an issue in having tested and thoroughly adapted the original CAMM research instrument (Appendix One). The first surprise was that only one student stated that they confidently understood the questions being asked at both pre-intervention and post-intervention stages of the study. One of the students who showed a decrease in CAMM score stated that he understood the questions much better after our discussion - this would have resulted in more progress being shown in aspects being assessed following the mindfulness intervention.

The second surprise was that all four students felt that their ability to act with awareness, particularly in being able to focus on the tasks at hand, had improved over the course of the mindfulness intervention. Students cited specific examples of how this faculty of attention had been enhanced: one student remarked that he was "now able to do larger projects and see them through to the end", while another student mentioned improved focus at school, partly due to needing good grades for entry to a course at college. Further, two of the students cited examples of improved attention with activities being pursued outside of school; in one, his performance in archery had "improved dramatically" with being able to focus on one thing at a time.

The other integral part of the CAMM research instrument was in evaluating the ability to accept internal experiences without judgement. Herein lies the third surprise as achieving this level of equanimity with the rising and falling of thoughts and emotions, some pleasant, some not, may take years, if ever, to fully achieve. Rather, interviews with students revealed an increasing ability to recognise and manage thoughts and emotions in increasingly mature ways. One student mentioned that he was "aware of having a bad day" on the snooker table, while another remarked that he had become "better at recognising anger in being able to feel the emotion in the body." Making that first step in developing an awareness of the internal environment is an important precursor in relating to difficult thoughts and emotions from different perspectives; a step that is difficult for many with ASC due to issues of impulsivity and problems with putting oneself in another person's shoes (theory of mind).

Insofar as managing difficult thoughts and emotions are concerned, the students interviewed were at various stages of letting be, letting go and being able to respond with varying degrees of perspective and spaciousness. While one student mentioned that he tries to "get rid of emotions he doesn't like", he also stated that he will often count to ten when angry, echoing comments from a number of students in their ability to focus on the breath in order to stay calm and "retain focus with the tasks at hand." Energy follows focus. Another student mentioned that he felt there was "more stuff" going on now and that he felt a need to "channel the energy constructively"; for example, "by hitting the gym if in a bad mood". He further remarked that he wasn't "keeping so busy as to block thoughts and emotions, but rather finding constructive outlets while still being aware of their presence." He also stated that he "may even use emotions such as anger to give him a boost. While many of these strategies may be tinged with judgement, what was impressive was the ability of these students, many of whom suffer from issues of anger, depression and anxiety, to demonstrate an ability to relate to internal experiences in more expansive and constructive ways, along with an ability to express such emotions in ways that are increasingly beneficial to themselves and others. This may be a more realistic and sensitive measure of emotional development in contrast to the much more difficult and long-standing ability to accept internal experiences without judgement...

Pause and Reflect
Three Minute Breathing Space

Becoming aware – Rest attention on sensations, thoughts and emotions using the question 'What am I experiencing right now?'
Gathering – Bring attention to the breath using slightly deeper breath to settle, perhaps to a count of three or four on the in and out breaths.
Expanding Outwards – Allow the breath to return to normal and rest attention on whatever arises in the body or mind, gradually expanding to an awareness of the space around you.

Pause and Reflect

One of the ways we adapted the Three Minute Breathing Space was to invite students to bring to mind a mildly irritating situation (e.g. being blamed for something that was not their fault) and to write down their immediate reactions to this situation. We then invited students to recall the situation once again, followed by practicing the Three Minute Breathing Space. They were then asked to write down their responses to this situation following the practice.

Would their *responses* to this situation be any different in having engaged the Three Minute Breathing Space?

These interviews were revealing and pointed out a number of potential weaknesses in using self-assessment research instruments such as the adapted CAMM:

- An assumption that questions are properly understood.
- Answering of pre and post-intervention research instruments from different levels of understanding, compromising a like for like comparison.
- In measuring more than one variable (e.g. acting with awareness and an ability to accept internal experiences without judgement), difficulty in ascertaining the effect and extent of the mindfulness intervention with respect to each particular aspect.
- The sensitivity of scales such as CAMM in measuring change, more successfully illustrated through qualitative approaches.

It is perhaps noteworthy that even the proponents who developed the original CAMM research instrument stated that further research was needed to examine the sensitivity of CAMM in detecting treatment effects, as well as its usefulness in identifying mechanisms of change (Greco et al, 2011). At the very least, it underscores the need to support the use of robust quantitative approaches with the more subtle and contextual approaches of qualitative techniques in working with students with ASC.

ASC AND THE MINDFULNESS INTERVENTION

A second objective to the study was to map key aspects of the mindfulness intervention against published development and learning needs of students with ASC. Key aspects of the mindfulness intervention were listed and grouped under three headings, namely structure to the intervention; content offered; and the intervention environment.

Category	Aspect
Structure	A Lesson template of *Play, Meditate, Share* and *Apply*
	B Consolidation of lesson materials over several sessions
	C Intensity of Intervention (one lesson per week + form times)
Content	D Mindful Eating of a Sweet
	E *Settling, Grounding, Resting* and use of Mindfulness *Supports*
	F Kindness Practice for Oneself and Others
	G Mindful movement
Environment	H Self-Awareness Room (location, ambiance, furnishings and equipment, facilitation)

Figure 7: Aspects of the Mindfulness Intervention by Category

In mapping key aspects of the mindfulness intervention against development needs, Figure 8 shows that five of the development needs were fully met while four were partially met using the criteria indicated.

The data may also be interpreted by looking down the columns. Within the structure category, intensity of intervention (C) was important in addressing or working with five of the development needs, while within the content category, the stock practice of settling, grounding, resting and use of mindfulness supports (E) was considered to be important in addressing all development needs. The table also indicates that creating the right environment (H) supports the majority of development needs in students with ASC.

Development Needs	A	B	C	D	E	F	G	H	Need Addressed?
1 Attention shifting			√	√	√	√	√	√	Fully
2 Preference for familiar	√	√	√	√	√	√		√	Fully
3 Reinforcer saliency				√	√	√	√	√	Fully
4 Arousal regulation			√	√	√			√	Partially
5 Perseveration	√		√	√	√	√	√		Fully
6 Perceptual inconstancy					√		√	√	Partially
7 Processing speed	√	√	√		√	√		√	Fully
8 Affiliative orientation					√	√	√	√	Partially
9 Theory of Mind	√				√	√	√		Partially

Need Addressed: Fully (≥ 5); Partially (2-4); Not at all (< 2).

Figure 8: Addressing Development Needs of Students with ASC

While this exercise represented a first pass at matching aspects of the mindfulness intervention against support for development needs, the amount of overlap became surprisingly evident.

INTERVENTION STRUCTURE

Much of the structure introduced in the mindfulness lessons served to build on the strengths of an autistic learning style, the hallmarks of which include a preference for habitual forms of learning and a resonance with routine, repetition, structure and predictability. As Siegel (2003) points out, the structured approach, such as that used with the template of Play, Meditate, Share and Apply (Greenland, 2010), is naturally reinforcing to routine-bound individuals, even where the content within that structure may be varied. Further, the use of routine structure and repetitive activities serve as important emotional restoratives in reducing feelings of anxiety and stress.

An integral component of all mindfulness practices is the opportunity for students to share their experiences. Also known as Enquiry, this phase represents a dialogue between facilitator and participants, aimed at drawing out understandings and insights from the practice. From the perspective of learning in students with ASC, this phase supports a number of learning and development functions. These include enabling social interaction, providing a forum for increasing understanding about oneself and others (theory of mind considerations), and an opportunity to develop communication skills in areas such as listening, turn taking, and the sharing of interests (Jordan, 2004).

With respect to intensity of intervention, a 'little and often' approach was the philosophy behind (a) offering instruction in mindfulness each week, (b) consolidating lesson materials over several weeks, and (c) providing opportunities to practice what had been learned during morning form times. In this way, strengths and needs inherent to an autistic style of learning (e.g. routine, preference for the familiar, arousal regulation using different supports) were taken into account, while adhering to a general principle that developing faculties such as attention from mindfulness benefit from sustained and cumulative practice.

One of the areas identified for improvement with the approach taken to mindfulness at the school was in the area of working more extensively with parents/guardians of students with ASC. Authors such as Siegel (2003) point to the importance of family support in successfully offering treatment interventions. Notable approaches in encouraging family support include offering mindfulness workshops and programmes for parents and making mindfulness materials available online in enabling home support.

INTERVENTION CONTENT

Apart from supporting many aspects of an autistic style of learning, the content of the mindfulness intervention provided a framework that supported (a) acting with awareness, and (b) accepting internal experience without judgement.

Attention shifting is addressed in practices such as the mindful eating of a sweet or raisin. When the mind wanders, it is gently returned to the taste and texture of the sweet. In students, including those with ASC, it also supports the generalisation of learned skills, namely, applying mindfulness to everyday activities such as eating, drinking and walking. An additional benefit of using a sweet as a mindfulness support is that it has a high reward saliency to students with ASC. As Siegel (2003) points out, food is well known as a classical reinforcer. Students who may be initially resistant to practicing mindfulness are therein able to do so when paired with eating a sweet – in other words, when paired with using something of real interest to them!

The foundation to all mindfulness and compassion practices offered at the school was in making use of a structured, sequential and routine approach that enabled students to move from a place of doing to being. Settling, Grounding, Resting and using Supports taps into all development needs of those with ASC, as well as adhering to best educational practices in offering systematic instruction, creating a structured learning environment, and providing support for the communications curriculum through sharing and discussion following mindfulness practice. Apart from its role in developing the faculty of attention, Greenland (2010) also points out that using the slightly deeper breathing associated with settling is an important way of self-regulating, while the progressive use of a range of different supports (e.g. visual, sound, tactile) is a valuable tool providing safe exposure to and assistance with arousal regulation and perceptual inconstancy. Further, using different supports enabled the mindfulness intervention to be tailored to the needs and inclinations of individual students, thereby increasing reward saliency by stimulating interest and motivation in students, along with supporting a single-focus sensory mode of learning characteristic of those with ASC (Lawson, 2011).

Judicially using a range of preferred and least preferred supports also enabled students to learn about habitual preferences and gradually develop an ability to understand, accept and relate to different stimuli and the perspectives they bring in seeing the world. Students are thus able to see that they are not bound to habitually react to arising thoughts and emotions and are able to relate to the world in different ways (Brach, 2003). In slowly gaining this insight, foundations were being laid for being able to accept internal experiences without judgement.

Kindness and self-compassion practices build on the template of Settling, Grounding, and Resting and work to address a range of development needs, most notably affiliative orientation and theory of mind. Kindness and compassion practices are designed explicitly to develop such attributes as sensitivity, non-judgemental perspective and empathy, all vital in gaining an awareness of self and others (Gilbert, 2009). In approaching inner experience with warmth, curiosity and openness, often from a place of safeness, these practices are also wonderful antidotes to manifestations such as anxiety, self-criticism and depression, commonly found in students with ASC (Neff, 2003). Although research in this area is in its infancy, the implication is that engagement in such practices will go far in addressing aspects of affiliative orientation and theory of mind considerations, as well as directly support an ability to recognise, manage and eventually accept internal experiences without judgement.

At its simplest level, mindfulness practices are attention training practices (Semple and Lee, 2008). In the case of mindful movement, the focus becomes the breath in relation to slow body movement and may have high reward saliency for students with ASC due to (a) its orientation towards proximal stimuli, and (b) if it can be related to other personal interests such as yoga, dance or even as a warm-up activity for a sporting exercise. Routine (perseveration) in using mindful movement practices also creates the conditions conducive to students taking turns in leading such exercises and allows for follow the leader type approaches. In one class, morning form times were typified by students standing in a circle routinely engaging these practices. Through leadership and imitation, these students were supporting their own learning and development through self-directed affiliative orientation.

The use of mindful movement also provides a good balance to more static (e.g. sitting, lying down) approaches used with mindfulness. Not only do we all have different inclinations, interests and learning styles associated with the practices, but they also work in different ways as emotional restoratives. While some students with ASC find solitude an effective means of relaxing, others need to release emotional energy by expressing it actively (Atwood, 2007). At our school, many students found it difficult to sit still for long periods of time and many students, particularly boys with excessive energy, gravitated towards the more action-orientated approaches. In the final analysis, mindfulness, like other educational interventions is best served by individuated approaches.

Pause and Reflect

Do different personalities gravitate to different forms of mindfulness practice?
Does gender influence accessibility to certain types of practice?
What is the relationship between compassionate action and mindfulness?

INTERVENTION ENVIRONMENT

With respect to the intervention environment, much effort went into creating a Self-Awareness room that was conducive to calming, communication and learning. This included the establishment of ground-rules for interaction, as well as attention to physical aspects such as the placement of chairs, use of neutral wall colours and carpeting to reduce noise. Managing sensory stimuli was important in addressing the development need of attention shifting, while the creation of a safe, familiar space provided the conditions that allowed the transition from doing to being in our students. Unfortunately, the location of the Self-Awareness room itself worked against these principles as it was located in a very busy area of the school. This made it difficult for students to settle, maintain attention and learn how to relate to their internal environment, free from external distraction. A consequence of this study was moving the Self-Awareness room to another, quieter part of the school.

Students very quickly formed preferences for where they wanted to sit and how they wanted to practice (e.g. on a chair, cushion, lying down). Over time, facilitators at the school learned what aids students needed in order to manage arousal levels. A number of our students regularly used stress balls during lessons in addition to engaging the practices on offer. Use of stress balls had an important repetitive element for those students as well as helping to regulate emotions (e.g. calming or channelling excessive energy) to the point where they could comfortably access the materials on offer in lessons. These preferences and the request for aids also provided important sources of reward saliency, judiciously used by facilitators in gaining the interest and motivation of students being taught (Siegel, 2003). Needless to say, facilitators had a vital role to play in creating the right learning environment in offering mindfulness to students with ASC at the school.

FURTHER ALIGNING MINDFULNESS TO LEARNING IN STUDENTS WITH ASC

In considering aspects of the mindfulness intervention in terms of structure, content and environment, it became evident that much of the instruction offered at the school tapped into the way students with ASC learn (e.g. use of single sensory supports in developing mindfulness) while also providing opportunities to develop wider faculties in areas such as theory of mind, arousal regulation and affiliative orientation. In so doing, the approach taken served to work with students from where they were, providing a basis for further learning, emotional development and enhanced self-awareness.

The limitations to the study were also noted, providing a basis for future improvements in offering mindfulness interventions. These included having different staff involved in administering and measuring the impacts of mindfulness, more involvement from parents/guardians in offering the intervention and refining the approach to be able to compare the effects of mindfulness on those with ASC to those students who have a range of other special needs. The need to use more than one research instrument was also identified, particularly as CAMM measured more than one variable and seemed to lack the ability to detect the subtler effects of mindfulness in students with ASC.

Recommendations of the study subsequently included developing a wider range of quantitative and qualitative measures of mindfulness, incorporating practices such as the three-minute breathing space into other curriculum subjects, developing a differentiated and progressive programme of mindfulness through the key stage years, along with conducting studies on the long-term effects of mindfulness, and exploring ways of gaining home support. As with all new journeys, much was learned on this one providing some essential insights and a foundation for further working with students with ASC. In the analogy of the Hero's Journey, it could be said that the development of the Self-Awareness Programme very much represented the Return in both personal and professional capacities, developing and sharing insights learned for the benefit of self and others.

POINTING IN NEW DIRECTIONS

After ten years, my own stars were beginning to realign and the compass needle began pointing in a familiar but slightly different direction. It was time for me to move on, leaving the Self-Awareness Programme in the capable hands of my colleagues at the school. New expressions of meaning and purpose were coming to the fore and resulted in me taking a sabbatical in 2014.

Circles within circles…Almost twenty years ago, I first read Bill Bryson's A Walk in the Woods (1997), an inspiring and hilarious account of Bryson's attempt to walk the Appalachian Trail in the Eastern United States. In 2014, this translated into my own four-month walk along that very trail, quickly followed by more than a year's worth of work in environmental conservation and youth development in Malaysia. Today, that path of engaged mindfulness continues to unfold in the current teaching of college students in the U.K. and a growing fascination with how mindfulness, nature and environmental education may combine in supporting the emotional development and wellbeing of young people, as well as contribute to addressing some of the serious environmental challenges we face today. The journey continues, with mindfulness always close in pointing the way home…

> **Pause and Reflect**
> **A Walk in Nature**
>
> Is there a link between nature and mindfulness?
> In what ways does mindfulness colour the way we see and interact with our world?
> How may the experience of nature and mindfulness contribute to wellbeing in students with ASC?

FURTHER RESOURCES

Child and Adolescent Mindfulness Measure
http://www.ruthbaer.com/academics/CAMM.pdf
Dialectic Behaviour Therapy for Adolescents (DBT-A)
https://www.researchgate.net/publication/23981243_Dialectical_behaviour_therapy_for_adolescents
Mindfulness-based Cognitive Therapy for Children (MBCT-C)
http://www.cebc4cw.org/program/mindfulness-based-cognitive-therapy-for-children-mbct-c/
Mindfulness-based Stress Reduction (MBSR) for Children
https://www.researchgate.net/publication/238609911_Mindfulness-Based_Stress_Reduction_for_School-Age_Children
Mindfulness in Schools Project (.b Curriculum)
https://mindfulnessinschools.org/

REFERENCES

ATWOOD, T., (2007). The Complete Guide to Asperger's Syndrome. London: Jessica Kingsley Publishers.
BERNAY, R., Using Mindfulness to Slow Down in Order to Speed Up Progress for Children with Special Needs. Paper presented at the conference "Double Blind Peer Reviewed Proceedings of the Making Inclusive Education Happen: Ideas for Sustainable Change", 28-30 September 2009, Te Papa, Wellington, New Zealand. Available:
http://www.imaginebetter.co.nz/downloads/IE_Conference/PR/4b_BernayPR.pdf [Date Accessed: 20/12/2010]
BRACH, T., (2003). Radical Acceptance: Awakening the Love that Heals Fear and Shame Within Us. London: Rider Books.
BRYSON, B., (1997). A Walk in the Woods. London: Doubleday.
CAMPBELL, J., (1949). The Hero with a Thousand Faces. Princeton: Princeton University Press.
COYNE, L.W., CHERON, D., and EHRENREICH, J.T., (2008). Assessment of Acceptance and Mindfulness Processes in Youth. In: S.C. HAYES and L.A. GRECO, eds., Acceptance & Mindfulness Treatments for Children & Adolescents: A Practitioners Guide. Oakland: New Harbinger Publications. pp. 37-54.
DHARMABNI, (2015). Photo Children Meditating. Available:
https://commons.wikimedia.org/wiki/File:Dharma_Primary_School_-_Children_Meditating_2015.jpg [Date Accessed 07/01/2019]
FRANKL, V., (2004). Man's search for meaning. Reading: Random House.
GILBERT, P., (2009). The Compassionate Mind. London: Constable & Robinson.
GORDON, D.M., (2012). Identifying a Suitable Research Instrument for Measuring the Effects of Mindfulness on Children with Special Needs. Professional Enquiry, MSc in Mindfulness Studies. University of Aberdeen.
GORDON, D.M., (2014). Effects of Mindfulness on Children with Autistic Spectrum Disorder (ASD). MSc in Mindfulness Studies. University of Aberdeen.
GRECO, L.A., BAER, R.A., and SMITH, G.T., (2011). Assessing mindfulness in children and adolescents: Development and validation of the Child and Adolescent Mindfulness Measure (CAMM). Psychological Assessment, 23 (3), pp. 606-614.
GREENLAND, S., (2010). The Mindful Child. New York: Free Press.
JORDAN, R., (2004). Meeting the Needs of Children with Autistic Spectrum Disorders in the Early Years. Australian Journal of Early Childhood, 29 (3), pp. 1-7.
LAWSON, W., (2011). The Passionate Mind: How People with Autism Learn. London: Jessica Kingsley Publishers.
MYRIAD, (2018). MYRIAD: My Resilience in Adolescents. Available: http://myriadproject.org [Date accessed: 14/05/2018]
NEFF, K., (2003). The Development and Validation of a Scale to Measure Self-Compassion. Self and Identity, 2, pp. 223-250.
NEFF, K., (2011). Self Compassion. New York: Harper Collins Publishers.
SEMPLE, R.J., and LEE, J., (2008). Treating Anxiety with Mindfulness: Mindfulness-Based Cognitive Therapy for Children. In: S.C. HAYES and L.A. GRECO, eds., Acceptance & Mindfulness Treatments for Children & Adolescents: A Practitioners Guide. Oakland: New Harbinger Publications. pp. 63-85.
SIEGEL, B., (2003). Helping Children with Autism Learn: Treatment Approaches for Parents and Professionals. Cary: Oxford University Press.
SINGHANIA, R., (2005). Autistic Spectrum Disorders. Indian Journal of Pediatrics, 72, pp. 343-351.
WEARE, K., (2013). Developing mindfulness with children and young people: a review of the evidence and policy context. Journal of Children's Services, 8 (2), pp. 141 – 153.
ZOOGMAN, S., GOLDBERG, S., HOYT, W., and MILLER, L., (2015). Mindfulness Interventions with Youth: A Meta-Analysis. Mindfulness, 6 (2), pp. 290-302.

APPENDIX 1 –
Adapted CAMM Research Instrument (adapted from Greco et al, 2011)

Children and Adolescent's Measure of Mindfulness Skills

We want to know what you think and how you feel.

1. Read each sentence.
2. Tick the one that's right for you.

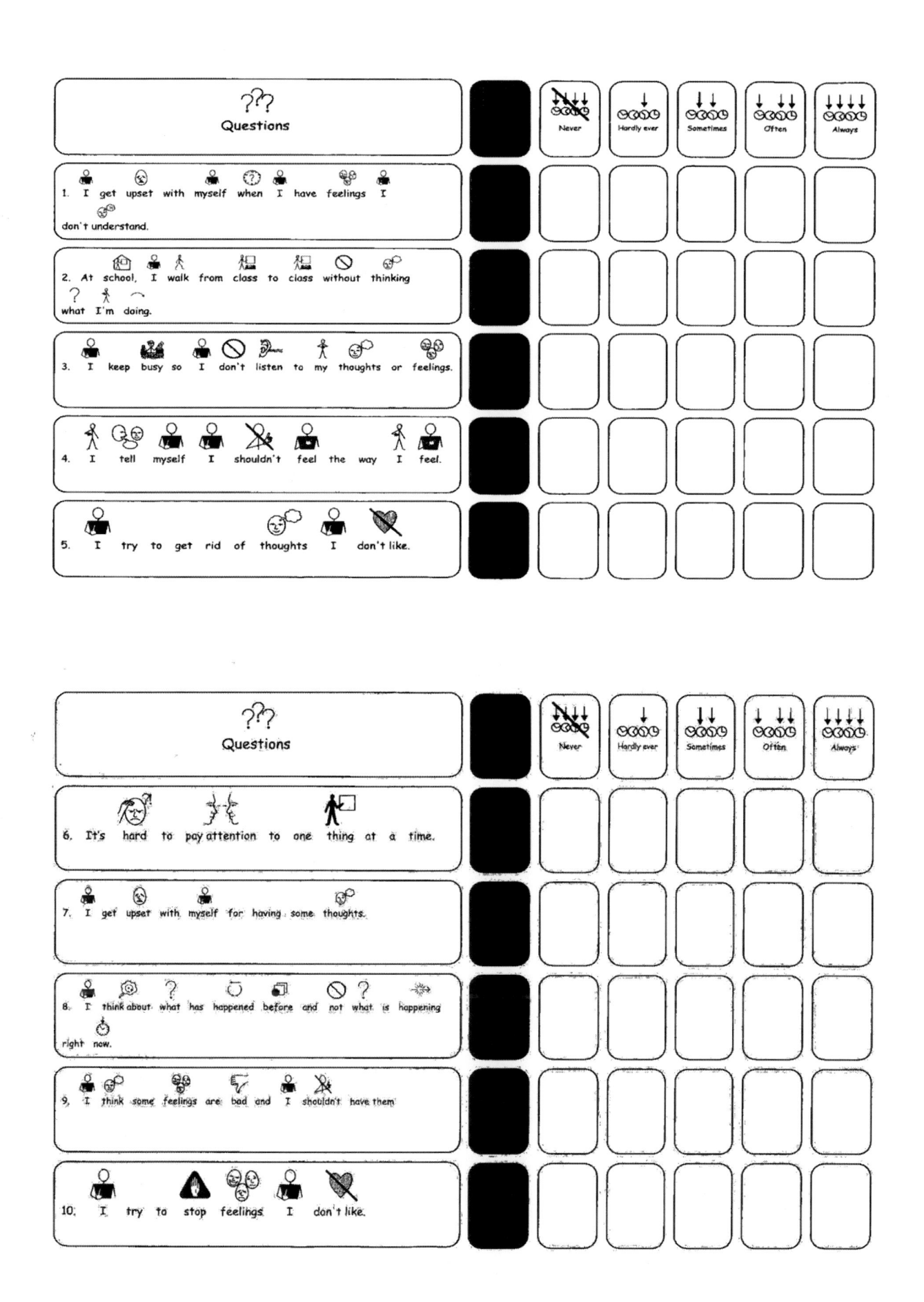

Questions		Never	Hardly ever	Sometimes	Often	Always
1. I get upset with myself when I have feelings I don't understand.						
2. At school, I walk from class to class without thinking what I'm doing.						
3. I keep busy so I don't listen to my thoughts or feelings.						
4. I tell myself I shouldn't feel the way I feel.						
5. I try to get rid of thoughts I don't like.						

Questions		Never	Hardly ever	Sometimes	Often	Always
6. It's hard to pay attention to one thing at a time.						
7. I get upset with myself for having some thoughts.						
8. I think about what has happened before and not what is happening right now.						
9. I think some feelings are bad and I shouldn't have them.						
10. I try to stop feelings I don't like.						

CHAPTER 6

DRAGONS AND WEEBLES: MINDFULNESS WITH ADOLESCENTS

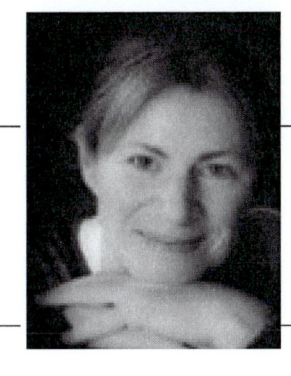

Heather Grace Bond

heather@heathergrace.co.uk

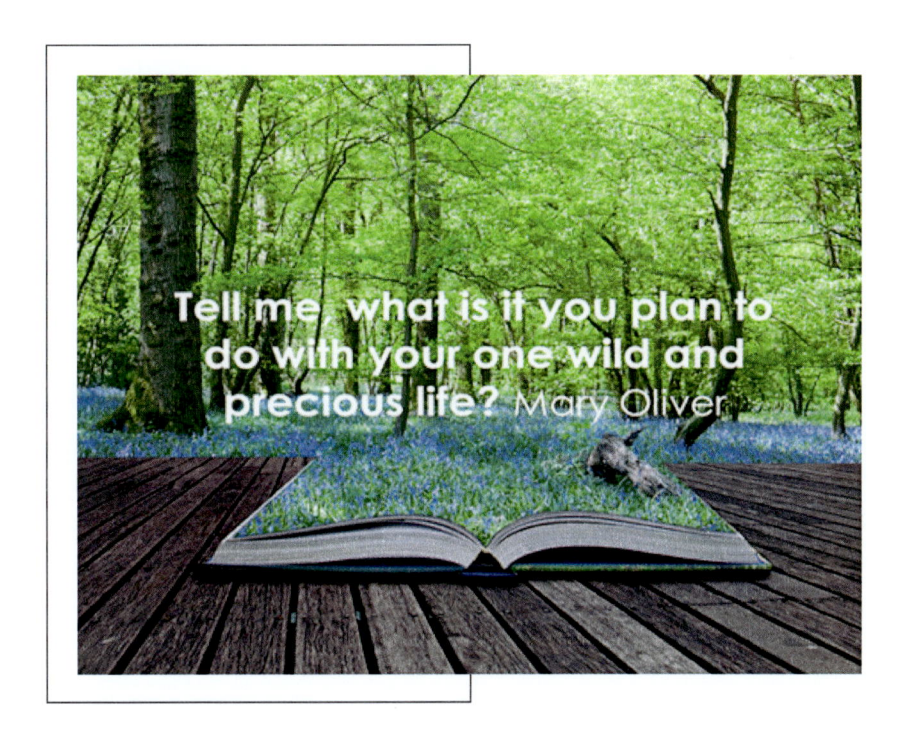

Figure 1: One Wild and Precious Life
Background image: Matt Gibson/Shutterstock.com

INTRODUCTION

I often reflect on how much suffering I might have managed to side-step if I had learned mindfulness and self-compassion as a child or teen! As young children, we are naturally very present, experiencing the world in an embodied way through our senses. How my heart leaps with joy to see a toddler listening to a blade of grass or sniffing a pebble – activities that many people might consider non-sensical. The magical qualities of innocence, curiosity and wonder that we mindfulness teachers refer to as 'beginner's mind' are naturally present within us, rather like a brightly shining light that gradually gets covered over as 'expert's mind' kicks in. Suzuki (1979) describes expert's mind as being one that is closed to the newness of the present moment, believing there is nothing fresh to be learned.

> **Pause and Reflect**
> **Raisin Exercise**
>
> Begin this practice by placing a raisin in the palm of one hand and taking a moment to notice the weight of it, as well as any sensations of what we might label as 'contact' or 'pressure'.
>
> Take some time to use all your senses to engage with the raisin as if you've never experienced one before. You might wish to then close your eyes for the rest of the practice so that your other senses may feel enlivened.
>
> Use your nose to inhale the aroma as if for the first time you have explored scent, and then use your ears to listen for any sounds that it might make. Is your body responding in any way to this exploration? Perhaps some anticipation around eating the raisin that's causing production of saliva in the mouth and maybe some interesting sensations to be noticed in the stomach area.
>
> As you bring the raisin up to your lips and place it onto your tongue, notice how it feels to have the raisin just sit there for a moment. Any urge to move the raisin so that you can bite into it – if so, what does that urge actually feel like? Any feelings or thoughts arising in this moment for you to notice?
>
> Deciding now to chew the raisin, feel the flesh of the raisin parting as you bite, noticing any sound as you do so and any flavour that might be being released into the mouth. Very slowly, beginning to chew and experiencing what that feels like; swallowing from time to time and experiencing what that feels like.
>
> Keep paying attention to the raisin until the moment that the last piece has been swallowed down and has disappeared from inner view, and then take a moment to experience any lingering flavour in the mouth.
>
> Finish the practice by sensing in to the whole of the body, as it is right now.

We commonly write-off present-moment experiences that seem familiar because on some level we feel that there's merit in freeing up the mind to concentrate on more pressing matters. For example, going over past events, perhaps believing that if we just go over them one more time then we'll gain the insight that we so desperately seek, or imagining a pleasant or not-so-pleasant future for ourselves. We ruminate, relive past memories and feelings and try to rewrite them, plan, analyse, predict, worry, daydream and live our lives so often from this place of not-really-hereness. We have travelled the roads of distraction so often in our lives that by adulthood they are more like super-highways! Where did it all go wrong?

As children, we begin to learn that adults have certain expectations of us in relation to our behaviour and that the world seems to consist of a lot of shoulds, should nots, musts and must nots. To keep ourselves safe – which consists of being accepted by our 'tribe' (or family and friends) – we learn to conform and to make constant judgements about how we're doing. Disapproval, to a child, often feels like the removal of love and consequently the disappearance of safety. Perhaps it's a little like learning to walk along a fairly narrow path that our parents or carers have set out for us, taking care not to veer too far from the path for fear of encountering the 'dragons' of their disapproval.

In my story, I have more to say about dragons, but perhaps I should start at the beginning…

BEGINNINGS

I had what could be described as an isolated upbringing on a farm on the Scottish Isle of Islay. My mother, wrestling with her own demons following the death of my father when my sister and

I were very small, was not a source of presence in my life and neither was she consistently able to give me the kind of warmth and acceptance that I yearned for. As a teenager I was shy, anxious and withdrawn. The experiences described to me by young people in the course of my work feel quite familiar - that desire to fit in, yet still feel somehow 'special'; the desire to be seen and heard when we want to be, and conversely sometimes the desire to be invisible; the desire to feel attractive and wanted; the desire to be accepted; ultimately, the desire to love and to be loveable.

At the age of seventeen, after thirteen years of longing to be a doctor so that I might rid the world of dreadful diseases such as the one that had taken my father, I made a foray into medical studies, but it quickly became clear to me that the Western view of medicine didn't really fit with how I saw the world. Even at that relatively tender age, I had a sense that addressing physical symptoms made little sense if the mental, emotional and spiritual dimensions were ignored. I knew that if I was to become a medical doctor, I would have to close off various parts of myself to meet the requirements to pass the exams; I chose instead to leave medical school and find out what else life might have in store for me. Little did I expect the winding path that would bring me to the present moment. It will perhaps suffice to summarise that after many years in an IT-related career, my growing interest in health and wellbeing (prompted by my rather notable lack of it in a high-pressure role) led me in 2008 to become a health-shop owner, then a complementary therapist and then a mindfulness teacher. Most of my training has been with the Mindfulness Association but I also trained as a Mindful Self-Compassion teacher with the Center for Mindful Self-Compassion and as a Mindfulness in Schools Project teacher of both the '.b' (11-18 year-old) and 'Paws b' (7-11 year-old) curricula.

DEPARTING INTO UNKNOWN TERRITORY

In 2013 I embarked on the MSc in Studies in Mindfulness at the University of Aberdeen. I can't overstate the fear for me of that first step into the wilds of the unknown; I hadn't undertaken any academic study since leaving Glasgow University with a Bachelors Degree in Science, fifteen years earlier. Moreover, study of the natural world generally involves an objective view of reality and the nature of being – the truth is 'out there' to be discovered and we just have to design the right experiments to get at that truth, then we can update our knowledge. Social science, however, encompasses a broad range of worldviews, ranging on one end of the spectrum from the scientific view to a position at the other end that purports there is no external truth – reality is created entirely by the mind. Learning of this broad range of potential worldviews was to me, like realising that all my life I'd been playing chess without realising there were other games that could be played. My goodness, I was scared, but I was also exhilarated.

During my time on the programme, home life inevitably had to transform a little to accommodate this learning endeavour. The changes were at times difficult for me, my husband, my three children and my two step-children to deal with. It sometimes felt like I was taking two steps forward and then one back as I successfully faced one challenge only to be confronted by another, but as the process continued, I began to recognise the role that my mind was playing in how I moved through them. Some challenges would hit my Achilles heel (for me, the story of, 'I'm not clever enough/good enough') and these were the challenges that felt like wading through deep bog; I would nearly give up. Other challenges felt more manageable and had more of a sense of, "I don't know what I'm doing here, but I'll allow myself to rest like a fool in the midst of it all, try to gather necessary resources to fill in the blanks, and trust that whatever transpires is perfect for my learning". These types of challenges were like having to navigate unknown territory while knowing there was a map out there somewhere and I simply had to trust that I would find it, or that it would find me.

Having reflected on what kept me going when I was so close to giving up, I can tell you that a large piece of the jigsaw puzzle was a healthy dose of self-compassion, since I was clearly experiencing difficulties and by far the most appropriate response was kindness. I think it's safe to say that, since being introduced to the concept of self-compassion, my growing capacity to recognise inner difficulties and pour the salve of self-kindness on them has completely transformed my experience. No doubt it has also affected the experience of those around me who might otherwise have felt the ripples of my inner difficulties erupting outwards! "When you find peace within yourself, you become the kind of person who can live at peace with others" (Peace Pilgrim, quoted in Friends of Peace Pilgrim, 2004, p. 132).

> **Pause and Reflect**
>
> What is your felt response to the words, 'finding peace within yourself? Perhaps you could imagine breathing in the words and then watch in a gentle way to see how (if at all) the body responds.

In addition to keenly recognising the value of self-compassion, I chose to acknowledge that the story of, "I'm not good enough", was just that – a story. It might be true, but equally it might not be. The clear-seeing of mindfulness, combined with self-compassion, are what pulled me through, and at the end of two years of study on the MSc Programme (exiting with a Postgraduate Diploma in Studies in Mindfulness), I opted to embark on the even-more-terrifying journey of a PhD. I am still on that journey, aiming to submit my thesis by September 2020, and my research explores the potential role of self-compassion in the context of secondary school education in Scotland.

The phase of life that is known as adolescence is, with its different fronts of biological development that take place on different trajectories, potentially fraught with inner difficulties. In my studies, I became very interested in exploring whether self-compassion might be a valuable way for young people to self-relate, and the capacity for it to be grown in adolescents. Self-compassion is an integral part of the Mindfulness Association's 8-week Mindfulness Based Living Course for adults. So I conceived the idea of developing an adolescent version of the course and then exploring the effects (if any) on around two hundred teen lives in a PhD study; the Mindfulness Association was wholeheartedly supportive of the idea, and so the new journey began.

My hero's journey then is really a story of bringing home the treasures of my journey, to birth a curriculum known as the Mindfulness Based Living Course for Young Adults (MBLC-YA). One day, I would love to tell you about my discoveries resulting from my research. Right now, however, I'd love to share some of the treasure of my journey by telling you about the curriculum. Before I do that, and so that we can place the curriculum in some kind of context, I think it may be helpful to share a little of my interpretation of the current landscape of education.

THE PURPOSE OF EDUCATION (IS THERE A PURPOSE?)

> The one continuing purpose of education, since ancient times, has been to bring people to as full a realization as possible of what it is to be a human being. Other statements of educational purpose have also been widely accepted: to develop the intellect, to serve social needs, to contribute to the economy, to create an effective work force, to prepare students for a job or career, to promote a particular social or political system. These purposes offered are undesirably limited in scope, and in some instances they conflict with the broad purpose I have indicated; they imply a distorted human existence. The broader humanistic purpose includes all of them, and goes beyond them, for it seeks to encompass all the dimensions of human experience (Foshay, 1991, p.277).

To look at whether there is any role for mindfulness and self-compassion within our schools, it is perhaps necessary to first consider the nature of education itself and deliberate what outcomes, if any, we might expect from our education system. Although the 18th century philosopher, Jean-Jacques Rousseau, in his well-known book 'Emile, or On Education' broadly uses the term 'education' to denote the dispositions conferred to us, "from nature, from men and from things" (2015, p.6), I use the term in the remainder of this chapter to more specifically refer to the capabilities and dispositions cultivated (or intended to be cultivated) in an individual through schooling. It is right to ask philosophical questions such as whether education should necessarily involve schooling and, if so, whether schooling in its current form is likely to achieve any of its potential aims, however we would need rather more than a book chapter to fully unpack the issues surrounding such questions!

Most children and adolescents in modern societies are routinely schooled in order to receive an 'education', and we can therefore infer that such societies have assessed there to be at least one purpose of education – at least for the type of education that happens in schools. For Biesta (2010) the very nature of education is such that it is a process that has both direction and purpose, and "the question of good education – the question of what education is for – is not optional but always poses itself when we engage in educational activities, practices and processes" (p.2). The worldview of a philosopher of education clearly has significant impact upon notions of what dispositions and capabilities education should endeavour to cultivate, why they should be cultivated, and the how they should be cultivated, but Biesta (2010) echoes Postman's (1995) concerns that considerations of what and why rarely seem to appear in discussions about education; the focus tends to be almost solely on the means by which dispositions and capabilities might be cultivated, and the effectiveness of those means.

I summarise as themes the views of some of those who have offered suggestions as to what education is for.

Theme – 'Education for...'	Example author(s)
the creation of an effective labour force and economic prosperity	Gibb 2015
preparation of individuals to lead a productive life	Foshay 1991, Gibb 2015
wise-governing and wisdom	Plato, as cited by Barrow (1976)
socialization into existing cultural, political and social order	Biesta 2010, Freire 1970
status - since the relative 'success' of pupils in tests from international comparative organisations such as PISA can be thought of as conferring status upon a country	Biesta 2010
its own sake, since knowledge is a good thing in and of itself	Gibb 2015
flourishing/wellbeing	Aristotle, as cited by Barrow 1976, Seligman, 2011

Figure 2: Purposes of Education

For Ancient Greek philosophers such as Socrates, Plato and Aristotle, the purpose of education was to foster the cultivation of aretai or excellences (what we now term 'wellbeing' or 'flourishing') and its ultimate aim was 'the good'. Aristotle's view of 'the good' is happiness or living well (eudaimonia) but this 'living well' doesn't refer to living a life filled with hedonistic pleasures but rather one that may yield a certain kind of contentment through engaging in activities that utilise and cultivate a person's excellences and dispositions.

Aristotle's musings, over two thousand years ago, highlight that the debate about what education is for was just as alive and pertinent then as it is now, and that the content of the debate is relatively unchanging:

> At present opinion is divided about the subjects of education. People do not all take the same position about what should be learned by the young, either with a view to excellence or with a view to the best life; nor is it clear whether their studies should be directed mainly to the intellect or to moral character. If we look at actual practice, the picture is also confusing; and it is not clear whether the proper studies to be pursued are those that are useful in life, those that make for

excellence, or those that are non-essential. Each kind of study gets some support. Even about those that make for excellence there is no agreement, for men do not all honor the same excellence, and so naturally they differ about the proper training for it (Frankena, 1965, p.63, quoting Aristotle).

The good life that was referred to by Aristotle may be understood as a direction of travel rather than a destination to be arrived at, and as activity rather than state. It was Aristotle's view that the highest purpose of man is the realisation of human potential, achieved through excellent activity. In the realm of psychology, this is referred to as 'self-actualisation'. Martin Seligman, commonly referred to as the founder of the positive psychology movement, which he launched in 2000, terms this 'human flourishing'. In his book, 'Flourish: A visionary new understanding of happiness and well-being', Seligman distinguishes between the gratifications, which he frames as eudaimonistic, and the pleasures, which he frames as hedonistic. The pleasures tend to be fleeting and are easily habituated so that increasingly greater stimulus is needed to achieve the same thrill, and if we cannot build a life of lasting happiness based on the pleasures, then instead we must build a life of lasting contentment by attending to the gratifications; in this way, we may flourish and achieve long-term wellbeing.

Interest in education for wellbeing (or flourishing) has birthed a positive education movement that aims to blend positive psychology with best teaching practice and has spawned organisations such as the International Positive Education Network (IPEN). Positive education endeavours to cultivate positive psychology virtues such as humanity (spanning the character strengths of kindness, love and social intelligence), courage (with accompanying character strengths of integrity, bravery, persistence, vitality and zest), transcendence (spanning the character strengths of hope, gratitude, appreciation, humour and spirituality), temperance (resting on the character strengths of self-control, humility, prudence, forgiveness and mercy), justice (encompassing the character strengths of leadership, citizenship and fairness), and wisdom and knowledge (including the character strengths of innovation and creativity, open-mindedness and curiosity, perspective and love of learning).

White & Murray (2015) list three forms in which programmes of positive education appear in schools:

1. scientifically-informed wellbeing interventions that have been empirically validated,
2. pro-active strategies for whole-school mental health – again, scientifically-informed, and
3. character-based lessons, specifically for the development of certain virtues and strengths.

Whether you are an experienced mindfulness practitioner or new to the subject, you might by now have a sense of a potential fit for mindfulness and self-compassion in the realm of positive education. Positive education though, like mindfulness, has not been without its critics. Criticisms of positive education include suggestions that:

- it distracts from more important matters of maintaining and improving academic teaching and learning
- it has become too focused on scientism – relying too heavily on empirical evidence at the expense of underlying philosophy, and
- its focus on positive mindset may be considered suppressive, ignoring the darker side of human experience and encouraging a 'glossing over' of difficulties.

Such criticisms must be addressed by the research community if positive education is to gain greater traction in schools.

MINDFULNESS IN SCHOOLS: THE IMPERATIVE

Our children can tell us the various merits of different operating systems for electronic devices, but are rarely in touch with how different emotions are experienced in the body, or how it feels to bring kindness to a moment of difficulty (MacKenzie, 2016, p.24).

There has been a veritable explosion of interest in mindfulness and self-compassion in the research world. In the year of 2015, just before I embarked on my PhD journey, a Google Scholar search for 'mindfulness adolescent' articles in that year returned approximately 5,700 results and 'self-compassion adolescent' returned approximately 1,310 results. In 2017, these figures are 7,710 and 2,140 respectively. The number of mindfulness articles related to adolescence is increasingly rapidly each year, but the number of self-compassion articles is almost doubling year-on-year, such is the level of interest. This is encouraging for someone exploring this nascent area of research!

> It is one of our culture's most significant tasks, one for which our schools have a special responsibility, to provide the tools and to develop the skills through which the child can create his or her own experience (Eisner, 1988, p.15).

This quote from Elliott W. Eisner points to the idea that as human beings we have a role in creating our subjective experience rather than simply experiencing life 'as it is'. Firstly, we can note how our subjective experience is not simply a flow of experiencing things exactly as they are in some kind of objective reality – if this were the case, sensory experiences would be the same for each person, and a glass of warm water would always feel warm to the touch to everyone, rather than warm to those whose hands are colder than the temperature of the glass, and cold to those whose hands are warmer than the temperature of the glass. In order to make sense of the world around us and communicate our subjective experience, we must create symbols such as words that point to actual things. For example, the word 'apple' is a pointer to an object that has certain properties, such as shape and colour. We cannot eat the word 'apple', hence it is simply a pointer – not the actual thing itself.

Similarly, in order to understand the world, we must make schema, or 'mental maps' as a way of organising categories of information. When new information arrives that fits with the current worldview, it is easily assimilated, however when it challenges the current schema, there is a disturbance in equilibrium until the schema is adjusted to integrate the new information. The work of Taylor and Crocker has advanced the theory that – at least in adults - rather than using our senses to gather information with which to test against our current schema, human beings have a consistent and strong tendency use the current schema to determine which information to process. Clearly, this results in a problematic propensity to see the world as we prefer to see it, rather than as it really is.

Referencing the work of Eisner, Ergas (2017) frames education as "a mind-making process" (p.viii), but since educational theory and practice were born of human minds in the first place, it follows that any problems with education reflect problems with the minds that created it. So, if the untrained mind has a strong preference to only process data that fits with its current worldview, I argue that mindfulness training in the school system not only fits well with the current wave of enthusiasm for 'education for flourishing' or 'positive education' but that it is imperative if education is ever to achieve whatever it sets out to do, and imperative if human beings are ever to reach their full potential. If we cannot see all of the mental barriers that we erect between ourselves and those we deem 'other', how are we ever to transcend them? If we cannot see that our preoccupation with self and having our preferences met causes suffering to others and to the planet, how are we ever to learn to do things differently?

WHY BOTHER WITH SELF-COMPASSION?

"It is likely that adolescence is the period of life in which self-compassion is the lowest." (Neff, 2003, p.95). Interest in the subject of self-esteem in the field of education has been enthusiastic since Nathaniel Branden's book, 'Psychology of Self-Esteem' was first published in 1969; for quite some time, educators strived to raise the levels of self-esteem in their pupils so that pupils would feel better about themselves and do better academically. However, towards the end of the twentieth century, Swann Jr (1996) highlighted that levels of self-esteem tend to be quite resistant to change. Self-esteem involves comparison between self and other; those with high self-esteem evaluate themselves as superior to others and those with low self-esteem evaluate themselves as inferior to others. Those high in self-esteem are more likely to project their faults onto others in order to maintain their superior sense of self. Those low in self-esteem are more likely to blame themselves when something goes wrong, rather than see others at fault. It seems that the desire in an individual to maintain and enhance levels of self-esteem can be a significant barrier to having a realistic and healthy sense of self (Baumeister, Heatherton and Tice, 1993; Vignoles et al., 2006).

Because of the difficulties and perils of raising self-esteem, prominent self-compassion researcher,

Kristin Neff, has offered the construct of self-compassion as a healthier way to self-relate. Neff defines self-compassion as a construct containing the three dimensions of mindfulness (with its opposite of over-identification), self-kindness (with its opposite of self-criticism) and common humanity (with its opposite of isolation). Studies with adults to-date have shown a significant causal link between self-compassion and wellbeing. Studies with adolescents to-date have demonstrated self-compassion to be positively associated with social connectedness (Neff and McGehee, 2010), life satisfaction (Bluth and Blanton, 2014), executive function (Shin et al., 2016), self-esteem (Barry, Loflin and Doucette, 2015), emotional wellbeing (Neff and McGehee, 2010; Bluth and Blanton, 2012, 2014), emotional intelligence (Castilho et al., 2016), greater ability to tolerate distress (Bluth et al., 2017), and a reduction in depressive symptoms (Neff and McGehee, 2010; Muris et al., 2015; Castilho et al., 2016; Bluth et al., 2017), levels of anxiety (Neff and McGehee, 2010; Muris et al., 2015; Bluth et al., 2017), perceived stress (Bluth and Blanton, 2012, 2014; Bluth et al., 2017), negative affect (Bluth and Blanton, 2012, 2014), vulnerable narcissism (Barry, Loflin and Doucette, 2015) and bullying victimisation (Gonynor, 2016).

Barry et al. (2015) have warned that, "High levels of overidentification and isolation may be particularly problematic in adolescents" (p.122) and may be linked to issues such as depression and anxiety. Self-compassion invites us to hold our inner difficulties in a clear awareness, recognising the moment of difficulty without over-identifying with it and making it part of 'our story' – the story of who we think we are. Further, it invites us to recognise that difficulties are part of the human experience and that there will be many others around the world experiencing a very similar difficulty in this moment. We can then choose to direct kindness towards ourselves in this time of difficulty, not necessarily to change our experience (although this often happens) but simply because we are suffering. Self-compassion would therefore seem a particularly helpful way for adolescents to relate to themselves and their experience. In many aspects of adolescent life, from personal life in terms of relationships to school life in terms of performance - academic, sporting or otherwise - there is plentiful potential to experience a sense of failure, whether this is 'real' or mentally-constructed. Mindset theory suggests that non-identification with failure is key to an individual achieving his or her full potential. Identification with failure is where, "I failed at something" becomes, "I am a failure" and is the hallmark of shame, which Professor Paul Gilbert frames as highly toxic because of its destructive and debilitating nature. Kristin Neff positions self-compassion as the antidote to shame. Since learning, schooling and adolescence afford many opportunities to experience failure and personal difficulty, perhaps secondary schools are a fertile ground to explore how a training in self-compassion affects participants' experience of school life, and what the mechanisms are that enable and hinder the learning of it in a school environment.

#WEEBLEISM

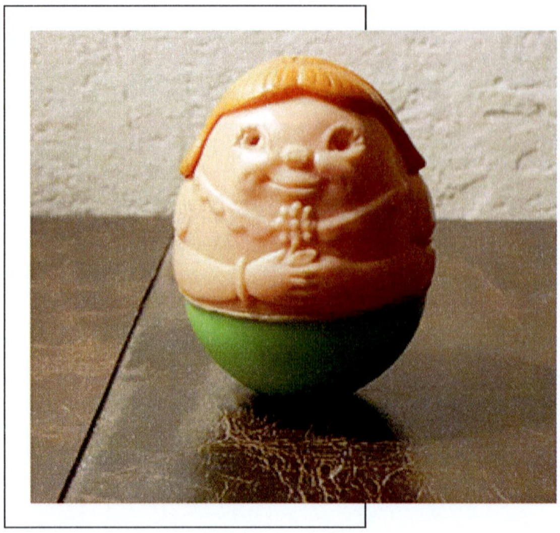

Figure 3: A Weeble.
Photo © Heather Grace Bond 2018

As a child, I loved Weebles and the tagline of, 'Weebles wobble but they don't fall down' was ingrained in my memory from an early age. When I became a mindfulness teacher and began exploring through the process of supervision how it feels to be fully embodied, the relevance of this simple child's toy became more apparent. I realised that the shape of the Weeble could be a metaphor for our attention – with most of our attention in our heads, we are like upside-down Weebles, but by deliberately grounding our attention down into our bodies we can become like right-way-up Weebles. When I became a Mindfulness in Schools Project teacher, I was delighted to discover that I wasn't alone in seeing the link between mindfulness and Weebles and I was keen to use them as a metaphor for a different way of being in the materials that I created for my adolescent version of the MBLC. I wasn't sure how they would be received but I had a feeling that teaching about becoming more Weeble-like (or mountain-like) could be acceptable in the classroom if delivered in a light way. And this is the story of the birth of #weeblism, as one MBLC-YA pupil hash-tagged it when summarising their experience of the course.

The MBLC, upon which the MBLC-YA is based, is founded on the work of Rob Nairn, whose training in psychology in conjunction with a deep immersion in Buddhist teachings has enabled him to skilfully convey much of the wisdom of Buddhist dharma in a secular manner so that it can be accessible to all. The MBLC is also informed by Professor Paul Gilbert's work, which brings together theoretical underpinnings of attachment theory, social mentality theory and evolutionary psychology to explain compassion as a psychological construct. The emphasis of the MBLC is on experiential learning – concepts and theories are introduced in a minimal way and then participants are offered the opportunity to explore experientially how the teaching 'lands' with them.

The MBLC-YA is a 10-session course that has been designed to be delivered within a time slot of 40-60 minutes. In creating the course, I have opted to retain most of the core elements of the MBLC except for the 'RAIN' practice which is intended to afford the opportunity to explore an inner difficulty in some depth; in the interests of ethical considerations, I decided to omit this practice and also to change the 'Lovingkindness for Self and Other' practice in a way that might feel more approachable for adolescents. The resulting 'Full Circle Lovingkindness' practice was inspired by the moving 'Kindness Boomerang' YouTube video by wellness organisation *Life Vest Inside*.

> **Pause and Watch**
>
> Go to https://youtu.be/nwAYpLVyeFU and watch the short 'Kindness Boomerang' video. At the time of writing, it has over twenty-nine million views!

Now that you've seen the video, you might want to try it out the Full Circle Lovingkindness practice yourself to see how it lands for you.

> **Pause and Practice**
>
> Go to www.mindfulnessassociation.net/site-gallery/mblc-ya-audio/media/full-circle-lovingkindness/ and listen to the 'Full Circle Lovingkindness' practice.

The following pages attempt to give you a flavour of the MBLC-YA sessions.

Introduction

In this introductory session, which sets out to explain a little about mindfulness and self-compassion in ways that are relevant to young people, participants are urged to consider what it is to live well – a question that has occupied philosophers for millennia! Mindfulness is framed as exercise for the mind, helping to keep it healthy in the same way that physical exercise helps to keep the body healthy. Video clips explain the concepts of mindfulness and self-compassion in an engaging way and the short practices of 'Noticing the Unsettled Mind' and 'Settling the Mind' are then introduced.

Session 1	*Your Amazing Mind.* This focus of this session is on the adolescent brain and its different trajectories of development, and a discussion on the effects of stress. A short body scan practice is introduced, where participants learn to move attention through different areas of the body with a curious and allowing attitude. A language of present-moment experience is offered such that participants can begin to recognise the possibility of noticing thoughts, emotions, body sensations and sensory perceptions and holding these with a lighter perspective.
Session 2	*Staying Present.* Training in mindfulness is explained in a little more depth as a combination of technique (returning a wandering mind back to the present moment) and attitude (curious, patient, open, kind). This session includes the 'Weeble Mode' practice as a way of building resilience – participants can learn to steady themselves by becoming more Weeble-like or more mountain-like when there's a wobble. Initial steps towards growing kindness are taken with the 'Memories of Kindness' practice.
Session 3	*Dropping Anchor.* In this session, participants explore the storminess of life in pairs or small groups, with the aim of drawing out the concept of common humanity – the shared experience of oftentimes messy experience of being human. The notion of a mindfulness support is introduced as a way of 'dropping anchor' and participants are given the opportunity to practice using sound as a support to enable the mind to stay more present and notice more quickly when it has wandered off.
Session 4	*Distraction.* The theme of this session is something that most of us are experts in and we explore the potential role of technology in fuelling the habit of distraction. In this session we look at distraction into the three times (past, future and present – daydreaming) and participants are encouraged to talk in pairs or small groups about the kinds of things that pull their attention away, and whether or not this is a good or a bad thing. Once there is some consensus in the group that distraction can be problematic, there is a further opportunity to practice using a mindfulness support (this time, the breath) to counter the habit of distraction.
Session 5	*Undercurrent.* This session introduces Rob Nairn's 'Undercurrent/Observer' model of mind, encouraging participants to recognise the content of the mind a little more clearly. In simplest terms, there is a part of us that is aware (the observer, and this part is self-aware so can observe itself) and there is the 'stuff' or 'content' of the mind that the observing part is aware of. This 'stuff' includes thoughts, emotions, body sensations and sense perceptions. Separation of experience from experiencer offers the possibility of greater perspective and a disentanglement from thoughts. 'I am not my thoughts' can be a powerful thing to learn!
Session 6	*Attitude.* Participants learn in this session that we can't change the content of the mind directly – we can simply learn to train the attitude of the observing part of us. Participants learn that the attitude through which we view our experience has much greater effect on the quality of our inner life than the content of the undercurrent. Difficult thoughts/feelings + resistance = horrible experience Difficult thoughts/feelings + non-resistance = much less horrible experience

Session 7	*Self-acceptance*. This session on the subject of self-acceptance builds on the previous session on attitude and introduces Professor Paul Gilbert's 'Three Circles Model' as a way of understanding emotion regulation. Participants are introduced to the practice of 'Self-Compassion Break' as a way of intending to bring kindness to inner-experience that feels difficult and facilitating a shift from the red circle of threat to the green circle of soothing.
Session 8	*Appreciation*. There is a growing body of research that suggests happiness and contentment are linked to gratitude and appreciation. The theme of this session is appreciating and taking in the good, with participants being offered the opportunity to eat chocolate or strawberries mindfully - really savouring the experience. The session also builds on the theme of kindness through watching the 'Kindness Boomerang' video clip and engaging in the 'Full Circle Lovingkindness' practice.
Session 9	*A Mindful Life*. The final session involves a review of the course, revisiting key teaching points. There is an opportunity to reflect on what character attributes pupils admire in others that they would like to develop in themselves and on what, if anything, has felt of value during the course. The course concludes with a short ending ceremony since rituals have an important role in marking transitions – in this case, the end of the course and the beginning of the rest of their lives. A small gift is given to each participant to remind them of this time of learning to live well.

MBLC-YA sessions are much shorter than the 2hr MBLC sessions and the materials have been carefully put together to be developmentally appropriate in terms of the language, images and video clips chosen to present the chosen concepts. Each session is accompanied by a PowerPoint presentation and the course is supported by a comprehensive Student Manual and an app for Android and iOS devices (with mp3 files of the practices also available on the Mindfulness Association's website).

Teacher-training for the MBLC-YA commenced in 2017 at Samye Ling and it makes my heart sing to hear of fellow teachers now taking this work out into schools and communities. I shall never tire of seeing photographs of students engaging in practice together or of materials they have co-created during the course. I am filled with appreciation for the opportunity to share this work and filled with gratitude that others are being drawn to teach it, bringing with them their unique gifts and inspirations around using the materials in creative ways to bring an alive sense of mindfulness and compassion to the classroom.

FOLLOWING MY BLISS: WHERE DRAGONS FLY

Following our bliss is where the magic happens, or so the hero's journey goes. When we let go of striving and struggling to move towards what it is that we think we want, we can then arrive at the place where the magic is happening all on its own. Over the years, I have found that getting out of my own way is the most successful way to be where the magic is at; I have learned to give my heart priority over my head. Fear lies in one direction; love lies in the other. One example of following my bliss in the past was creating a holistic therapy business called 'WhereDragonsFly' and you will probably have noticed thus far in my writing that dragon symbolism holds a particular fascination for me.

As our tutorial group gathered around our table at our writers' retreat for this book and we discussed developments in my writing, two dragonflies flew over us. We burst into joyful laughter, sharing a sense of wonder at the unfolding of life. This, we easily agreed, was a pretty special moment. The aspiration of the Hero's Journey, as Vin Harris said earlier in Chapter 2, is a reflection of the common desire to know ourselves – to find out who we really are. In journeying to find out who we are, perhaps we learn as much about who we are not, as we learn about who we are. We learn that we are not our thoughts, or the sum of them. More surprisingly, we learn that we are not our experiences, although there may have been long periods of our life where we've allowed them to define us. We learn that we are not the roles that we play. And once we have seen the man behind the curtain in the Wizard of Oz, pulling all of the levers, suddenly there is freedom to discover our true nature.

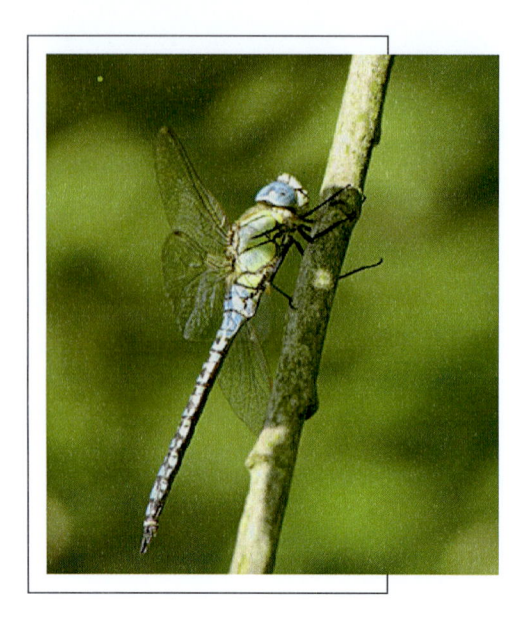

Figure 4: Dragonfly
Photo by Andreas Eicher

Mythical creatures that confront us on our hero's journey are a perfect metaphor for the challenges that we must face. If I had to sum up what I have learned over these past few years, then I would say this: the dragons we encounter are not our enemies. When we learn to befriend them, we find that they are full of wisdom and can help to guide us home to our true selves.

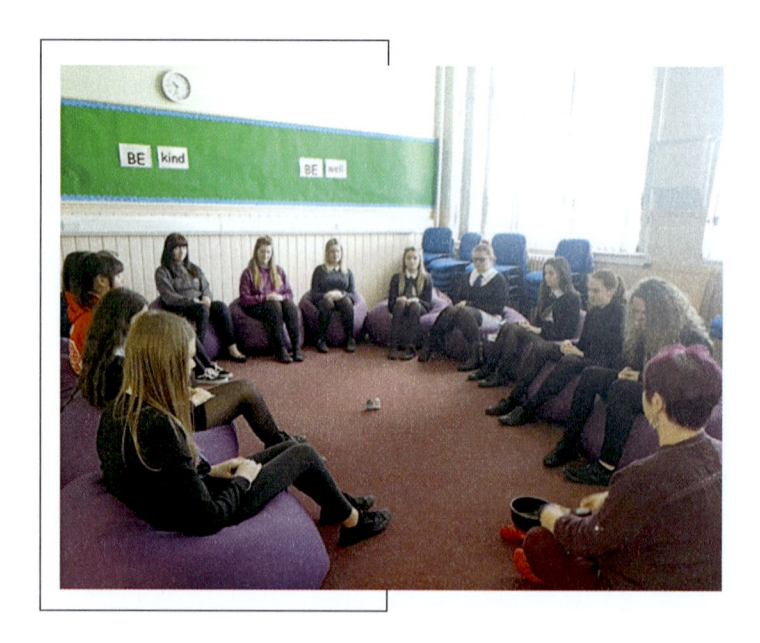

Figure 5 : Zana Lamont working with pupils from Carrick Academy, Maybole.
Photo © Lindsay McBain 2018. Photo used with permissions.

May our children be free from unnecessary suffering and the causes of it.

May our children learn to recognise and turn toward their difficulties with courage and kindness.

May our children learn to be good dragon-whisperers, since this is the best kind of magic.

FURTHER RESOURCES

MBLC-YA Teacher Training Info
www.mindfulnessassociation.net/teacher-training/teaching2-mblc-ya/
MBLC Info on the Mindfulness Association's website
www.mindfulnessassociation.net/courses/mblc/
My website
www.heathergrace.co.uk

REFERENCES

BARRY, C.T., LOFLIN, D.C., and DOUCETTE, H., (2015). Adolescent self-compassion: Associations with narcissism, self-esteem, aggression, and internalizing symptoms in at-risk males. Personality and Individual Differences [online]. 77, pp. 118-123. Available from: http://dx.doi.org/10.1016/j.paid.2014.12.036
BAUMEISTER, R.F., HEATHERTON, T.F., and TICE, D.M., (1993). When ego threats lead to self-regulation failure: negative consequences of high self-esteem. Journal of personality and social psychology. 64 (1), pp. 141-156.
BIESTA, G., (2010). Good education in an age of measurement: Ethics, politics, democracy. Paradigm Publishers.
BLUTH, K. and BLANTON, P.W., (2012). Mindfulness and self-compassion: Exploring pathways to adolescent emotional well-being. [online]. Available from: http://link.springer.com/article/10.1007/s10826-013-9830-2 [Accessed 11 Dec 2018].
BLUTH, K. and BLANTON, P.W., (2014). The influence of self-compassion on emotional well-being among early and older adolescent males and females. The Journal of Positive Psychology [online]. 10 (3), pp. 1-12. Available from: http://www.pubmedcentral.nih.gov/articlerender.fcgi?artid=4351754&tool=pmcentrez&rendertype=abstract.
BLUTH, K., CAMPO, R.A., FUTCH, W.S., and GAYLORD, S.A., (2017). Age and Gender Differences in the Associations of Self-Compassion and Emotional Well-being in A Large Adolescent Sample. Journal of Youth and Adolescence [online]. 46 (4), pp. 840-853. Available from: http://link.springer.com/10.1007/s10964-016-0567-2.
CASTILHO, P., CARVALHO, S.A., MARQUES, S., and PINTO-GOUVEIA, J., (2016). Self-Compassion and Emotional Intelligence in Adolescence: A Multigroup Mediational Study of the Impact of Shame Memories on Depressive Symptoms. Journal of Child and Family Studies [online]. pp. 1-10. Available from: http://dx.doi.org/10.1007/s10826-016-0613-4.
EICHER, Andreas (2013) Dagonfly Photo Wikimedia. Creative Commons Share-Alike 3.0 https://commons.wikimedia.org/wiki/File:2013.07.16.-2-Kirschgartshaeuser_Schlaege_Mannheim-Suedliche_Mosaikjungfer-Maennchen.jpg
EISNER, E.W., (1988). The Primacy of Experience and the Politics of Method. Educational Researcher [online]. 17 (5), pp. 15-20. Available from: http://edr.sagepub.com/cgi/doi/10.3102/0013189X017005015.
ERGAS, O., (2017a). Schooled in our own minds: mind-wandering and mindfulness in the makings of the curriculum. Journal of Curriculum Studies [online]. 0272 (August), pp. 1-19. Available from: https://www.tandfonline.com/doi/full/10.1080/00220272.2017.1363913.
ERGAS, O., (2017b). Reconstructing 'Education' through mindful attention: Positioning the mind at the center of curriculum and pedagogy. Springer.
FOSHAY, A.W., (1991). The Curriculum Matrix: Transcendence and Mathematics. Journal of Curriculum and Supervision. 6 (4), pp. 277-293.
FRANKENA, W.K., (1965). Three historical philosophies of education: Aristotle, Kant, Dewey.
FREIRE, P., 1970. Pedagogy of the Oppressed. Rprnt 2017. Penguin Classics.
FRIENDS OF PEACE PILGRIM (2004) Peace Pilgrim Sante Fe, New Mexico: Oak Tree Press
GIBB, N. Rt H., (2015). The purpose of education - GOV.UK. GOV.UK [online]. Available from: https://www.gov.uk/government/speeches/the-purpose-of-education [Accessed 8 May 2017].
Artist: GIBSON, Matt. (undated) Image title: Contents of magical book containing bluebell woods spills over and blends into background Source: Shutterstock.com
URL: https://www.shutterstock.com/image-photo/contents-magical-book-containing-bluebell-woods-77690716
Date of purchase of licence: 4th November 2018
GONYNOR, (2016). Associations Among Mindfulness, Self-Compassion, and Bullying in Early Adolescence.
MACKENZIE, H.G., (2016). Awakening Child: A journey of inner transformation through teaching your child mindfulness and compassion [online]. John Hunt Publishing. Available from: http://amzn.eu/5eggB59.

MURIS, P., MEESTERS, C., PIERIK, A., and KOCK, B. de, (2015). Good for the Self: Self-Compassion and Other Self-Related Constructs in Relation to Symptoms of Anxiety and Depression in Non-clinical Youths. Journal of Child and Family Studies 25[online]. pp. 607-617.

NEFF, K.D., (2003). Self-compassion: An alternative conceptualization of a healthy attitude toward oneself. Self and identity 2 [online]. pp. 85–101. Available from: https://pdfs.semanticscholar.org/b357/87b9b21486d00458e85f8bcdf84d44e83c7c.pdf.

NEFF, K.D. and MCGEHEE, P., (2010). Self-compassion and psychological resilience among adolescents and young adults. Self and Identity. 9 (3), pp. 225–240.

POSTMAN, N., (1995). The end of education: Redefining the value of school. 1st Edition. Vintage.

ROUSSEAU, J.-J., 2015. Emile, or On Education. Kindle. Some Good Press.

SELIGMAN, M.E.P., (2011). Flourish: A visionary new understanding of happiness and well-being. Kindle. Nicholas Brealey Publishing.

SHIN, H.-S., BLACK, D.S., SHONKOFF, E.T., RIGGS, N.R., and PENTZ, M.A., (2016). Associations among dispositional mindfulness, self-compassion, and executive function proficiency in early adolescents. Mindfulness [online]. pp. 1377–1384. Available from: https://link.springer.com/article/10.1007/s12671-016-0579-8.

SUZUKI, S., (1979) Zen Mind, Beginner's Mind. New York: John Weatherhill.

SWANN JR, W.B., (1996). Self-traps: The elusive quest for higher self-esteem. WH Freeman/Times Books/Henry Holt & Co.

VIGNOLES, V.L., REGALIA, C., MANZI, C., GOLLEDGE, J., and SCABINI, E., (2006). Beyond self-esteem: influence of multiple motives on identity construction. Journal of personality and social psychology [online]. 90 (2), pp. 308–33. Available from: http://www.ncbi.nlm.nih.gov/pubmed/16536653.

WHITE, M.A. and MURRAY, A.S., (2015). Building a Positive Institution. In: Evidence-Based Approaches in Positive Education [online]. Dordrecht: Springer Netherlands. pp. 1–26. Available from: http://link.springer.com/10.1007/978-94-017-9667-5_1.

CHAPTER 7

COMBINING POETRY AND MINDFULNESS: STORIES OF CREATING NEW SPACES IN HIGHER EDUCATION

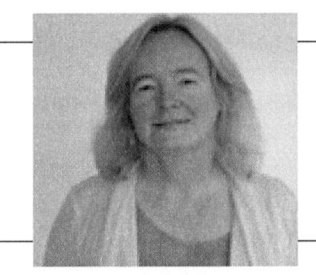

Terry Barrett

terry.barrett@ucd.ie
terrybarrett500@hotmail.com

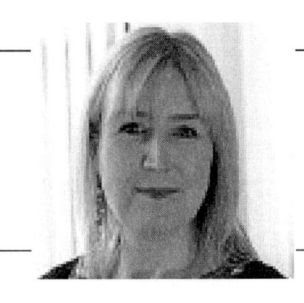

Naomi McAreavey

naomi.mcareavey@ucd.ie

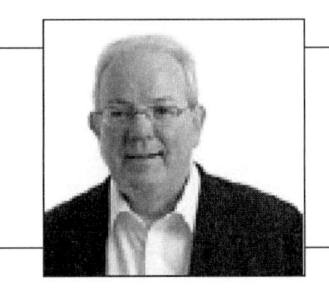

Larry McNutt

larry.mcnutt@itb.ie

INTRODUCTION

I (Terry) narrate this chapter. When I was a child we lived in a big old drafty house in Ireland. Some Saturday mornings I got into my parents big double cosy bed and we read poems aloud to one another. As a young child my father would sometimes read *The Owl and the Pussy-cat from A Puffin Book of Verse*

> The Owl and the Pussy-cat went out to sea
> In a beautiful pea-green boat,
> They took some honey, and plenty of money,
> Wrapped up in a five-pound note (Lear, 1983).

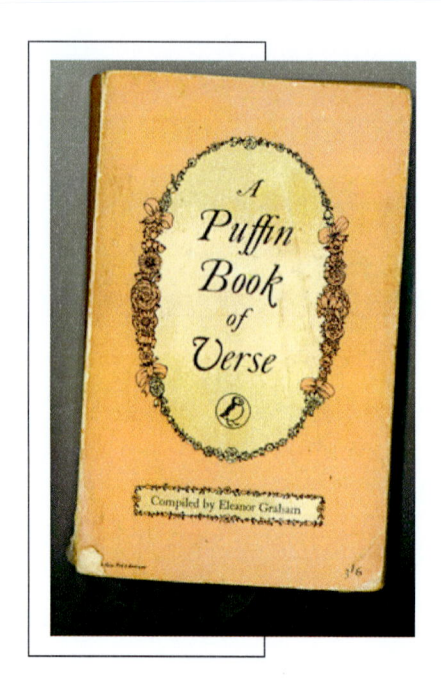

Figure 1: One of the my prized possessions - a book my father read from
Photo © Terry Barrett 2018

Sometimes as a young teenager I would read Composed Upon Westminster Bridge (Wordsworth, 1802)

> Earth has not anything to show more fair:
> Dull would he be of soul who could pass by
> A sight so touching in its majesty:
>
> …
>
> Ne'er saw I, never felt, a calm so deep!
> The river glideth at his own sweet will:
> Dear God! the very houses seem asleep;
> And all that mighty heart is lying still!

Pause and Reflect

What is one of your favourite poems? Pause to enjoy reading it now, silently or aloud, whichever you prefer. What is your felt response to the poem?

For a long time, poetry and meditation have been close to my heart. Separately and together they have helped me savor the beauty of nature, the warmth of friends and family and my inner strength and courage. They give space and self-compassion for feelings of anger and sorrow that have led sometimes to a sense of common humanity and compassion for others. Poetry and mindfulness give me a deeper, more heartfelt perspective of what is happening on my hero's journey.

The return part of the hero's journey (that Vin Harris talks about in Chapter 2) resonates with me. Having benefited from spaces of guided mindfulness meditation practice on the MSc Studies in Mindfulness programme (as described by Graeme Nixon in Chapter 3), I wanted to help to provide a similar place for others. So I coordinate a weekly lunchtime guided mindfulness practice for staff at University College Dublin. When guiding I regularly end the practice with a poem.

My current professional context also includes facilitating mindfulness and mindful learning workshops for academic staff. I use poetry in my faculty development and research work (Barrett, 2011; Barrett, 2017). My interest in exploring the interrelationship between poetry and mindfulness is in order to enhance my personal and professional practice.

This chapter presents stories about three different ways that lecturers combine poetry and mindfulness, namely, 1) using mindful reading to teach poetry (any poem) to students and to create egalitarian spaces for poetry exploration 2) creating mindful spaces for reflection, personal transformation and thanks through reading, writing and performing poetry, and 3) listening to poetry to resonate with the nature of mindfulness and connecting with inner spaciousness, values and creativity.

DIFFERENT PERSPECTIVES ON THE INTERRELATIONSHIP BETWEEN POETRY AND MINDFULNESS

The idea (elaborated by Vin Harris in Chapter 2) of poetry being an expression of "penultimate truth" as near to the truth as words can express, really resonates with me. A mindful learning approach encourages us to see things from different perspectives (Langer, 2000; Barabazet and Bush, 2014). I therefore review what a cognitive scientist, a Nobel prize-winning poet, a professor of medicine, a mindfulness leader and an English literature scholar have to say about the interrelationships of mindfulness and poetry.

TEXT	PERSPECTIVE	Conceptual Understanding of the Interrelationship of Poetry and Mindfulness
Gibbs, R.W. (1994) The Poetics of Mind.	Cognitive Scientist	"human cognition is fundamentally shaped by various poetic or figurative processes" p.1. "figuration is not merely a matter of language but provides much of the foundation for thought, reason and imagination" p.435.
Heaney, S. Crediting Poetry: Nobel Lecture (1995)	Poet Nobel Prize Winner for Literature	"I credit poetry…for making possible a fluid and restorative relationship between the mind's centre and its circumference… for its truth to life, in every sense of that phrase" p.450. "poetry's credit..the power to remind us that we are hunters and gatherers of values" p.467.
Connelly, D. (1999) Being in the Present Moment: Developing the Capacity for Mindfulness in Medicine.	Professor of Medicine Co-director Program for the Humanities in Medicine	"the power of poetry to insist on immediacy and attention to the present moment. Poetry can both illustrate the state of awareness through the response it elicits in the reader and act as a powerful means for developing the capacities for attentiveness" p.120. "There is a kinship between poetry's ability 'to be in the present' and physicians need to overcome distractions, to achieve poetry's simultaneity through some form of mindfulness" p.123.
Kabat-Zinn, J. (2003) Coming to our Senses.	Mindfulness Leader, Teacher, Researcher	"Our greatest poets engage in deep interior exploration of the mind and of words and of the intimate relationship between inner and outer landscapes" p.27.
Ullyat, G. (2011) "The Only Chance to Love the World" Buddhist Mindfulness in Mary Oliver's Poetry.	English Literature Scholar, Mindfulness Practitioner	" Mary Oliver's poetry lends itself to mindfulness, her usage of simple ordinary language, together with poetic devices such as adequation and correspondence, inform all three corollaries of mindfulness: Beginner's Mind, Mindful Awareness and Nowness, the ability to be fully present in the here and now" p.128.

Figure 2: Perspectives on the Interrelationship of Poetry and Mindfulness

I consider that this theoretical literature helps us to understand two questions: How is poetry mindful? and How is the mind poetic? From the literature, I have identified four types of interrelationships between poetry and mindfulness in terms of the question "How is poetry mindful?" These are poetry as: a focus for and developer of attention, a device for connecting us to our senses and to the present moment, a restorer of the relationship between the mind's centre, the mind's circumference and outer landscapes and as a gatherer of values.

What about the question "How is the mind poetic?" A key interrelationship between the mind and poetry is the understanding that human thinking and imagination is shaped by figurative and poetic processes, that is, the mind is essentially poetic. Gibbs (1994, p.1) asserts that:

> Metaphor, metonymy, irony and other tropes are not linguistic distortions of literal mental thought but constitute basic schemes by which people conceptualise their experiences and the external world.

Despite the fact that Kabat-Zinn (2003, p.153) highlighted the need for more review and research on "the poetry of mindfulness and the appropriate use of the poetic imagination within mindfulness-based interventions", very few empirical studies have investigated this. The few that have focus on the question: What impact does the use of poetry in structured mindfulness courses have on participants? I review three studies.

Name of Study	Research Method	Main Findings
Santorelli, S. (1999) Week 5 In Heal Thy Self: lessons on Mindfulness in Medicine. New York: Three Rives Press p.146-152	Case study of week five of a Mindfulness Based Stress Reduction course and a teacher's account of participants' responses to the poem The Guest House	Positive impact of understanding the "how" of allowing whatever arises in awareness "to be held in an open, noncensoring, nonjudgemental manner." p.50. Also shows variety of responsive impact to the poem, The Guest House.
Shapiro, S.L. (2001) Poetry, Mindfulness and Medicine. Family Medicine 33 (7) p. 505-507	Case study of the use of poetry in a 7-week mindfulness course for undergraduate medical students	Positive impact on openness to acknowledging emotions, body awareness, expression of intentions and sense of connection with others.
Black, A.L. (2009) Does poetry matter in the teaching of mindfulness-based interventions? Bangor University, Masters Dissertation	Interviews with mindfulness teachers who teach structured MBSR or MBCT courses.	a) Positive impact as many teachers spoke about how the participants "loved the poetry" p.69. " A poem can open a door for some participants and give them the words to verbalize their own experience as they identify with what the poet says" p.69. b) Negative impact when it is a hindrance to presence and practice. c) Optional extra to MBSR and MBCT rather than essential component of these courses

Figure 3: Impact of poetry on structured mindfulness courses

In Week 5 in Heal Thy Self: Lessons on Mindfulness in Medicine. Santorelli (1999) recounts how he read The Guest House (See Appendix 1) aloud three times. He discusses how individual participants responded to the poem with very moving stories. He summarises their reported impact of the poem as giving them an understanding of the "how" of allowing whatever arises in awareness "to be held in an open, non-censoring, nonjudgemental manner" (Santorelli, 1999, p.50). These narratives are vey helpful for understanding the interrelationship of poetry and mindfulness in terms of seeing poetry as a trigger for understanding both the nature of mindfulness and the 'how-to' of mindfulness. This study has the strength of rich thick description of participant stories and the limitation of being a case study of one mindfulness teacher's account of the response of one class group to one poem. In contrast this chapter focuses on lecturers' perspectives of the interrelationships between poetry and mindfulness, in more general and less structured contexts than a structured 6-8 week mindfulness course.

Shapiro (2001) in *Poetry, Mindfulness and Medicine* presents a case study of the use of poetry in a 7-week elective mindfulness course for undergraduate medical students. This paper is very useful for people considering using poetry in mindfulness courses as it gives examples of specific poems used, the rationale for the choice of poem and participants' response to the poems. The conclusion of this case study is that "In the class, reading and discussing poetry appeared to provide students with an alternative route to learning, allowing them to feel, listen and discover in different ways" (Shapiro, 2001 p.505). She argues that poetry offers an alternative way of knowing to cognitive knowing. This study has the limitation of being a teacher's reported account of students' responses to poetry. In the study reported in this chapter, I decided to ask my participants to read one or two poems they use in higher education contexts and talk about how they use the poem, as I found the discussion of the choice of and response to specific poems in this paper very illuminating.

Does poetry matter in the teaching of mindfulness-based interventions? is the title of a masters dissertation that researches MBSR and MBCT teachers perspectives' on the use of poetry in these two specific courses (Black, 2009) through interviewing teachers. Naomi concludes that "poetry offers much of value to a class" (Black, 2009, p.77) and documents case studies of teachers stories of the beneficial impact of poetry on participants. However, she also cautions that poetry "can also be a hindrance if the poetry becomes "more essential than the essential presence and practice of the teacher, the presence and practice of the participants" (Black, 2009 p.77). She concludes that poetry in these two mindfulness courses "is an optional extra that can be helpful but not essential" (Back, 2009, p.77). This chapter explores lecturers' (faculty) perspectives on the interrelationships between poetry and mindfulness not from the perspective of structured mindfulness programmes but from the perspective of their role as lecturers in higher education. This paper prompted me to add a question on lecturers' perception of any cautionary comments they would make about combining poetry and mindfulness in higher education contexts (See Appendix 2 for Interview Guide).

RESEARCH DESIGN: FINDING A RESEARCH APPROACH COMPATIBLE WITH POETRY AND MINDFULNESS

The literature review also helped me to clarify and refine the research questions and interview guide.

> **Research Questions**
>
> 1. How do lecturers (faculty) use poetry and mindfulness practically together in higher education?
>
> 2. What are the perceived conceptual interrelationships between poetry and mindfulness for lecturers (faculty) who practice both in higher education?

I conducted the research from the perspective that knowledge is constructed socially. The perspective is built on the assumption that some knowledge comes from *"affective and embodied aspects of human experience"* and all knowledge is *"ideological, political and permeated with values"* (Schwandt, 2000, p.198, my emphasis). This study focuses on three interviews with academic staff (faculty) about how they use poetry and mindfulness together in different ways. I agree with

Way, Zwier and Tracy (2015) who argue that if reality and knowledge are socially constructed then we should view the interview space as one of shared dialogue and meaning making. In this regard, I aimed to be open-minded and to foster the interview as a space of expression, storytelling, acceptance, discovery, connection and meaning-making. I agree with Bolton (2006, p.218) that: "All professional and personal experience is naturally storied; telling or writing stories are prime human ways of understanding, communicating and remembering". I therefore chose a narrative form of enquiry and to write about how the lecturers used poetry and mindfulness together as stories. This type of enquiry " that precisely in virtue of being attuned to the poetic figuration of life itself - both as lived and as told - opens the way toward an enlarged understanding of self and the world" (Freeman ,1993, p.231 quoted in Sherman, 2014, p.114).

I deliberately wanted the interviews to be infused with a mindfulness-based approach, to have congruity between the process and topic of the research. The interviews began by sitting together in silence in mindfulness meditation for 15 minutes. This is what Stelter (2010, p.863) refers to as "clearing the space." I found the guidelines on experience-based body anchored interviewing (Stelter, 2010) namely; present moment focus, bracketing and non-judgemental attitude, descriptive questioning and moving to connecting experience to thoughts, emotions and actions, were very helpful in informing the shape and detail of my interview guide (see Appendix 2). Merleau-Ponty's understanding of embodiement: "Consciousness, is being toward-the-thing through the intermediary of the body" influenced my approach to the research (Merleau-Ponty, 1962, p.138-139). As I was interested in embodied educational practice, the key question was about how interviewees used poetry and mindfulness together in higher education. To this end, the interview started with an invitation to the interviewee to read a poem that combined poetry and mindfulness, that they used with students or staff. Then the interviewer asked them about how they experienced reading the poem now, followed by how they used the poem with students/staff. I video-recorded rather than merely audio-recording the interviews so I would have an embodied recording to review and this helped me recapture an "aesthetic and visceral connection, " with the interview (Cooper and Hughes, 2015, p.30).

The sample was a convenience sample of three lecturers (faculty) who practice both poetry and mindfulness separately and together. I interviewed two lecturers who I knew and who had not undertaken the MSc Studies in Mindfulness programme. I got someone to interview me, so I was the main interviewer. the third research participant and a student on the MSc Studies Mindfulness programme at the time of the interviews. Naomi is an assistant professor in English specialising in Renaissance literature. Larry was Head of School of Informatics and Engineering and a member of a development team for a new technological university for Dublin at the time of the interview. I am an assistant professor in education development and have completed a Postgraduate Diploma in Studies in Mindfulness and I am a trained mindfulness teacher.

I narrate the stories. I did a mindfulness meditation before viewing each video as a way to help me view the videos in a mindful and embodied way. The purpose of doing a mindfulness meditation before viewing a video is to "cultivate the capacity to simply listen with minimum intrusion of the conceptual mind and pre-formulated ideas" (Crane et al 2015, p.1106). I watched each video in turn, immersing myself in the video. Then I took notes with quotations to make an overview of the interview. Then I looked at the video again adding to my notes. I watched the video again a number of times noticing new things and adding to my notes.

In the following sections the narratives begin with a poem that the interviewee chose to read or an extract of the poem. Then the reflective stories of how they used these poems with students and/or staff in ways that combine poetry with mindfulness are presented. Each narrative is followed by a discussion of the wider educational significance of these stories recounted as recommended by Kim (2008), in terms of how other lecturers might adapt these approaches and the links with educational theories. The conclusion summarises the findings of the two explicit research questions as suggested by Kvale and Brickmann (2009).

USING MINDFUL READING TO TEACH POETRY (ANY POEM) TO STUDENTS AND TO CREATE EGALITARIAN SPACES FOR POETRY EXPLORATION

Naomi is an assistant professor in English specialising in Renaissance literature. She uses a specific mindfulness practice (mindful reading) to teach poetry to literature students. Her primary aim as an English lecturer is to teach students to become more *critical* readers of poetry/literature, and for her mindful reading, with its focus on emotional, bodily and social responses, starts this process. Students then have to critically analyse the text, considering the poem's form, its politics etc. She does not think mindful reading can get students to this level on its own, but it does get them closer to it than other pedagogical methods because it gets them to fully and openly engage with the poem, both as individuals and a group, and helps to develop confidence in their ability to read poetry.

After 15 minutes of meditation with her body very still and her eyes closed, Naomi read a poem by Sir Philip Sydney, *Sonnet 9* from Atrophil and Stella that she teaches her second year English students. She read it from a well-used book on a Renaissance Literature course that had some post-its sticking out.

> Queen Virtues court, which some call Stellas face,
> Prepar'd by Nature's chiefest furniture,
> Hath his front built of Alabaster pure;
> Gold is the covering of that stately place.
>
> The doore by which sometimes comes forth her Grace,
> Red Porphir is, which locke of pearl makes sure:
> Whose porches rich (which name of cheekes endure)
> Marble mixt red and white do interlace.
>
> The windows now through which this heav'nly guest
> Looks over the world, and can find nothing such,
> Which dare claime from those lights the name of best.
>
> Of touch they are that without touch doth touch,
> Which Cupid's selfe from Beauties myne did draw:
> Of touch they are, and poore I am their straw.

In describing how she had just experienced reading this poem Naomi commented that she had some mindful moments when reading the poem where she noticed her emotional and bodily responses to reading the poem.

Naomi described the way she facilitates mindfully reading this poem with her English literature class. She follows a well-established mindful reading practice (Barbezat and Bush, 2014, p.115, See Appendix 3). Firstly, she "gets her students to sit in a circle" (*hands gesturing to make a circular movement*). Then, she spends time getting students and herself to settle the body and mind. She explained that she needs the settling time for herself as sometimes her heart is pounding at the start and then she relaxes. Then she gets each of the students in turn to read a line of the poem aloud. Then one minute of silence. The students read the poem aloud again followed by another period of silence. Next the students are invited "to share a word or two about their physical or emotional response to the poem." She invites them to "say anything at all" (*putting arms up in the air and open*) After this the poem is read again followed by a minute of silence and students are invited to share a longer response to the poem. She encourages the students to "Let the poem speak to you." Naomi also shares her response in each round but does so as the last person. It involves "taking time and being present."

Following this, when the space for poetry exploration opens up Naomi then uses this "open space" to get the students to think about literary form together with historical context and therefore more critically engage with the poem. She uses the full fifty minutes of a class to do the mindful reading and critical analysis of one poem.

This approach has encouraged "deep listening" to the poem. It is a "more egalitarian way" where "everyone contributes" more or less to the same degree. The mindful reading of the poem, "sitting with the poem" facilitates students "really getting into the poem" and " realising that the skills they have are more sophisticated than they thought", rather than reading the notes about the poem first. This "egalitarian, more democratic " approach means that student hear "different voices" reading the poem and get "different perspectives." This way the "teacher is not the foundation of knowledge" and students respond and build on one another's responses rather than the dynamic being individual students making responses and looking to the teacher for validation of those responses. Mindfully reading a poem helps students "to get there quickly and more deeply and together. We all get there." (*making a sweeping movement with her hands*). As a teacher, she "enjoyed it." She uses mindfulness as "an alternative teaching method" rather than "teaching mindfulness." Her personal mindfulness practice helps her " to be comfortable with silence" and to be aware of her own emotions.

SIGNIFICANCE

The wider education implications of this mindful reading approach is that most academics are not trained mindfulness teachers but they can facilitate the mindfully reading and exploration of a short text in their discipline. The protocol of instructions for mindfully reading a text (See Appendix 3) used by Naomi is detailed in *Contemplative Practices in Higher Education* (Haskell in Barbezat and Bush, 2014, p.115). Mindful reading as opposed to speed-reading;

> slows down the reader and the reading and that alone changes the student experience. It is a process of quiet reflection, which requires mindful attentiveness, a letting go of distracting thoughts and opinions to be fully in the moment with the text. It requires patient receptivity and an intention to go further, and it moves the reader into a calm awareness, allowing a more profound experience and understanding (Barbezat and Bush, 2014, p.113).

This approach is used not only in English literature but also in other disciplines. Naomi facilitated a mindful reading of this same poem with a group of lectures from different disciplines so they could experience this approach and adapt it for their disciplines. She noticed on this occasion how many related the poem to the physical surroundings of the room and hotel we were in. A science lecturer said she would use this approach for reading an abstract of a scientific paper with her class. I have facilitated lecturers reading a quotation from Freire about dialogical knowing (learning through discussion with others) as part of a module on curriculum design.

A key significance of mindfully reading a text is that it is a way of operationalising the democratic social relations and dialogical process needed to facilitate co-elaboration and co-construction of knowledge (Barrett and Moore, 2011). What did Freire mean by democratic social relations and dialogical knowing?

> What is dialogue in this way of knowing? Precisely this connection, this epistemological relationship, the object to be known in one place links the cognitive subjects leading them to reflect together on the object. Dialogue is the bringing together of the teacher and the student in the joint act of knowing and reknowing the object of study. Then instead of transferring the knowledge *statically*, as a fixed possession of the teacher, dialogue demands a dynamic proximation towards the object (Shor and Freire, 1987 p.10).

Moving from the practical to the conceptual, Naomi discussed how poetry is just one object for mindfulness and would not privilege it over other objects for mindfulness practice: "Anything can be mindful, mindful cookery, mindful running." What distinguishes Naomi's approach is that she does not use poems about mindfulness but uses the mindfulness practice of mindful reading to teach her discipline of English literature.

> **Pause and Reflect**
>
> What texts would you like to invite your students to read mindfully in class?

CREATING MINDFUL SPACES FOR REFLECTION, PERSONAL TRANSFORMATION AND THANKS THROUGH READING AND WRITING POETRY

Larry was a lecturer, Head of School of Informatics and Engineering at the then Blanchardstown Institiute of Technology and a member of a development team for a new technological university for Dublin, at the time of the interview. After practicing mindfulness meditation in silence for 15 minutes, Larry responded to the invitation to explaining his choice of poem *The Uses of Not*. For the ten-year anniversary of a new institution of higher education Larry was asked to put together his recollections of the ten years. He decided to do a personal reflection of the poems that meant the most to him during the ten years and why, rather than a professional procedural review. This was later published as a booklet entitled "Institutional Review." It highlights that what we do as educators is about the body, mind and soul, not just the mind. He read one of those poems in an absorbed manner.

The Uses of Not   By Lao Tzu

Thirty spokes
Meet in the hub
Where the wheel isn't is
Where it's useful
Hollowed out.
Clay makes a pot.
 Where the pot's not
 Is where it's useful

Cut doors and windows.
To make a room
Where the room isn't,
There's a room for you

So the profit in what is
Is in the use of what isn't

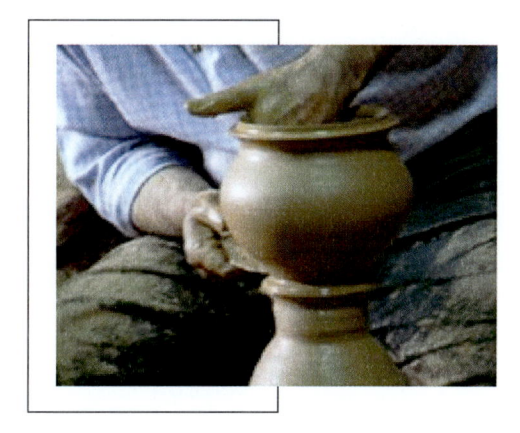

*Figure 4: Man Shapping Pottery
Photo by Oostdyk*

In describing how he had just experienced reading this poem. Larry commented: "It cries out to me all the time. Spaces in the wheel is where it is useful…It would not turn without the spaces." Larry elaborated how the higher education system values the spokes of the wheel but not the spaces between the spokes. The poem "recaptures the importance of space." It counters "the need to be always busy." It raises the questions: "Where do we give space to learners? (*hand moving outward and opening up*) Do we encourage them to create their own spaces?" This poem counters the notion that "If it's not counted it doesn't count." Mindfulness practice includes "valuing spaces and gaps." (*hands parting and opening out*). In higher education this means tackling the current issue of "over-assessment" and helping students to see "a gap in the timetable is not a bad thing" and the space is what they need. The spaces can be used for student and staff reflection after an assignment and to process their experiences. This can become "a personal transformation space." The creation of these type of spaces is very important as "education is in danger of just being a transaction and the concept of your personal transformative space is being squeezed out." He argues that if we allow that to continue "everyone will suffer, the students and the communities they return to."

Larry chose a second poem from that booklet that resonates with him personally that he reads on occasion to acknowledge how people in the college are interconnected and the importance of saying "thanks". The poem is *Those Winter Sundays by Robert Hayden*. The poem starts:

Sundays too my father got up early
And put his clothes on in the blueback cold,
Then with cracked hands that ached
From labor in the weekday weather made
Banked fires blaze. No one ever thanked him.

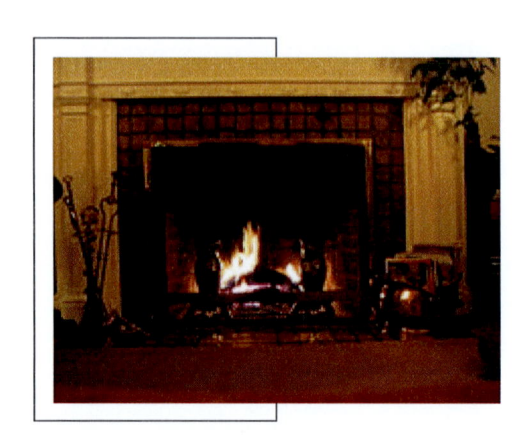

Figure 5: The Fireplace
Photo by Sproule

He discussed how this poem challenges us to think about who we are not thanking and taking time to say thanks: "If you are busy, busy, taking time out to say thanks can disappear." The poem may prompt the mindfulness practice of being aware, noticing and being grateful for all those who help us in daily life in college: the cleaners that clean the classrooms, the IT support people, the security staff etc. In addition to practicing mindfulness and poetry for himself, Larry said in his management role: "At meetings I would deliberately choose poetry or images that resonate on a personal level first to centre the conversation."

Larry then talked about another way in which poetry and mindfulness come together in the college was that first year students had the opportunity to work with a poet and to write and perform a collective poem about starting college. The writing of the poem was "a concrete, personal way of making space," It was a way of saying to students: "What is in there we value." Working on the collective poem was a way for students to reflect on and " process their life experiences" and to share their experiences, diversity and collective strength." Shortly after the interview these first year creative digital media students performed their poem *Here We Come* at a conference.

Pause and Watch

For the text and performance of the students' poem *Here We Come* see
http://www.ahead.ie/connectedvoices

Larry sees the interrelationship between poetry and mindfulness is in poetry's distilling ability : "Poetry distil it down, like an essential oil, the nugget you need. There is nothing around it, no noise" There is "just space". He sees a poem as a signpost: " Where is the signpost asking you to go?"

SIGNIFICANCE

This view of the potential of reading and writing poetry to create mindful spaces for reflection, personal transformation and thanks has a wider educational significance. It recognises the need to process the major transition experience that is the first year of college (Tinto, 1975) by providing spaces that have the time, media and creativity to express these lived experiences. Moreover, reading and writing poetry can help students to realise that they do not have to separate the personal from the educational and they can be encouraged to connect themselves with their learning and their disciplinary knowledge (Barbazet and Bush, 2014).

Savin-Baden (2008) discusses the creation of different types of learning spaces in higher education. Larry's two ways of combining mindfulness and poetry are some practical ways of doing this. These spaces are:

> 1) primary spaces of reflection of thinking about experiences e.g. the daily routine of timetabled activities and gaps in the timetable
> 2) transitional spaces of responding to a challenge e.g. who am I not thanking and
> 3) transformational spaces of collectively reflecting and naming emerging issues and identities e.g. in relation to being a first year student

Creating spaces that prompt people to increase their gratitude is important in light of Wood et al's (2010) review of 12 studies that suggests that interventions specifically designed to increase gratitude are effective in improving wellbeing. Larry's stories give rise to questions for all staff in higher education.

Pause and Reflect

What type of reflective and transformative spaces do you want to create in your educational context?
How could reading, listening to, writing or performing poetry have a role in creating these spaces?

LISTENING TO POETRY TO RESONATE WITH THE NATURE OF MINDFULNESS AND CONNECTING WITH INNER SPACIOUSNESS, VALUES AND CREATIVITY.

I (Terry) am an assistant professor in education development. I have completed a Postgraduate Diploma in Studies in Mindfulness and I am a trained mindfulness teacher. After sitting together in silent mindfulness meditation with the interviewer for 15 minutes I explained my choice of poem: "It's a poem I use in my own practice. I use it in my own personal practice as well as when I am guiding a practice." I read the last part of Doha: Spiritual Song of Realisation by Gendun Rinpoche (undated) very slowly with long pauses.

> Wanting to grasp the ungraspable, you exhaust yourself in vain.
> As soon as you relax this grasping, space is there,
> open, inviting and comfortable.
>
> So, make use of it. All is yours already.
> Don't search any further.
> Don't go into the inextricable jungle looking for the elephant
> who is already quietly at home.
>
> Nothing to do
> Nothing to force
> Nothing to want
> And everything happens by itself.

Responding to how I experienced reading the poem I commented:

> Sitting in silence with you and reading the poem, spaciousness is there, that is resonating with me now. In the middle of busyness I can feel spaciousness… Reading the poem I could feel my chest expanding and being more spacious and in touch with something deep in me. It is comfortable and comforting. It is physically spacious and emotionally comforting and calming (*putting my hand on my heart*).

The context in which I use this poem in higher education is that I coordinate a mindfulness group for staff in our university that meet once a week at lunchtime to do a guided mindfulness meditation practice together. I use mindfulness and poetry together by sometimes reading part of this poem at the end of a meditation, when I guide a practice with this group. The poem is "part of the practice". I then described how I regularly guide Lovingkindness practice (Barrett, 2015). I invite you to do this practice now and to listen to the poem I read at the end of the practice.

Pause and Practice

In Lovingkindness practice we wish happiness and wellbeing for ourselves and others.
Become aware of your breath coming in and out. Feel yourself grounded your bum on the chair, your feet on this floor.
Say the following phrases silently to your self and if it suits say them on the out breath:
May I be happy.
May I be wel.l
May I be at ease.
May I take care of myself happily.

Repeat this for a few minutes.

Now bring to mind someone you have a natural warm connection with, maybe a friend or a family member and then repeat the following phrases for them for a few minutes:
May you be happy.
May you be well.
May you be at ease.
May you take care of yourself happily.

Then say these phrases for a group of people close to you or for a group of people you work with, then for someone you are having a little difficulty with and finally for all beings.

Recite the short poem Fluent by John O' Donohue (O'Donohue, 2000, p.30).
Watch and Listen to Terry reading Fluent in Wicklow Ireland
https://www.facebook.com/themindfulnessassociation/videos/2153941074857418/

We dedicate this practice that it may result in small acts of kindness, caring, welcome and warmth for ourselves and for others whose lives we touch.

I discussed how these lines of poetry are my wish for myself and for others. I talked about how I find it so inspiring and that is "always calling me to tap into my inner being, values and creativity," and for others "their own creativity, their own way" (*moving my hand from touching my heart to moving outwards in an arc*). This links with Heaney's (1995, p.467) understanding of the power of poetry "to remind us that we are hunters and gatherers of values". For me this poem captures the essence of mindfulness, that is, that it is good "to live from the inside-out." I often read it at the end of guiding a Lovingkindness practice.

In terms of the practical interrelationship between poetry and mindfulness I use poetry to capture some aspects of mindfulness: "I think poetry can do that." For some people poetry is a way into mindfulness if someone combines mindfulness and poetry. I discussed the resonating quality of mindfulness:

> The spaciousness and comfortableness is here (*my hand on heart*). The poem is out there (*my hand moving outwards*). The poem resonates with my inner being, my inner experience. (*my hand moving from being out there to touching my heart*). And it is inspiring me to be aware of that and to be grateful for that.

In terms of the conceptual relationship between poetry and mindfulness both are "less is more". Poetry has "no excessive words" but contains just a "nugget" to help your practice or resonate with "what is happening inside". It has a "naming quality" and helps us to be in touch with our heart and soul. Both mindfulness and poetry have "a stripping away" quality. Both mindfulness and poetry are "practice-based." Poetry is a practice "It is personal, embodied and deeply meaningful." Both are about the senses and the body: "You can only experience your senses in the here and now."

SIGNIFICANCE

My view resonates that a poem can invite us "to connect with what is already there". This links with Connelly's (1999, p.120) view of poetry's power to trigger our "attention to the present moment", and to Ullyat's (2011, p.128) assertion of the ability of some poems to draw us towards "Beginner's Mind, Mindful Awareness and Nowness". Poetry can be used to capture the essence of mindfulness or an aspect of mindfulness. O'Donohue (2000) would meet Kabat-Zinn's (2003, p.27) criteria of a great poet as he prompts us to engage in deep reflection "of the intimate relationship between inner and outer landscapes," with the poem *Fluent*.

More widely it is important for teachers in higher education to consider the timing of the reading of a poem in the context of a mindfulness practice group. Research (Black, 2009, p.67) suggests that the timing of reading a poem at the end of a practice is effective. The end of a practice was popular because the participants were settled and receptive to a poem's meaning. (Burack, 1999; Shapiro et al, 1998).

There is a need for mindfulness practice groups for staff as well as students in higher education. Mindfulness for staff can be a tool for self-care and for more student-centred reflective work with students and colleagues. Kernochan et al (2007, p.71) discuss how their mindfulness practice has "shifted them toward student-centred teaching" and becoming "more sensitive to our students". Zanjonc (2013) said the following inspirational words: "We need to calm ourselves...Open up... Certain things begin to show themselves....We bring all of who we are to all that the world is".

CONCLUSION

The first research question was: How do lecturers (faculty) use poetry and mindfulness practically together in higher education? The lecturers in this study used poetry and mindfulness together in three different ways namely 1) using mindful reading to teach poetry (any poem) to students and to create egalitarian spaces for poetry exploration, 2) creating mindful spaces for reflection, personal transformation and thanks through reading and writing poetry, and 3) listening to poetry to resonate with the nature of mindfulness and connecting with inner spaciousness, compassionte values and creativity. These approaches suggest possibilities that some faculty might wish to adapt to their educational contexts. For all lecturers the use of mindfulness and poetry together in professional contexts was linked to their personal mindfulness practice. We are aware of the limitations of reflecting the experiences of the interviews within the structure and somewhat hard edges of a book chapter. As Larry put it we "hope that the reader will be able to experience the soft edges of the acts of sharing poetry, the quiet moments these interactions engender and the risks of putting personal in public places."

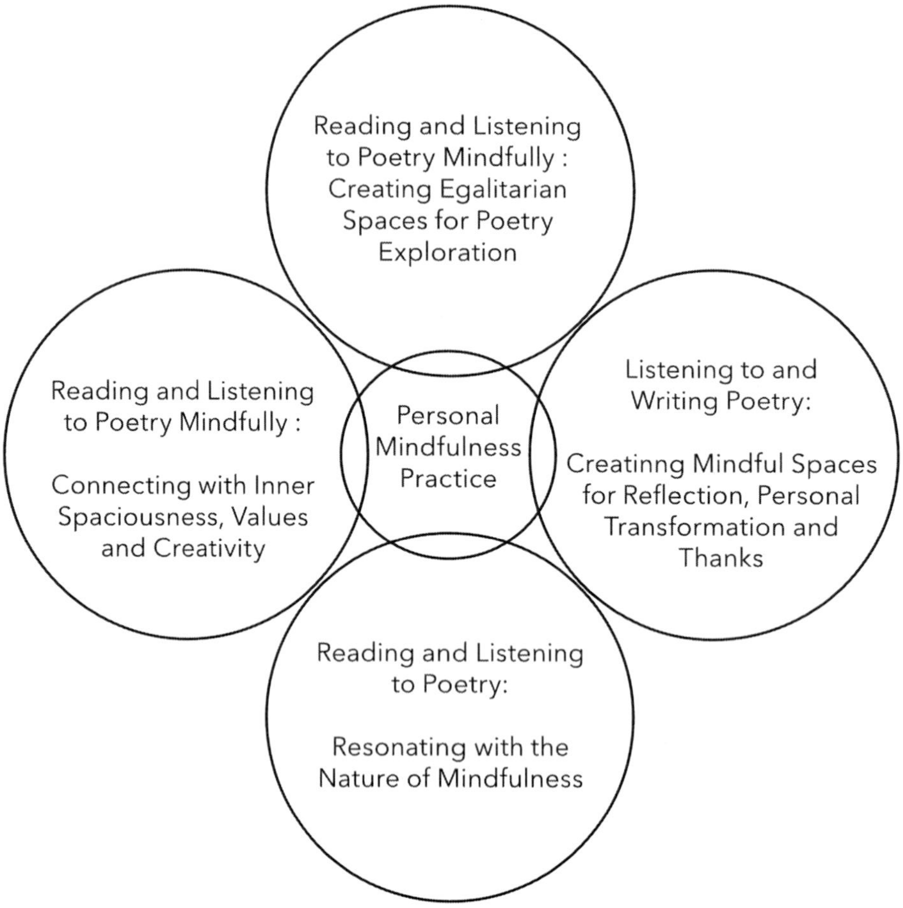

Figure 7: A model of ways lecturers (faculty) use poetry and mindfulness practically together in higher education

This model may be a generative trigger for lecturers and other educators to develop these and other approaches for combining poetry and mindfulness in their own contexts.

The second research question was: What are the perceived conceptual interrelationships between poetry and mindfulness for lecturers (faculty) who practice both in higher education? Participants highlighted the particular sensual, distilling, resonating, naming, centering, inspiring and signposting qualities of poetry. However, one lecturer did not privilege poetry especially. She commented that you can do anything mindfully e.g. mindful cooking, running or poetry, and that poetry is just one of many possible objects for mindfulness practice. The following figure summarises these perceived conceptual interrelationships with quotations from the participants.

POETRY **MINDFULNESS**

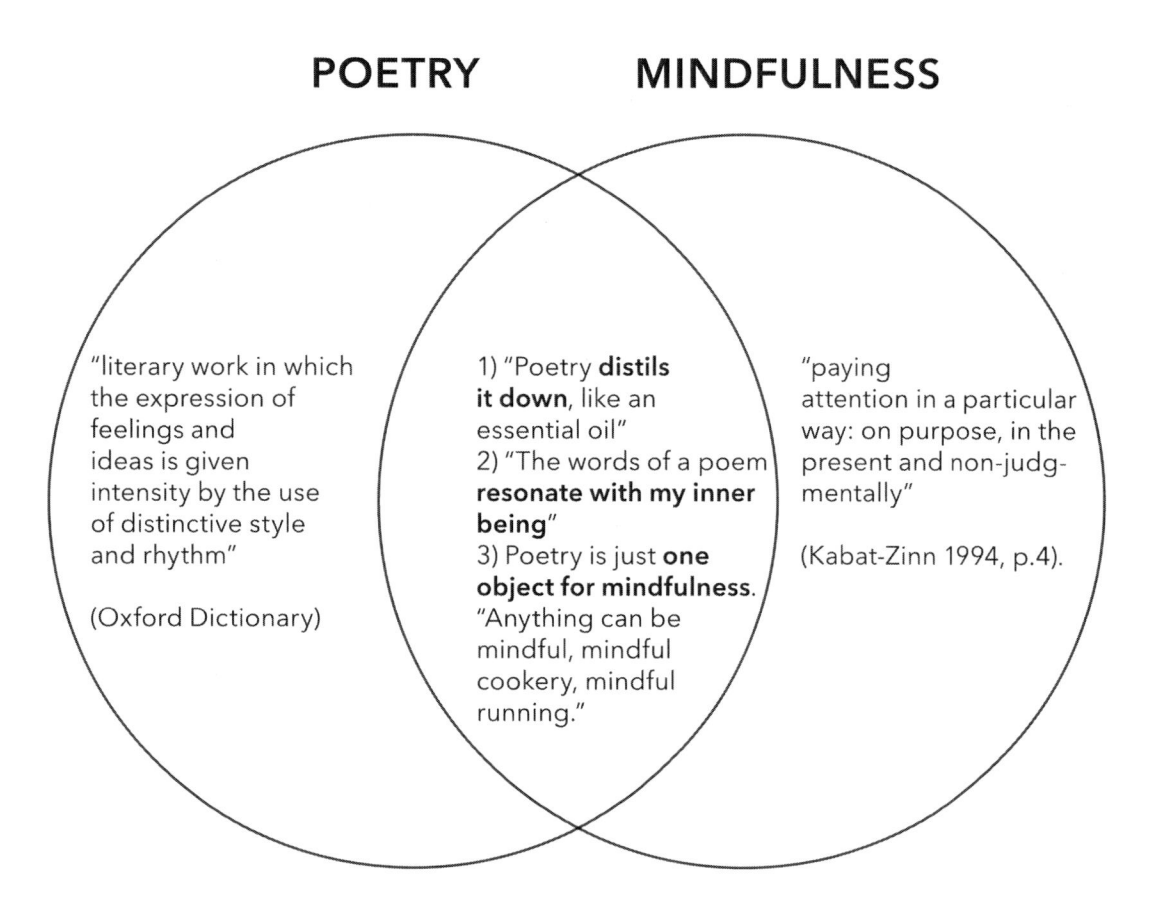

"literary work in which the expression of feelings and ideas is given intensity by the use of distinctive style and rhythm"

(Oxford Dictionary)

1) "Poetry **distils it down**, like an essential oil"
2) "The words of a poem **resonate with my inner being**"
3) Poetry is just **one object for mindfulness**. "Anything can be mindful, mindful cookery, mindful running."

"paying attention in a particular way: on purpose, in the present and non-judgmentally"

(Kabat-Zinn 1994, p.4).

Figure 8: Lecturers perceptions of the conceptual interrelationships between poetry and mindfulness

In terms of cautiousness about using mindfulness and poetry together, all three lecturers highlighted that it may bring up personal issues for people. In this context it is important that the purpose and structure of the session is clear and that people are made aware of the resources they have within themselves and the wider supports and resources available on campus.

Lecturers' initiatives in creating new spaces through combining poetry and mindfulness, and the wider social context of national and international developments in contemplative pedagogies, played interrelated roles in lecturers' meaning-making of these initiatives. They linked these initiatives to "contemplative pedagogies" and Daniel Barbezat who gave a keynote and workshop in Ireland (ICEP 2015; Barbezat and Bush, 2014). The research questions were explored in ways that made connections between the stories of the interviewees and wider educational practices in different higher education contexts. These stories of using poetry and mindfulness together in higher education contexts in Ireland to create new spaces is part of world-wide developments in the growth of the use of mindfulness and contemplative pedagogies in higher education (Barbazet and Bush, 2014). I see my role in promoting contemplative ways of knowing through combining poetry and mindfulness as part of the return phase of my journey as a mindful hero. Contemplative ways of knowing can powerfully complement rational-scientific ways of knowing for students and staff.

> The contemplative mind is opened and activated through a wide range of approaches-from pondering to poetry to meditation - that are designed to quiet and shift the habitual forms of chatter of the mind to cultivate a capacity for deepened awareness, concentration and insight (Hart, 2004, p.29).

FURTHER RESOURCES

Mary Oliver reads Wild Geese
https://www.youtube.com/watch?v=lv_4xmh_WtE

Mindfulness Poetry for Transformation
Mindful Living Programs
A collection of poems with mindfulness themes
http://www.mindfullivingprograms.com/resources_poetry.php
Sharon Salzberg's website
This includes guided audio and video mindfulness, compassion and Lovingkindness meditation practices
www.sharonsalzberg.com

REFERENCES

BAER, R. A., SMITH, G.T., HOPKINS, J., KRITEMEYER, J. and TONEY, L. (2006). Using Self-Report Assessment Methods to Explore Facets of Mindfulness. Assessment 13 (1), pp. 27-45
BARBEZAT, D. and BUSH, M., (2014) Contemplative Practices in Higher Education: Powerful Methods to Transform Teaching and Learning. San Fransisco: Jossey Bass.
BARRETT. T. (2011) Breakthroughs in action research through poetry. Educational Action Research Vol 19, No. 1, 5-12
http://dx.doi.org/10.1080/09650792.2011.547393
BARRETT, T. (2015) Lovingkindness Caring for Others and Self: The Heart of Higher Education. Voice of the Educator: Self Care and Contemplative Practices. International Conference for Engaging Pedagogies, College of Computing Technology Dublin, 3-4 Decemeber
http://icep.ie/paper-template/?pid=141
BARRETT, T. (2017) A New Model of Problem-based learning: Inspiring Concepts, Practice Strategies and Case Studies from Higher Education. Maynooth: AISHE. The full book or individual chapters can be downloaded freely at http://bit.ly/2qHv5gB
BLACK, A.L. (2009) Does poetry matter in the teaching of mindfulness-based interventions? Bangor University, Masters Dissertation
BURACK (1999) Rethinking Meditation in Education - Educational Uses of Meditation. Tikkun Magazine.
BURR, V. (2015) Social Constructionism. London: Routledge
BOLTON, G. (2006) . Narrative Writing: Reflective Enquiry into Professional Practice. Educational Action Research 14 (2, pp.: 203-219
CONNELLY, D. (1999) Being in the Present Moment: Developing the Capacity for Mindfulness in Medicine. 74 (4), pp.420-423
COOPER, K.A and HUGHES , N. R., (2015) Thick Narratives: Mining Implicit, Oblique and Deeper Understandings in Videotaped Research Data. Qualitative Enquiry 21 (1),pp. 28-35
CRANE, R.S.,STANLEY,S., ROONEY,M., BARTLEY, T., COOPER,L. and MARDULA,J. (2015) Disciplined Improvisation: Characteristics of Inquiry. Mindfulness 6 (5), pp. 1104-1114.
FIRST YEAR CREATIVE DIGITAL MEDIA STUDENTS, Blanchardstown Institute of Technology, Here We Come For text and performance of the poem see
http://www.ahead.ie/connectedvoices
FREEMAN, M. (1993) Rewriting the self: History, memory, narrative. London : Routledge
GIBBS, R.W. (1994) The Poetics of Mind. Cambridge; Cambridge University Press
GENDUN RINPOCHE, (undated) Doha: Spiritual Song of Realisation
Available at http://www.peterrussell.com/Odds/Gendun.php
HAYDEN, R . (1996) Those Winter Sunday.s. Collected Poems of Robert Hayden edited by Frederick Glaysher. Liveright Publishing Corporation Available at
https://www.poets.org/poetsorg/poem/those-winter-sundays
HEANEY, S. (1995) Crediting Poetry: Nobel Lecture. In Heaney, S (1998) Seamus Heaney Opened Ground Poems 1966-1996. London: Faber and Faber
HART, T. (2004) Opening the Contemplative Mind in the Classroom. Journal of Transformative Education, 2 (28), pp. 28-46
ICEP (International Conference on Engaging Pedagogies) (2015) Voice of the Educator: Self Care and Contemplative Practices. College of Computing Technology, Dublin, 3-4 December
KABAT-ZINN, J. (1994). Wherever you go, there you are: Mindfulness meditation in everyday life. New York:Hyperion.
KABAT-ZINN, J. (2003) Mindfulness-based Interventions in Context: Past, Present and Future. Clinical Psychology 10 (2), pp.144-155.

KERNOCHAN, R.A., MCCORMICK. D. W., and WHITE, J.A. (2007) Spirituality and the Management Teacher : reflections of Three Buddhist on Compassion, Mindfulness and Selflessness in the Classroom. Journal of Management Inquiry, 16 (1), pp. 61-75

KIM, J.-H. (2008) A Romance with Narrative Inquiry: Towards an Act of Narrative Theorizing. Curriculum and Teaching Dialogue 10 (1 and 2): 251–267.

KVALE, S., AND BRICKMAN, S., (2009) InterViews: Learning the Craft of Qualitative Research Interviewing. London : Sage

LANGER, E. (2000) Mindful Learning Current Directions in Psychological Sciences 9 (1) pp. 220-223

LEAR, E, (1983) The Owl and the Pussy-cat. The Puffin Book of Verse Compiled by Eleanor Graham (1967) p.167 Harmondsworth: Penguin Books Ltd

LEWIN, K. (1951). Field theory in social science: Selected theoretical papers (D. Cartwright, Ed.). New York, NY: Harper & Row

MERLEAU-PONTY, M. (1962) Phenomenology of perception. London: Routledge and Kegan Paul

O'DONOHUE, J. (2000) Fluent p. 30 Conamara Blues London: Doubleday

OOSTDYK, R. (2006) Man shaping pottery in Cappadocia, Turkey. Photo taken by Randy Oostdyk, and released under GFDL.Wikimedia Commons.
https://en.wikipedia.org/wiki/File:Makingpottery.jpg

SANTORELLI, S. (1999) Week 5 In Heal thy Self: Lessons on Mindfulness in Medicine. New York: Three Rives Press p.146-152

SHAPIRO, S.L., SCHWANTZ, G.E and BONNER, G., (1998) Effects of MBSR on Medical and Pre-Medical Students. Journal of Behavioural Medicine, 21 (6), pp.581-599

SHAPIRO, S.L. (2001) Poetry, Mindfulness and Medicine. Family Medicine 33 (7) p. 505-507

SHERMAN, G.L.., (2014) Refocusing the Self in Higher Education: A Phenomenological Perspective. New York: Routledge

SPROULE, R. (2004) The Fireplace Phot taken by Robbie Sproule. Creative Commons 2.0 license
http://www.flickr.com?Flickr.com

STELTER, R. (2010) Experience-Base, Body-Anchored Qualitative Research Interviewing. Advancing Qualitative Methods 20 (6), pp. 859-867

SCHWANDT, T. (2000). Three Epistemological Stances for Qualitative Inquiry: Interpretivism, Hermeneutics and Social Constructionism. In Handbook of Qualitative Research. N. Denzin and Y. Lincoln (eds) London: Sage Publications, pp.189-214

SYDNEY, P. Sonnet 9 Astrophil and Stella The Penguin Book of Renaissance Verse 1509-1659, selected and with an introduction by David Norbrook and edited by H.R. Woudhuysen (London: Penguin, 2005), p. 201.

TINTO,V. (1975) Dropout from Higher Education: A Theoretical Synthesis of Recent Research"Review of Educational Research 45, pp.89-125.

TZU , LAO"The uses of not" (Book One, Chapter 11) by from Lao Tzu: Tao Te Ching: A Book about the Way and the Power of the Way, translated from the original Chinese by Ursula K. Le Guin (Shambhala Publications, 1998 edition).
http://www.ayearofbeinghere.com/2015/06/lao-tzu-uses-of-not-book-one-chapter-11.html

ULLYAT, G. (2011) "The Only Chance to Love the World" Buddhist Mindfulness in Mary Oliver's Poetry. 27 (2), pp. 115-131

WAY, A.,K. ZWEIR, R.K. and TRACY. S.J. (2015) Dialogic Interviewing and Flickers of Transformation: An examination and Delination of Interactional Strategies that Promote Participant Self-Reflexivity. Qualitative Inquiry 21 (8), pp. 720-731

WOOD, A.M., FROH, J.J.and GERAGHTY, A.W.A., (2010) Gratitude and well-being: A review and theoretical integration. Clinical Psychology Review 30 (7), pp. 890-905

Wordsworth, W (1802) Upon Westminster Bridge
https://www.poets.org/poetsorg/poem/composed-upon-westminster-bridge-september-3-1802

ZAJONC, A (2013) Radio Interview with Krista Tinet. On Being 12th Sept
http://www.onbeing.org/program/arthur-zajonc-holding-life-consciously/109/audio?embed=1
Date of purchase of licence: 4th November 2018

GONYNOR, (2016). Associations Among Mindfulness, Self-Compassion, and Bullying in Early Adolescence.

MACKENZIE, H.G., (2016). Awakening Child: A journey of inner transformation through teaching your child mindfulness and compassion [online]. John Hunt Publishing. Available from: http://amzn.eu/5eggB59.

Appendixes
Appendix 1 Guest House by Rumi
Appendix 2 Interview Guide
Appendix 3 Protocol of Instructions for mindfully reading a text (Haskell in Barbezat and Bush, 2014. p. 115).

Appendix 1 The Guest House by Rumi

This being human is a guest house.
Every morning a new arrival.
A joy, a depression, a meanness,
some momentary awareness comes
as an unexpected visitor.
Welcome and entertain them all!
Even if they are a crowd of sorrows,
who violently sweep your house
empty of its furniture,
still, treat each guest honorably.
He may be clearing you out
for some new delight.
The dark thought, the shame, the malice.
meet them at the door laughing and invite them in.
Be grateful for whatever comes.
because each has been sent
as a guide from beyond.

Appendix 2 Interview Guide

1. As I mentioned before I thought we would start by sitting in meditation in silence together to settle ourselves, clear some space and arrive at this interview
2. Would you like to begin by reading a poem or two through which you have made connections between poetry and mindfulness?
3. What is your experience of reading the poem now?
4. How do you use this poem with students or staff?
5. How do you use poetry and mindfulness together in higher education?
6. What is your sense of the practical interrelationships between poetry and mindfulness?
7. What are you cautious comments (if any) about issues in combining poetry and mindfulness in higher education?
8. What for you are the conceptual interrelationships between poetry and mindfulness?
9. Any other comments, about poetry and mindfulness, this interview or anything else.

Appendix 3 Protocol of Instructions for mindfully reading a text David G Haskell in (Barbezat and Bush, 2014. p.115).

- Sit quietly and relax your minds and bodies for one minute
- Read aloud, slowly the entire text, each person reading one or two sentences, 'passing along' the reading to the left to the next reader
- One minute of silence and reflection
- One person reads aloud a short passage that is chosen in advance
- Another minute of silence and reflection
- Each person shares a word or short phrase in response to the reading-just give voice to the word without explanation or discussion
- Another person reads the short passage
- One minute of silence and reflection
- Each person shares a a longer response to the text- a sentence or two. All listen attentively to one another without correcting or disputing
- Another person reads the short passage one last time, followed by another minute of silence

CHAPTER 8

INTRODUCTION TO STORIES OF MINDFUL HEROES IN HEALTH SETTINGS

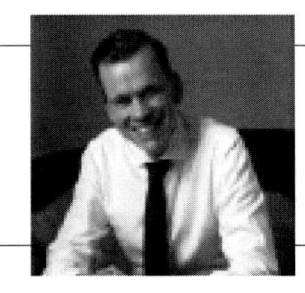

Paul D'Alton

paul.dalton@ucd.ie

Our hospitals and community healthcare facilities share one thing in common – people turn up to them because they are suffering, and they want to suffer less. Across the world, on any given day many millions of suffering human beings cross the threshold of our healthcare facilities seeking one thing: healing.

Jon Kabat-Zinn referred to hospitals as 'dukkha magnet zones' and this is probably true of other community heath care facilities also. Human suffering is writ large in the consultation rooms, the endless corridors and lonely wards. The great paradox is that our healthcare facilities are exactly the same places where heartbreaking acts of compassion happen, where acts of untold tenderness and human intimacy defy description. Where human acts of kindness are sometimes too painful to recall. These compassionate, tender and intimate acts are unsung; they rarely make the news and sadly, the processes we have to 'measure' the quality of healthcare seem incapable of capturing them.

I have had the privilege and the pain, the joy and the frustration of spending most of my working life as a clinical psychologist in healthcare. For more than a decade I worked full time in oncology at a large teaching hospital in Dublin, Ireland. Suffering on an oncology ward takes many different forms. For many people the oncology ward is an utterly unwanted home of uncertainty - will my treatment work, has my cancer spread, how long do I have?

Paradoxically the oncology ward is a sanctuary of hope; a place we seek literal and metaphorical healing. We turn up to the oncology ward afraid of and for our lives; we turn up with the hope of healing.

As a young clinician I harboured a frustrated and frustrating, ill-articulated and half-formed intuition that we as clinicians needed some other way to help manage the plague of human misery and suffering, we encountered on a daily basis. The traditional psychotherapy tools of the day were useful, they were impacting on peoples lives and in no small way reducing human suffering. However, I often found these tools were blunted and wondered about the durability of the changes they seemed to bring about.

A wise and searching supervisor handed me Jon Kabat-Zinn's (2013) Full Catastrophe Living and said I might find something in that tome useful. I did - I came to know the radical act of changing the relationship I had with suffering. I began the letting go of the illusion that a life could be lived without suffering, without dis-ease, dissatisfaction and imperfection.

Over the course of my career I have been blessed to find environments where this radical act of turning up to suffering is encouraged and supported. I have taught the 8-week Mindfulness Based Cognitive Therapy (MBCT) programme to close to 500 patients in acute care at the hospital where I am Principal Clinical Psychologist and Head of Department. I am also an Associate Professor at University College Dublin where I founded and co-direct the MSc in Mindfulness Based Interventions. I am the external examiner at the Centre for Mindfulness at the University of Bangor, Wales.

As healthcare providers we inhabit a world made up of enormous expectations and persistent human suffering. We voluntarily walk into the very heart of human suffering on daily basis when we cross the threshold of our hospitals and healthcare facilities. Our lives as healthcare providers are dedicated to reducing human suffering, to reducing the disease burden of those who come to us in need. But sometimes we can do little with the disease, sometimes there is no cure, the disease will end someone's life.

To care for a living can be costly. It can also be the most alive, potent and fertile ground for mindfulness practice. The stories told in the following three chapters vividly testify to this. The mindfulness teachers in these chapters make the radical and courageous step into this potent and fertile ground whole-heartedly. The stories in this section tell vivid and memorable stories of lives lived in the face of enormous suffering. As mindfulness meditation practitioners we know this is exactly where our practice comes to life, where the rubber hits the road.

I was struck by two common threads that seemed to weave their way across each of the three chapters – firstly the relationship we have with ourselves which seems to be the source of so much suffering and secondly the concept of suffering as a result of the impact of the unavoidable first arrow, and the suffering brought about by the impact of the second arrow, where we may have a little more wriggle room in how we show up. The stories told are stories where these fundamental tenets of mindfulness practice are the organic soil from which so much else is cultivated and flourishes.

I was equally struck by the wider social lens adopted by the writers. There is sometimes a naive attempt for mindfulness to be used to plaster over the systemic issues in healthcare that cause suffering; funding cuts, exclusion of people who challenge, the ever increasing soul destroying bureaucracy, the preoccupation with measurable outcomes - with product as opposed to process.

In adopting a wide social lens each of the three writers did the opposite of spiritually by-passing the issues of social and economic injustice and inequality that romantic mindfulness has a tendency to do. There is maturity and solidness in the work presented here that prevents any spiritual bypassing of the inequity that perpetuate human suffering.

The Dalai Lama says there are 7.5 billion of us humans on this earth and we share one thing in common – we want to live a happy life. We want to suffer less, we want to feel better, and to live better, we want to be at peace. Our hospitals and community healthcare facilities are often the frontier lands of this desire to suffer less, to be healed. The stories told in this section are beautiful stories of radical acts of changing the relationship we each have with suffering, dis-ease, dissatisfaction and imperfection that make us beautifully human.

FURTHER RESOURCES

MSc Mindfulness Based Interventions, University College Dublin
https://sisweb.ucd.ie/usis/!W_HU_MENU.P_PUBLISH?p_tag=PROG&MAJR=W323

REFERENCES

Kabat-Zinn, J. (2013). Full Catastrophe Living : Using the wisdom of your body and mind to face stress, pain, and illness. New York: Bantam Books

CHAPTER 9

THE ROAD TAKEN: EXPLORING LIVED EXPERIENCES OF MINDFULNESS IN PEOPLE ON SUBSTANCE RECOVERY JOURNEY

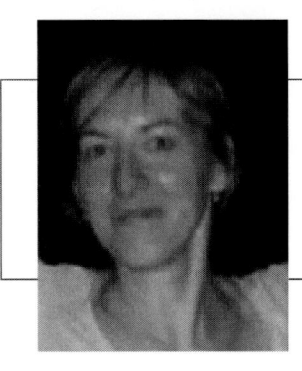

Jana Neumannova

dzama@post.cz

> Two roads diverged in a yellow wood,
> And sorry I could not travel both
> And be one traveller, long I stood
> And looked down one as far as I could
> To where it bent in the undergrowth.
>
> (Frost, undated)

INTRODUCTION

There are many roads to travel and numerous opportunities for adventures. However, the purpose of this chapter is to take you on a journey exploring lived experiences of mindfulness in heroes, both male and female, recovering from substance misuse. But before I do, I will describe my own journey into this meditative practice and how I started teaching mindfulness in a substance recovery environment. Before moving to Scotland, I worked as a physiotherapist in a large regional hospital in the Czech Republic where my main task was assisting patients to establish an optimal level of physical wellbeing. My prime focus was 'the physical body' and by using a variety of physiotherapeutic techniques I had a clear goal, which was to develop individual treatment plans for patients and support them in recovering their physical strength and abilities.

However, I soon realized that focusing all treatment towards the body is an incomplete approach and patients' psychological wellbeing, attitudes to their health conditions and to the actual healing processes of their body plays a crucial part in a successful recuperation too. Needless to say, as a practicing physiotherapist in a well-established medical institution I had a limited opportunity to explore my patients' attitudes and background stories to establish how they came to seek help from a physiotherapist. Regarding the journey theme of this book, I was not exactly unhappy being a physiotherapist, nor was I facing any difficult challenges in life but the prevailing sense that *'there is more to life than this'*, as Vin Harris talks about in Chapter 2, was eventually responsible for my departure. When, in 2002, I was offered the opportunity to provide physiotherapy support to a patient suffering from Multiple Sclerosis living in Edinburgh, I did not hesitate. This was not only a possibility to provide in depth one-to-one physio service but also to explore what more there is to life in an unfamiliar location.

Shortly after settling in the city I started volunteering in an organisation offering information, advice and support to stimulant drug users. What appealed to me most about this opportunity was working with recreational stimulant drug users directly at dance events across Scotland. During this time, I was exposed to multiple stories of how people came to use legal or illegal substances. By reflecting on these stories what stood out for me most were the extremes of problematic drug use when the highs were too high, and the lows were too low. That is to say, to achieve the initial pleasure, higher and more frequent doses were needed, while the comedowns, the after-effects from taking stimulants, became more intense and unpleasant. The extreme polarities of repeatedly experiencing these states negatively impacted on people's quality of life and had damaging effects on their body as well as the mind. However, through these experiences I was reminded that the body has an incredible power to regenerate and although the mind can be whimsical, it too has a great potential for healing, given the right treatment. I empathise with recovering addicts who face their demons inflicted by their drug addiction on daily basis, and I have a respect for them seeking help to deal with their issues.

My observations fed my curiosity to learn more about the human mind and as a result I decided to study psychology. Learning about the nature and the complexity of the human mind enhanced my understanding of this subject. However, the familiar sense of 'something is missing', when the focus in narrowed down to observing or treating only 'the mind', soon emerged again. This gap was finally filled by the practice of mindfulness, which I was introduced to, by a close friend during my studies and I became a regular attendee of these meditative gatherings. From the outset, the mindfulness approach positively resonated with me and I found it reassuring that through paying attention to embodied experiences in a specific way one can eventually experience stability and peace of both, in the mind and the body, and mobilise my own resources for healing. It suddenly made perfect sense to me and I felt that mindfulness is an effective approach to address the 'being human' in a holistic way.

After completing my studies in psychology, I was certain that I wanted to continue developing my mindfulness practice. I began volunteering in a small local charity offering support to adults with moderate mental health issues, where I started co-facilitating group sessions for clients aimed at improving their psychological wellbeing. One of the courses provided by the charity was also Mindfulness Based Cognitive Therapy (Segal et al., 2013), a program designed to help people suffering from depression, or as a relapse-prevention for depression. This was a great opportunity to enhance my own practice and share my knowledge and experience of this approach with clients as well as advancing my facilitating skills under the guidance of my supervisor in the charity.

This experience reaffirmed my belief in the efficacy of the mindfulness approach and I felt that I would benefit from my formal education in the discipline. Subsequently, my attention was caught by the University of Aberdeen's MSc Studies in Mindfulness promising to combine the academic element with the experiential practice, as well as offering the expanded curriculum covering compassion and insight. This novel academic pursuit also represented a further challenge and adventure in exploring mindfulness. When planning my dissertation project, I decided to use my experience of teaching mindfulness and helping people effected by drug use, to offer sessions in substance recovery settings. My aim was to share the mindfulness approach with recovering drug addicts, hoping to contribute to their wellbeing and offering an alternative way of coping with life's struggles. My goal was to offer guidance on their journey to recovery and provide effective coping strategies tailored to their individual needs in order for them to gain more clarity and stability in life.

ADDICTION, RECOVERY AND MINDFULNESS

> When you can stop you don't want to, and when you want to stop, you can't …
> (Davies, 1998, p. 35)

Some of you might be familiar with substance addiction and recovery settings, whether it is through reading, personal experience or work, but for others this territory may be completely new. Substance abuse is a complex problem often negatively impacting on lives of addicts, their significant others as well as the wider community. Substance addiction has been described as developing compulsive behavioural habits to seek pleasing activities or override negative experiences (Bien, 2009). Initially, such temporary escapes from one's reality offer satisfaction and increase the desire to continue experiencing the pleasurable effects of substances, or avoid the unpleasant ones. However, the body becomes desensitised and develops a tolerance, causing the person to take drugs more frequently and in increased doses. When people become accustomed to taking drugs under certain conditions (i.e. in a specific time or place) they establish a habitual pattern and experience compulsive urges, otherwise known as cravings, to use a substance. Their lives become dominated by the cycle of drug use in order to get the next fix. The main purpose of drug misuse then, is to avoid discomfort from withdrawals and potential dissatisfaction with life, which is often accompanied by a deterioration in personal circumstances and relationships (Hsu et al., 2008). Recovering from substance misuse is not a straightforward process and it is often characterised by recurrent relapses (Witkiewitz et al., 2012).

In recent years, mindfulness has been applied in substance recovery settings. Through mindfulness techniques people learn to pay attention to different layers of their present moment experiences in a non-judgemental way. If you think of substance addiction as a way of escaping or suppressing challenging experiences, then encouraging individuals to experience the present reality through mindfulness may sound like a harsh thing to do. On the contrary, although the mindfulness approach makes people more aware of their reality, they may also recognize that their experiences are impermanent, and can be experienced without acting on them. This way people gain a greater insight into their habitual patterns and at the same time learn to approach uncomfortable inner states (physical sensations, emotions and thoughts) and urges connected to substance misuse, and other life events, in a more effective way (Bien, 2009).

The research regarding substance addiction, and how mindfulness influences individuals' drug use or prevent relapse, tends to be quantitative (Fattore et al., 2014; Katz and Toner, 2013; Garland et al., 2012; Wu et al., 2010). However, there are limited studies in the field exploring the first person's perspective. I believe that our lives are shaped by different stories and experiences and the meanings we assign to them. Through shared narratives we can deepen our understanding of our own lived experiences and the those of others. In line with the idea underlying this book, every journey has a story and when this is acknowledged and shared with others it provides a unique viewpoint of how individuals experience the world and their position in it.

MY RESEARCH PROJECT

As a result of my thinking described above, I adopted a qualitative approach to my work-based project. From my experience of working with recovering drug addicts I can also see that those in recovery still have hope for a better life and that we can alter the course of our lives no matter how difficult this may be. It is for this very reason that I have chosen to address the participants in my study as heroes.

Building on this idea, as part of my MSc, I delivered a Mindfulness Based Living Course - MBLC (Mindfulness Association, 2013) to recovering drug addicts. In the case of the substance recovery, when people identify themselves as 'recovering addicts', rather than 'addicts', the new position supports their decision to seek help and improve their wellbeing (Buckingham et al., 2013). Taking this into consideration, the premise of my study was that individuals who are already taking an initial step to improve their substance-misuse situation are more likely to persevere on their journey to recovery.

Further, my belief was that when individuals do not associate mindfulness only with attaining specific targets (i.e. sobriety), they have greater flexibility to apply it to other areas of their functioning. Along with exploring the general principles of mindfulness, the MBLC also allows the participants to engage more in practices of kindness and compassion, which I believe is an important therapeutic element in substance recovery settings. Most recovering addicts are not only recovering from substance abuse but may be facing other challenges in life, such as improving physical and mental health, amending disrupted relationships and their social functioning, pursuing education and employment and many more. Therefore, offering strategies for kindness and compassion may provide a skillful way of dealing with challenging situations and a way of approaching difficulties with an open attitude rather than a fear of failure.

Only candidates who were over 18 years; spoke English; had no previous experience of MBLC; were recovering from any substance misuse and for any length of time; and were already participating in supportive programmes within relevant recovery organisations were included in the sample. Those with suicidal tendencies or psychotic episodes within past 6 months prior to the start of the course, as well as people with severe learning difficulties were excluded. This was to ensure that the participants were psychologically stable and able to understand the course content. The figure below shows overall number of participants at different stages of the project.

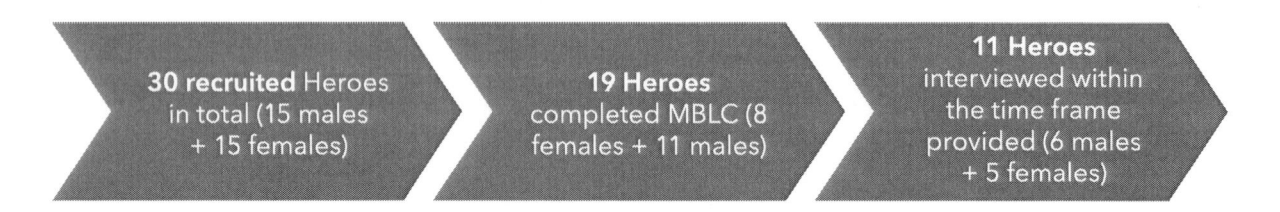

30 recruited Heroes in total (15 males + 15 females) → **19 Heroes** completed MBLC (8 females + 11 males) → **11 Heroes** interviewed within the time frame provided (6 males + 5 females)

Figure 1: Number of Participants

The main reasons for participants dropping-out were unstable health or changes in circumstances, followed by other life priorities (i.e. new employment or childcare). Ultimately, only participants who attended minimum of 6 sessions were included in the final data analysis. Despite the evidence pointing out that even a ten-minute mindfulness intervention affects people's emotional reactions (Erisman and Roemer, 2010), novice practitioners may benefit from being exposed to mindfulness practices for a longer period in order to fully understand the concept of mindfulness (Williams, 2010). My intention was to allow the participants to engage in a broad variety of topics and practices connected to mindfulness throughout the course before exploring their experience of it. Seventeen participants met these criteria but only 11 were able to meet for the final semi-structured interview within the time frame provided.

Despite the effort to capture as broad a sample as possible, all participants were of White European origins aged 27 to 62 with an average age of 44. Occupations included support worker, artist, student, counsellor, chef and a pharmacy dispenser. Three were unemployed and two retired. The main substance people were recovering from was alcohol, followed by methadone, diazepam, cannabis and poly-drug use (alcohol, diazepam, cannabis).

THE HEROES' STORIES

> If we were not equal we could not understand each other or those who came before us. If we were not distinct we would not need to understand each other. (Maykut and Morehouse, 1994, p. 27).

After each MBLC course I conducted a semi-structured interview and analysed the stories by using Interpretative Phenomenological Analysis (IPA), which is an "approach that attempts to describe an individual's experiences from their own perspective as closely as possible but recognises the interpretive influence of the researcher on the research product." (Coolican, 2004, p. 241). Phenomenologists argue that we can never know the real world, but we can only interpret it through our experience of it (Spinelli, 2005). I adopted a constructivist point of view which promotes the idea that our knowledge about the world is relative and socially constructed through our interactions with the world. This means that I inevitably brought my own characteristics, as well as cultural-educational-social background and values, into the process of data analysis and I had to be aware of my own assumptions about the world when I was interpreting the collected narratives. Such a process, otherwise known as a reflexivity in research, is a critical view of researcher's own involvement within the researched process and brings depth into **What** kind of knowledge is produced and **How** it is being accessed (Berger 2015). As the mind can set itself quickly into habitual patterns, in order to create an effective distance from my assumptions about the narratives, I applied mindfulness, in particular a regular pausing as described by Kramer (2007), to monitor my own involvement with the narratives.

This process led to producing six final themes:

1) Balanced life and management of substance misuse
2) Barriers to recovery progress
3) Value of social contact and connections to self and others
4) Developing a structure in life
5) Learning and discovering in recovery
6) Support in recovery and its nature.

1. BALANCED LIFE AND MANAGEMENT OF SUBSTANCE MISUSE

This reflects on the position of people on their recovery path at the time of our journey together and their desire for stability and balance in life. The participants in my sample were all aware of the extent of their drug abuse and openly identified the issues leading them into addiction, which were often associated with disrupted relationships or personal identity. This often led to increased levels of stress and anxiety and even greater substance misuse making the initial problems even worse. The heroes also identified the need to create balance in their life focusing specifically on effectively organising their physical environment; regulating an optimal level of meaningful activities on a daily basis, and their need to explore new techniques for managing sobriety and improving their mental health wellbeing. Some examples are presented below:

> So I had all these responsibilities and I could manage them very badly. I did them but they were like chores ... I was in real conflict with myself because I was unhappy and trying to control everything and manage everything to keep up the appearances ... I was functioning supposedly well but inside ... I felt totally different. I was just creeping by and it was just hell.

> I've had periods where I started taking on or doing too much. And then it has an effect on me big time. And my mood drops and I get stressed. I don't deal with stress very well. I've gone the other way and done not enough. And it equally has really a detrimental effect on me...

Overall, the heroes' circumstances suggest that their lives span out of control, which reflects the more general patterns of addiction identified earlier. Three participants summarise the main reasons people accessed the MBLC course were:

> when I get all stressed out, want to find a way, kinda, bringing myself down

> almost like putting a degree of control around thinking

> I've been interested to give it a shot but I've never heard of it before

---

Pause and Reflect

Take a moment to notice any current challenges in your life.
How do you respond to difficult moments?

2. BARRIERS TO RECOVERY PROGRESS

Practicing awareness of present moment experiences allowed the heroes not only to notice more about themselves but helped them to monitor the responses to their experiences. By learning to notice more and react less, people were able to recognize some of their automatic behaviours and potential triggers leading to substance use. By training attention to Here and Now the participants were gaining greater awareness of their circumstances and were able to respond more skilfully to challenges. Some observations they made were also perceived as obstacles preventing them from progressing successfully on their recovery. They identified internal obstacles related to individual negative attitudes towards their thoughts, behaviours and their relationships. The external barriers included elements such as practical arrangements of supportive group sessions; personality of other participants, and the structure of provided support. Two heroes expressed the following:

> Obstacles would probably be just my own brain, really. You know, it's not the way it used to think ... I think I got to the point where I was overwhelmed with stress and dealt with it by shutting it out

> Just tied to the chemist, so, it's just like ongoing thing. Lie a vicious circle, like going around in a washing machine ... I just need to jump of that machine ... And that's the way I feel about it

Facing obstacles often led to increased levels of stress, feelings of being stuck and an inability to move forward. These barriers only added a negative spin to people's already disturbed social functioning. For this reason, dropping into a moment, recognizing an obstacle or a potential trigger of maladaptive habits proved to be a useful strategy in cultivating stability in the moment. In other words, the triggers become less overpowering and manageable. The enhanced awareness of obstacles in the heroes' lives did not necessarily lead to them reversing these behavioural patterns but participants' attitudes of relating to difficulties has changed to being more accepting and tolerant.

Observations

- The idea that 'Thoughts are not facts' often caused a considerable relief to the participants and encouraged them to revise their relationship not only to their thinking but to challenging emotions too.

- Dropping into a moment and practicing regular pausing in and outside of the mindfulness sessions let to increased awareness of the present moment and gaining a better stability.

Figure 2: Facilitator's observations

3. VALUE OF SOCIAL CONTACT AND CONNECTIONS TO SELF AND OTHERS

The need for social contact and connections was the strongest theme. It became clear that a regular and stable social contact in a drug-free environment was a highly important and empowering element for people recovering from substance misuse. The majority of the heroes mentioned that creating a distance from actively using peers and the sense of collectiveness and sharing experiences within the recovery-focused activities was important and provided them with stability, purpose and a sense of belonging. The participants often experienced the notion 'I'm not alone with my problems' and were provided with the space to relate to their issues in a non-judgemental way. They mentioned:

> having met people initially right at the very start made me realised what my problem was
>
> the meditation itself, it works for me more in the group than at home, which I was very surprised
>
> it was just to be able to relax in other people's company
>
> I feel more, more relaxed, more connected with myself when I was in the group
>
> like actual ... social contact and being in room with other people ... it was, kind of, I'm not the only one this is happening to

The heroes also realized that re-connecting with significant others and restoring broken relationships is essential for their wellbeing. Considering the individuals' disrupted social functioning and relationships with others, it is not surprising that they were lacking a sense of clarity and stability within their lives. Mindfulness turned out to be a useful approach enabling people to pause and experience moments of stillness. Being aware of different layers of own experiences, the heroes became more competent in recognising their own needs. For some, it was the need to connect on a deeper level with the present moment experience, with themselves and others:

> I'm having a struggle making sense of my situation ... my life ... myself and my relationships in particular... I'm in real conflict with that every day ... So coming here was really good to have that time ... and connect with yourself and be present ... Whereas, if you're with people taking drugs, you know, you're not really with them, they're not really there at all

By practicing moment-by-moment awareness and allowing oneself to be connected to whatever is happening in that particular moment, without necessarily identifying with it, provided the heroes with a choice to deal with difficulties more skilfully. In the context of substance recovery, the heroes were learning to deal with internal reactions leading to relapse in more effective way. Practicing awareness of minor difficulties in life was a necessary step for people to gain confidence in the technique before moving onto applying it to more intense situations in life.

Recognizing that one is experiencing a moment of difficulty and allowing oneself to stay with the challenge can be intimidating and hard to comprehend for some. Kindness was an essential element on such journey. Practicing kindness in this context allowed the heroes to take a better care of themselves throughout moments of struggle in an attentive and nurturing way. Responding to their own needs in a kind way can also be seen as a way of building inner strength and motivation to continue a journey.

Observations

- The concept of Kindness often sparked interesting debates and allowed the participants to reflect on their attitude to self and others.

- Expressing kindness to others was often perceived as an easier step than expressing kindness to oneself or receiving kindness from others.

- Being encouraged to express small gestures of kindness towards themselves the heroes gradually realized that they can provide a basic form of self-care.

Figure 3: Facilitator's observations.

4. DEVELOPING A STRUCTURE IN LIFE

The heroes also revealed their aspiration for having a certain structure in life and they pointed out three types of beneficial structures. Firstly, there was a call for developing a regular daily routine, which would provide people with a sense of purpose. Having somewhere to go was especially important for unemployed or retired individuals. Being occupied with a meaningful, non-drug-related activity on daily basis was also useful strategy to diverge from negative thinking and a potential drug misuse:

> Coming here has helped me a lot .... And I'm glad I've got [somewhere] to go ... I've got a purpose for that day

> The structure was definitely like a big help for me, especially at the end. Not being at work at the moment, I had kind of a big, vast, empty week

> Things to do ... things to keep me busy or I just ... I'll just end up ... blathering myself, you know

Considering that the onset of addiction impacts on individuals' social network, which can gradually narrow down to substance related groups, detaching from such an environment is crucial for successful recovery. In this sense mindfulness sessions in general provided a great opportunity for people to engage in a social framework where the aim was to reflect on internal embodied experience through which they could explore their attitude to life and society.

Secondly, the participants appreciated having a structure within the actual classes and workshops they were attending. Clear guidance through mindfulness practices also served as an effective anchor, which often correlated with their increased motivation to continue learning and attending the classes:

> It was very well structured, very well organized

> from what I can gather from mindfulness, you know, it was very structured. Very guided and it's quite step-by-step ... It can take you through when you're a complete beginner ... That really helped

> So the mindfulness class ... you never asked anything there ... Good not to have any pressure ... You can think your own thing ... I liked the breathing ... nice and even ... I canae do that in the house

Throughout the mindfulness sessions, the heroes were able to put the learnt theoretical aspects of mindfulness into immediate practice and were invited to share their stories afterwards. Such collective dialogue and reflection brought more clarity about their next direction. Through mindfulness and conversations people can observe closely their experiences and externalize them through narratives. In turn, this can lead to seeing challenging experiences as more fluid and impermanent, allowing people to detach themselves from personalised difficulties (Percy, 2008).

Some heroes also aspired to follow a philosophical system that would provide guidance through their recovery process but also reflected on their spiritual and personal needs. Such desire was evident particularly in socially isolated participants or those recovering from substance misuse for a long period of time. The need for an ideological structure reaching beyond practicalities of life rooted in people's desire to consolidate self-discipline on their journey through recovery and life is evident here, for example:

> I don't have a system that supports me spiritually, actually ... Because it gives some self-discipline, rather than randomising everything and using what you want. And that's not right ... You should really have something to work with

It is not seldom that people in addiction recovery often surrender to a Higher Power (individually defined God) in order to deal with their addictive behaviours as they admit they are powerless over their substance use (Alcoholics Anonymous, 2018). The secular form of mindfulness is not relying on acquiring any particular faith or beliefs and, as Graeme Nixon discussed in Chapter 3, it allows individuals to access and explore spirituality and various beliefs in their own ways. Gaining a deeper connection to their own experiences and attitudes may result in identifying a personal form of spiritual needs and guidance and seeking to develop in this area. In this way, the secular form of mindfulness can be seen as perhaps more inclusive as it does not rely on the acceptance of specific belief structures of others, or denying own beliefs, instead being open to a broad variety of personal concepts.

Observations

- Following the same structure each week in mindfulness classes worked well as an element of stability and reassurance.

- Enquiry in heroes' experiences served as a space to share their reality and to clarify potential confusion from experienced practices.

Figure 4: Facilitator's observations.

5. LEARNING AND DISCOVERING IN RECOVERY

Learning alternative, non-drug coping strategies and how to relate to unpleasant physical sensations of intense mental health episodes was an important part of the heroes' recovery journey. Mindfulness seemed to provide an effective platform for noticing and acknowledging various triggers and their negative effects on participants' moods and behaviours and the new discoveries served as a motivation to continue learning more about the self, mindfulness or other strategies. Below are some examples:

> it's just made me a bit more calm and, you know ... when I get annoyed I found other ways to deal with it rather than just to drink

> the difference just now is being aware that there are things that I can do to alleviate the physical pain, if you like, of anxiety. And going forward I do have this appetite for learning more

> If I'm having a sort of anxiety filled day, I'm sort of, every now and again doing things like, you know, sort of, 3-minute-breathing-space at ..., specific points when I'm realising or getting anxious

Such a level of awareness can be seen as an initial step of breaking the cycle of conditioned habits which is extremely important in substance recovery. By regular mindfulness practice the heroes had the opportunity to build up the awareness and reduce their reactivity to any internal or external triggers and unpleasant events. This is also supported by the idea that during mindful attention, the brain networks associated with triggers and cravings are less functionally connected (Westbrook et al., 2013), which allows for more cognitive freedom and individuals' increased ability to respond more skilfully to challenges.

The heroes also reported making positive progress in coping better with higher levels of stress and anxiety and were able to see a broader picture of their situation. They also recognised that self-care is an important element:

> I've always had problems with overthinking in a negative way...Thanking to mindfulness I stopped paying attention to all those things ... I know they are but it's not that important as life itself

> I look at it [recovery] in a different angle now ... A couple of years ago It's all been about bad things ... Now, I'm learning to really start loving myself. I basically do things which are good for me ... I'm doing it because it's good for me, my body and good for my mind as well

> something I want to avoid [intense thoughts]... But once I got the hang of it ... watching the thoughts and then moving onto, sort of ... kindness and compassion kind of idea ... it has become less unpleasant experience

Through mindfulness meditative practices people are encouraged to be more in tune with the experience of pleasant or unpleasant sensations in their body and mind, which allows for better recognition and understanding of their own suffering. By engaging with the idea of compassion and self-compassion the participants learned that they can gain a better control over their approach to their struggles and re-shape their relationship to themselves. Being compassionate to one's own suffering does not mean avoiding it or being overwhelmed by it, but rather exploring the nature of it and being committed to respond in a nurturing way (Gilbert and Choden, 2013). The enhanced interest in personal welfare may also result from changed individual priorities as people progress on their recovery journey. As people advance to more stable stages of their recovery, managing their own substance abuse may be less of a priority and physical and mental health may be more emphasised.

Through immediate application of newly gained information the heroes also discovered their own strengths and some even reached an insight (subtle, intimate discovery) while engaging in mindfulness practice:

> It was just appreciation, an insight ... And it came from nowhere ... Before, I could think it but not feel it. I felt it yesterday. It felt universal ... It's a bit psychological but I think my ego wasn't there. The ego, the sense of self wasn't there. I was a part of a whole, ehm, every person ... It wasn't a sense like an acid trip ... Nice to know that I'm not alone in this universe ... You know, feel that things are possible

Experiencing a state of diminished sense of ego was the case for one participant within the whole sample. This level of connection, or a state of awakening, as some may call it, can occur when people retrieve themselves from over-stimulating surroundings and attempt to focus their attention on a single object, such as breathing. Although, through enhanced awareness of a flow of experiences, and resting in the present moment, people can eventually access the essence of wholesome states and experience a non-conceptual self, it usually requires extended training. Reaching this stage of contemplation in only eight weeks is remarkable yet puzzling at the same time. A potential explanation for this finding is the person's affiliation to other contemplative practices or a higher pre-disposition to mindfulness.

Observations

Introducing and practicing compassion allowed the participants to acknowledge the intense struggles in life and offered a way to deal with these in a safer and calmer way.

Figure 5: Facilitator's observations

6. SUPPORT IN RECOVERY AND ITS NATURE

This was a more generic theme reflecting in a broader sense on certain characteristics of group recovery-focused interventions that determined whether, and to what extent, the heroes participated in such support. Many participants mentioned that **timing** of sessions was important for their regular attendance and preferred workshops scheduled from mid-morning to early-evening. The **availability** was a further element. The participants appreciated that the mindfulness course was available to them at a free-of-charge rate, as well as places on the course being available without long waiting times and minimal assessments prior to their participation on the course. Another characteristic was **accessibility**. The heroes mentioned that accessing support group programmes on a voluntary basis, rather than it being a mundane request by authorities, led to a higher retention in a program. The **quality and style** of the available support programmes was another crucial factor to be considered with the standard of intervention content, as well as the attitude of supporting staff being mentioned frequently. In general, the heroes seemed to take into account the nature of supportive sessions they considered attending, rather than randomly selecting what was on offer. The facilitator's attitude, knowledge, communication and presentation skills were also highlighted. What seemed to be important was not only the facilitator's knowledge but their ability to present this and skills to engage with the group. People's satisfaction with these factors correlated with regular attendance. The final characteristic the participants identified as crucial for their attendance was the **level and length** of group support. A step-by-step strategy followed by an immediate practical application of discussed topics was the preferred option, in comparison to a purely theoretical approach. The heroes stated that 8 weeks was an adequate length of time for them to acquire both, the theoretical and embodied new skills.

Examples of comments:

> I have appreciation of what's on offer … Because I couldn't afford to do this otherwise

> You see where it fits in a more practical application rather than just being a theory You go to some of these things, like, you can tell straight away that the person who is running the show has done just a 3 months crash course in anxiety management or, you know … They don't really know anything what they're talking about. Which is, you know, annoying and frustrating

> It's important to get someone, I think, who has got the right approach and the right manner

> I'd say 8 weeks is good, a good length of time to be able to, to get the hang of it as well

The heroes' reflection of the support provided in recovery settings corresponds with existing research exploring such interventions in general, as well as with the essence of mindfulness (Krug & Sandberg, 2013; Garland et al., 2012). A careful consideration of what, how and when to organise group recovery sessions is important for maintaining regular attendance of participants and their meaningful interactions. The embodied presence and attitude of the facilitators seems to also be relevant, as they determine the level heroes may engage in mindfulness practices.

THE JOURNEY CONTINUES

My journey through life can be summarized as one that appreciates the opportunity of an adventure, perhaps more than the final destination. My response to life is motivated by seeking connections to experiences, new ideas and, most importantly, people. As Vin Harris suggested in chapter two, "If the metaphor resonates why not respond?" In the recent years, mindfulness has been an important element on my path and through practicing, as well as teaching mindfulness, I have deepened my knowledge about myself. To me, sharing the mindfulness practice with people in recovery is about being there for them through difficult times and holding a space for people to connect to themselves and to others. My intention is to introduce more of the elements of kindness and compassion to the lives of substance recovering heroes through the medium of mindfulness practices.

I continue delivering the MBLC, as well as drop-in mindfulness sessions, in substance recovery settings and it has been a rewarding experience to date. The heroes come to mindfulness sessions for different reasons. Some are looking for new ways of coping, others are seeking connections, or are looking for a break from intense circumstances, and some are simply being curious. People in substance recovery benefit from mindfulness practices on number of levels. Firstly, they learn to connect to their experiences and build a closer connection to themselves and, eventually, to others. Secondly, by practicing connecting to the present moment experience the participants learn to identify their unhelpful habits, which helps them to avoid repeating them. Thirdly, people recognise that their strength comes from within and by using elements of kindness and compassion they build a sustainable level of inner strength. Mindfulness seems to be an effective way for people to learn from their experiences and provides them with tools to cope with life's challenges. The MBLC course retention is 40-50% and the participants seem to benefit from practicing mindfulness in the company of others. The longer their recovery path, the more committed the participants are to attending sessions and practicing mindfulness. It is important to respect the individual journey, to follow one's own pace and path. In the words of the poet Robert Frost (undated):

> I shall be telling this with a sigh
> Somewhere ages and ages hence;
> Two roads diverged in a wood, and I –
> I took the one less travelled by,
> And that has made all the difference.

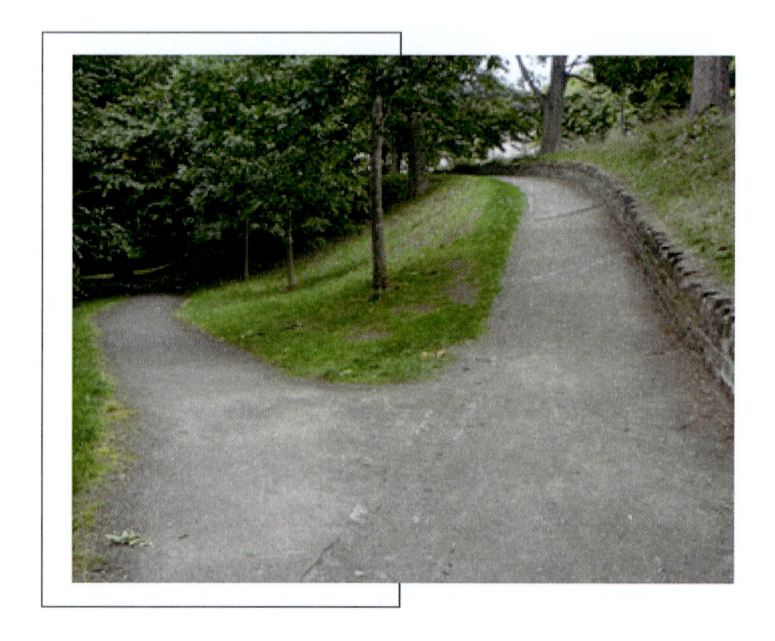

Figure 6: Diverged Road. Photograph © Jana Neumannova 2018

FURTHER RESOURCES

Brewer, J., (2015). Mindfulness, the Mind and Addictive Behavior. YouTube. 8th October 2015. https://www.youtube.com/watch?v=7a9sWI0vJzc
FRN. (undated). Mindfulness in recovery. Foundations recovery network. https://www.dualdiagnosis.org/treatment-therapies-for-dual-diagnosis-patients/mindfulness/
Garland, E.L. and Howard, M. O., (2018). Mindfulness-based treatment of addiction: current state of the field and envisioning the next wave of research. NCBI- National Center for Biotechnology Information. https://www.ncbi.nlm.nih.gov/pmc/articles/PMC5907295/
Hari, J., (2015). Everything you think you know about addiction is wrong. YouTube. 9th July 2015. https://www.youtube.com/watch?v=PY9DcIMGxMs
Osterlind, D. and Muradyan, A., (2017). What is Mindfulness, and how does it help with addiction? YouTube. 30th March 2017.
https://www.youtube.com/watch?v=R2XY0KQ5G_s

REFERENCES

ALCOHOLICS ANONYMOUS. (Undated). The 12-Steps of Alcoholics Anonymous. Great Britain: Alcoholics Anonymous (Great Britain) Ltd. Available: http://www.alcoholics-anonymous.org.uk/About-AA/The-12-Steps-of-AA [Date Accessed: 21st August, 2018].
BERGER, R., (2015). Now I see it, now I don't: Researcher's position and reflexivity in qualitative research. Qualitative research, 15 (2), pp. 219- 234.
BIEN, T., (2009). Paradise lost: Mindfulness and Addictive behaviour. In: F. DIDONNA, ed., Clinical Handbook of Mindfulness. New York: Springer Science and Business Media. pp. 289 – 297.
BUCKINGHAM, S.A., FRINGS, D., and ALBERY, I. P., (2013). Group Membership and Social Identity in Addiction Recovery. Psychology of Addictive Behaviours, 27 (4), pp. 1132 – 1140.
COOLICAN, H., (2004). Research Methods and Statistics in Psychology. 4th Edition. London: Hodder Arnold.
DAVIES, L., (1998). Candy: A novel of Love and Addiction. Sydney: Ballantine Books.
ERISMAN, S. M. and ROEMER, L., (2010). A Preliminary Investigation of the Process of Mindfulness. Mindfulness, 3, pp. 30-43.
FATTORE, L., MELIS, M., FADDA, P. and FRATTA, W., (2014). Sex differences in Addictive disorders. Frontiers in Neuroendocrinology, 35, pp. 272 – 284.
FROST, R., (undated). The Road Not Taken. Poetry Foundation. Available: https://www.poetryfoundation.org/poems/44272/the-road-not-taken [Date Accessed: 15/08/2018]
GARLAND, E.L., SCHWARZ, N.R., KELLY, A., WHITT, A., and HOWARD, M.O., (2012). Mindfulness-Oriented Recovery Enhancement for Alcohol Dependence: Therapeutic Mechanisms and Intervention Acceptability. Journal of Social Work Practice in the Addiction, 12, pp. 242 – 263.
GILBERT, P. and CHODEN (2013). Mindful Compassion. London: Constable & Robinson Ltd.
HSU, S. H., GROW, J. and MARLATT, A. G., (2008). Mindfulness and Addiction. In: M. GALANTER and L. A. KASKUTAS, eds., Recent Developments in Alcoholism. London: Springer Science and Business Media. pp. 229 – 249.
KATZ, D., and TONER, B., (2013). A Systematic Review of Gender Differences in the Effectiveness of Mindfulness-Based Treatments for Substance Use Disorders. Mindfulness, 4, pp. 318 – 331.
KRAMER, G., (2007). Insight Dialogue: The Interpersonal Path to Freedom. London: Shambhala.
KRUG, E., and SANDBERG, K., (2013). A home for body and soul: Substance using women in recovery. Harm Reduction Journal, 10 (39), pp. 1-16.
MAYKUT, P. and MOREHOUSE, T., (1994). Beginning qualitative research: A philosophic and practical guide. London: The Falmer Press.
MINDFULNESS ASSOCIATION, (2013). Mindfulness Based Living Course: Eight week mindfulness course curriculum update. UK: Mindfulness Association.
PERCY. I., (2008). Awareness and authoring: The idea of self in mindfulness and narrative therapy. European Journal of Psychotherapy and Counselling, 10 (4), pp. 355 – 367.
SEGAL, Z. V., WILLIAMS, J. M. G. and TEASDALE, J. D., (2013). Mindfulness-based Cognitive Therapy for Depression: a new approach to preventing relapse. 2nd ed. London: The Guilford Press.
SPINELLI, E., (2005). The Interpreted World: An Introduction to phenomenological psychology. 2nd ed. London: Sage Publishing Ltd.
WESTBROOK, C., CRESWELL, J.D., TABIBNIA, G., JULSON, E., KOBER, H., and TINDLE, H. A., (2013). Mindful attention reduces neural and self-reported cue-induced craving in smokers. SCAN, 8, pp. 73 – 84.
WILLIAMS, J. M. G., (2010). Mindfulness as a Psychological Process – Commentary. Emotion, 10 (1), pp. 1 – 7.
WITKIEWITZ, K., LUSTYK, M. K. B., and BOWEN, S., (2012). Retraining the Addicted Brain: A Review of Hypothesized Neurobiological Mechanisms of Mindfulness-Based Relapse Prevention. Psychology of Addictive Behaviours, 27 (2), pp. 351 – 365.
WU, L-T., LING. W., BURCHETT, B., BLAZER, D. G., SHOSTAK, J. and WOODY, G. E., (2010). Gender and racial / ethnic differences in addiction severity, HIV risk, and quality of life among adults in opioid detoxification: Results from the National Drug Abuse Treatment Clinical Trials Network. Substance Abuse and Rehabilitation, 1, pp. 13 – 22.

CHAPTER 10

FINDING MY BLISS: TOP TIPS FOR INTRODUCING MINDFULNESS TO HEALTHCARE STAFF

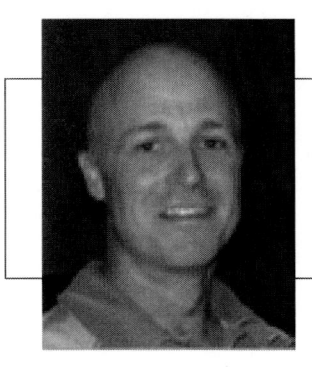

Ian Rigg

<u>riggif@hotmail.co.uk</u>

INTRODUCTION

The purpose of this chapter is to take you on a journey. I plan on sharing a little of the story of how I became a Mindfulness Facilitator; while at the same time demonstrating how mindfulness-based interventions (MBI) were launched within a Health Service setting in the County of Cumbria in the U.K. and offered to staff as part of a health and well-being initiative. My hope is that in sharing this story, you may pick up something that could be relevant and useful for you on your own journey. You may be attempting to set up similar interventions in a work setting or perhaps you are a member of staff who is curious about the benefits of mindfulness while juggling a busy schedule.

BACKGROUND

I have been working in a variety of health and social care settings in the U.K. and the U.S. since the early 90's and my main area of work was with difficult to reach children and young people. For the last 12 years of this period of my working life, I had specialised as a Young Person's Drug and Alcohol Counsellor and in the latter half of this role I was employed by the Health Service. At the beginning of the 1990's, I began training in TaeKwon-Do (TKD) (a Korean martial art) and opened up a TKD school upon returning to the U.K. in 2002. The relevance of sharing this last piece of information will become clear as the story enfolds.

I became interested in learning how to meditate because I thought that meditating was something that a martial artist should know how to do and as I look back, a seed had been sown much earlier, watching David Carradine in the T.V. series Kung Fu and the Jedi in the Star Wars movie. Would a Jedi ask the following question? Is the journey we find ourselves on already mapped out (kind of like a passenger) or is it just a collection of twists and turns in response to the randomness of life? I like the following answer to this type of question:

> You can have it as you like. You can distinguish in your life a pattern or see merely a chain of accidents. Explanations are meant to please the mind. They need not be true. Reality is indefinable and indescribable (Nisargadatta Maharaj, 1974, p. 274).

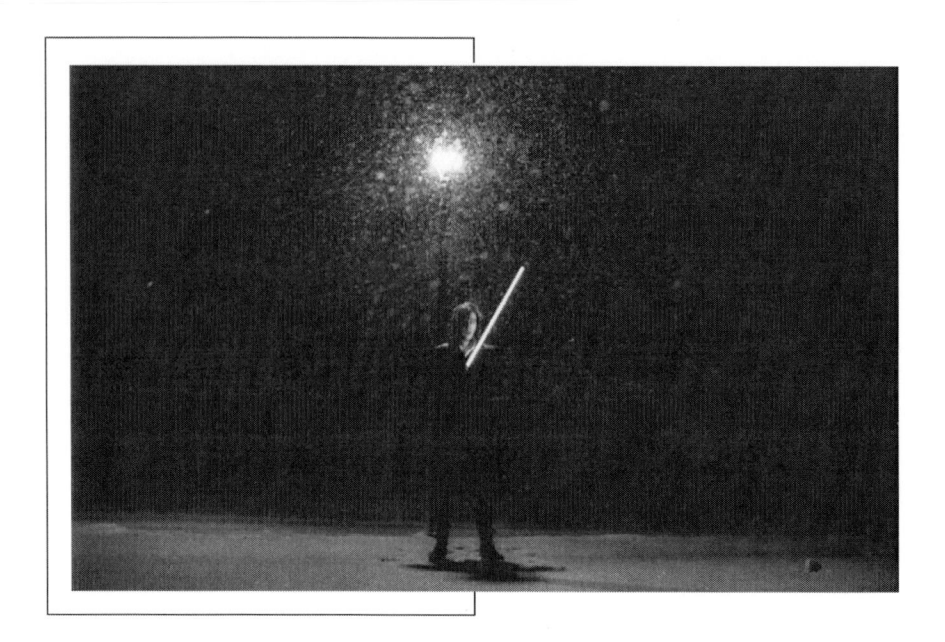

Figure 1: Jedi Training Photo by Ben Konfrst.

THE BEGINNING

I remember looking in martial arts books and seeing pictures of rows of students meditating or a picture of a monk sitting in quiet contemplation, however, there would be little, if any, instruction on how to meditate. Nor did any of my martial arts instructors teach meditation in the classes I attended. I have always been fascinated by the East and have spent a lot of time travelling around countries in Asia. While there I would always take time to visit temples and feel humbled while at the same time touched by the stillness and energy in these places. One of my friends at work (Des) was into meditation and for Christmas he bought me Rob Nairn's book, Tranquil Mind. This book ignited my curiosity to find out more and Des also told me a little about his meditation practice and how he lived in a community close to a Tibetan Buddhist temple in Scotland. At that time I did not realise that Samye Ling was the first and largest Tibetan Buddhist temple in Europe and that it was an hour from my home.

My style is to consider my options and then to jump in with both feet! My first experience of meditation was to attend an eight-day retreat at Samye Ling in 2004, aimed at providing the participant with an introduction to Buddhism and meditation. I vividly remember when I began to get a felt sense of what meditation may have to offer. On day three, I was standing outside by myself with a cup of tea and my senses began opening up to the moment. The warmth of the cup in my hand, the taste of the tea, the sound of cows and sheep in the distance and the feet on the ground. I heard the sound of a bee and looked down to find that the flowers around my feet were covered in bees going about their business and the colours of the flowers were vivid. I remember thinking I feel like I'm high and tasted the tea again to see if there was anything untoward in it. I thought there's something else going on here! All my senses were open, and I felt connected to everything around me. This is the moment the penny dropped for me and at that moment I resolved to continue practicing no matter what!

If we reflect on the stages of the hero's journey, we can see that the call to adventure comes up in the desire to learn how to meditate and that one of my initial helpers on this path was my friend Des. Now of course I could have refused to answer the call at this stage and chosen not to attend a meditation course, but this did not happen; therefore, I ventured forth and began the journey. Throughout this chapter, my journey can be looked at in two ways. The inner journey I made while embarking upon a meditation practice and the outer journey as far as engaging with and relating to the world.

After completing this retreat, I then attended a weekend course ran by Rob Nairn and I was blown away! Rob helped make sense of the process of meditation by presenting Buddhism in an accessible way while also looking at the psychological underpinnings of meditation from a western point of view. This was my first encounter with the protective figure of an old man "to supply the amulets and advice the hero will require" (Campbell, 2008, p.59), but of course at the time, I just thought of Rob similar to Yoda, the Jedi Master from the Star Wars movies; since I hadn't read any Joseph Campbell at that point. I then began attending weeklong retreats with Rob (in the same location) each year to deepen my practice. After about four years, while on a week retreat with Rob, I found out that Rob also ran one-month retreats in South Africa. It was August at the time and the next retreat was in November. After much negotiation at home and at work I secured a place on the month-long retreat. At this point I was officially "weird!" My partner, work colleagues, friends and family could not understand why I would use up most of my holiday time to go and "sit and do nothing!" Embarking on anything that is outside of the social norm requires courage, dedication and the willingness to be different or misunderstood.

TARA ROKPA CENTRE, SOUTH AFRICA

Rob took us on a graduated path of settling the mind, reflecting on our experience and gaining insights into and working with the deeper forces at play that obstructed us from seeing clearly. Rob gave a teaching in the morning, which framed the day's practice and each day followed a similar process of sitting, walking meditation, reflection and yoga. Up until this point I'd been trying to learn yoga by myself, so this regular tuition each day began to sow the seeds of more to come. As well as allowing me to be in my body without needing to achieve a goal. In the first week of the retreat my mind was very distracted, and my body was in a lot of discomfort from sitting on the floor all day. In week two my body began to get used to sitting and my mind began to move from random everyday distraction to the stories of my life that triggered a stronger emotional reaction. In week three I saw clearly the knots I tie myself in and struggled to accept the absurdity of the self-imposed suffering. In week four my body felt as strong as steel and my mind had begun to stabilise and allow and accept the randomness of my inner world without taking it and myself so seriously. Participants were also expected to maintain silence throughout the retreat outside of the normal teaching sessions, which for me was a welcome change to always having to listen and talk at work. This gave my mind more space to settle and also brought into focus the power of preferences and perceptions, i.e., how we are constantly making up stories about other people and situations based on our likes and dislikes.

At this stage I had well and truly crossed the threshold into "the regions of the unknown" (Campbell, 2008, p.65) and had embarked on the hero's journey proper.

UPHEAVAL (OR DESCENDING INTO THE BELLY OF THE WHALE AND EMBARKING UPON THE ROAD OF TRIALS)

2007 – 2010 were years of great upheaval and change for me. I came to the end of my psychotherapy training in 2007 and my meditation practice had led me to explore the relevance of mindfulness in counselling and psychotherapy. By this time I had been working as a Young Person's Drug and Alcohol Counsellor for a number of years and was transferring over to the Health Service and continuing in this post in 2009. Around the same time my long-term relationship was also coming to an end. While attending another of Rob Nairn's monthlong retreats in South Africa, Rob mentioned that he would be teaching on the first Studies in Mindfulness MSc in Scotland, a partnership between the University of Aberdeen and the Mindfulness Association. I didn't have a degree at that time and I doubted my academic ability to study at this level, however, I thought if I can get accepted onto the course then it would be a great opportunity to study with Rob more regularly; with the MSc a bonus should I even get that far.

In 2010, I enrolled on the first cohort of the Studies in Mindfulness MSc at Samye Ling. This was a unique opportunity to be taught mindfulness, compassion and insight training by Rob Nairn and other tutors from the Mindfulness Association; while at the same time being challenged on an academic level by the University of Aberdeen. I remember thinking I hope I can just scrape through the first assignment and then I'll see if it's possible for me to continue studying at this level. I got a good mark for my first assignment and my confidence in my academic abilities grew as each assignment and each year came and went. The parallels between attempting to meditate and study and write assignments were not lost on me. I spent many hours sitting at my kitchen table looking over the top of my computer into the garden trying to focus enough to begin an assignment and then getting up and doing anything but. Writing became a process of re-directing my attention back to the moment without getting caught up in over thinking and my overly analytical brain needed to relax to allow genuine creativity to emerge. In 2012, Rob announced that he would be taking a sabbatical from teaching and informed us (the retreat participants) that he would be inviting Donal Creedon to lead the end of year retreat at TRC in South Africa in 2013, in his place. Rob rated Donal very highly, therefore, in 2013 I began attending retreats with Donal Creedon and also with Drupon Rinpoche at Samye Ling.

In 2013, I graduated with an MSc and for my final year dissertation I decided to study the effects of the 8-week Mindfulness Based Living Course (MBLC) when delivered to a mixed group of health care staff in a work setting. My motivation for doing this was ignited by working in a job that at times could be highly stressful (Young Persons Drug and Alcohol Service) and also noticing that other workers I came into contact with from a variety of other agencies (Police, Social Services, Youth Offending, Teachers, Nurses etc) were also subjected to stress over the course of their working lives. Mindfulness Based Interventions were beginning to develop an evidence base within work settings at this time (Boellinghus, Jones, et al., 2012 and Irving, Dobkin, et al., 2009) and the opportunity to alleviate the suffering of stressed out staff seemed like a worthwhile project to embark upon for a dissertation.

Having carried out a literature review in preparation for the dissertation, it was clear that there were only a small number of similar studies that had been attempted in this area and the studies highlighted the difficulty of the retention of staff on an 8-week intervention in a busy work setting (Mackenzie, Poulin, et al., (2006), and Poulin, Mackenzie, et al., (2008). Because of the recent emergence of the Mindfulness Based Living Course (MBLC 2011) it had also not been studied as an intervention in a work setting before. So excited by this challenge, I decided to honour the integrity of the format of the MBLC and attempt to deliver it in full to mixed groups of health care staff.

MSC A PILOT STUDY

Throughout the remainder of this section I will offer what I call top tips, which will hopefully assist the reader in negotiating potential obstacles in the delivery of similar programmes. So how did I start? I first of all offered my own team the complete MBLC (An 8-week course consisting of 8 classes, which are typically two hours long, preceded by an introductory class before the 8-week course begins and I used a day of mindfulness as a follow up after the course had ended) and after receiving positive feedback from them, I was given permission to offer the intervention to other staff within the organisation.

Top Tip 1: Management Support. Get your immediate supervisor on board and practice your craft through the delivery of the intervention to a small group of willing participants or in research speak, conduct a pilot study with participants who are representative of the definitive sample. Then it was time to attempt to run the study and I remember thinking, I wonder if anyone will want to attend this course, but I was hopeful that I would at least be able to get around 8-15 participants to make it a viable group.

The promotional material for the course generated a large amount of interest in a short space of time and within one week I had enough participants to run two courses (31 staff across two groups). After the introductory sessions, I received further requests from staff to attend the course as an individual member of staff or to come and run a course for their teams. Because of time limitations and workload restrictions, the requests were recorded for future reference to build up an evidence base should permission be given to run the course again at some stage in the future. **Top Tip 2: Record Requests**

Both courses ran at the same time, in the same week, on separate days and participants were offered the opportunity to move back and forth between groups to increase the opportunities for participants to attend a session on a weekly basis. I also ran the courses in the morning, because I figured that this would be the best time to engage staff rather than when they were already involved fully immersed into the working day. I decided to use a mixed methods approach (see Rigg, 2013 for a more detailed description of methods used) to effectively capture a wide variety of data. **Top Tip 3: Capture a Mixture of Quantitative and Qualitative Data**

Participants recorded a variety of benefits from the course, which were also consistent with other studies (improved sleep, ability to focus, a marked reduction in perceived stress, able to handle challenges and difficulties, an improvement in the relationship and communication with others, improvements in the ability to manage and prioritise their own health and well-being, as well as achieving a better work / life balance, etc, etc) and the retention rate of 84% was more than I'd hoped given difficulties noted in retention from the literature review. One participant commented on the positive impacts of the training:

> I found myself able to relax and de-stress. I am now more aware of my well-being and have made a conscious decision to eat more healthily resulting in a healthy weight loss. I am also sleeping much better and find that I am more focused at work and not getting as stressed and bothered regarding office politics. I am also kinder to myself."

It didn't take long for the Team Leaders of the participants to hear about and see the tangible benefits of the course. Participants were very keen for their managers to experience these benefits first hand. The participants were also hopeful that their managers would then be less stressed, understand the benefits of the MBLC and in turn allow other staff to participate. For this reason, I was keen for managers to attend the courses and also because they may then be able to unlock doors within the organisation for further training to be carried out.

TEACHING MINDFULNESS

> The hero comes back from this mysterious adventure with the power
> to bestow boons on his fellow man (Campbell, 2008, p.23).

Teaching mindfulness had never been something I'd considered, however, once I began delivering courses at work for the MSc I quickly realised that this work had the capacity to be of significant benefit to others. At this time (2012) I began working as a Mindfulness Facilitator for the Mindfulness Association (MA) (teaching on the MA's one-year courses) and, as my confidence grew I also began offering mindfulness courses in my local community.

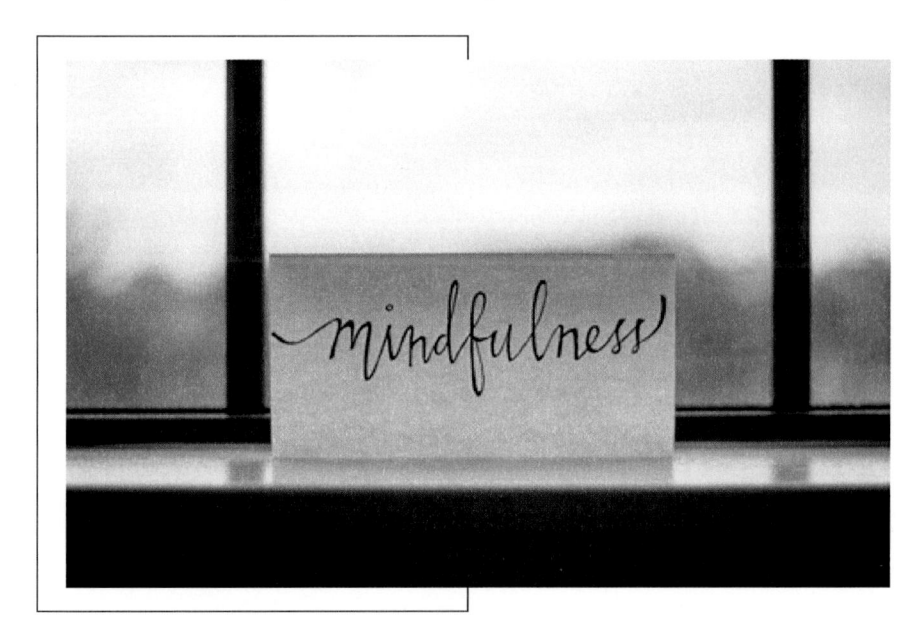

Figure 2: Mindfulness. Photo by Lesly Juarez.

I was still employed full time as a Drug and Alcohol Counsellor in the Health Service and by now I had received a number of requests to run more mindfulness courses for staff. After a period of time, I was given permission from my manager to run two more courses (one with a group of managers) and this bore similar results from the first round of training. I then began campaigning within the Health Service about the benefits of mindfulness and I had the real time evidence to back up my claims of the positive benefits of mindfulness, which I presented in report and presentation format. I spoke with anyone who would listen within the organisation, targeting strategic leads, and used the backing of the participants and group of managers to good effect. **Top Tip 4: Get the Backing of Strategic Leads**

After about two years of campaigning, I was growing tired of feeling like I wasn't getting anywhere. I was considering dropping out of the Health Service and exploring and offering the benefits of mindfulness on my own. I spoke with Rob Nairn about my frustrations and he commented that good mindfulness facilitators are also needed within the Health Service and he thought I should persevere a little more. By now I had completed four 8-Week MBLC with around 50 staff and the evidence I had collected and reported on clearly highlighted the benefits of the intervention. My campaigning finally began to pay off and I was invited to write a proposal about how mindfulness-based interventions could be launched in the Health Service in my area. This meant taking a look at the existing health and well-being initiatives for staff and researching the availability of other Mindfulness Based Interventions in health care settings. At the same time, the drug and alcohol service that I was part of was being disbanded because of financial cutbacks and members of our team, including myself were offered a redundancy package.

Mindfulness was put forward as part of a staff health and well-being initiative. The opportunity then arose to interview for the job of a Mindfulness Facilitator within the same organisation (a 3-day a week post, rather than full time) and after being successful at interview I was suddenly at a cross roads. Work for myself and the Mindfulness Association as a Mindfulness Facilitator and / or take a 3-day a week job as a Mindfulness Facilitator or take a redundancy package and look for another job similar to the one I had been working in for 20 years. After careful consideration, I decided to take the three-day Mindfulness Facilitator job and supplement this by continuing with my weekend work teaching for the Mindfulness Association. In addition to this I also continued to run a martial arts school on a couple of evenings a week.

THE LAUNCH OF MINDFULNESS BASED INTERVENTIONS IN A HEALTH SERVICE SETTING

Initially I found myself in the Human Resources Department, while also being supported from a manager in Organisational Development (OD) and after the first year I transferred fully into the OD Team. In the early stages of development, discussion was had around who to deliver the courses to and where and what time etc. My idea was that we should direct our attention to the well-being of staff in the first instance, so that they could take better care of themselves and, in turn the clients they served. We could discuss client interventions at a later date. I wanted to run the courses during work time and argued that we should treat Mindfulness Based Interventions the same way as we would any other course and schedule them during work hours and allow staff to attend without expecting them to take holidays or time off in lieu. These proposals were supported, although I had no budget for room rental etc and, therefore, had to use the meeting and training rooms on-site.

I began the role in August 2015 and after getting my promotional material together I scheduled three 8-week MBLC (15 staff on each course) to begin in September. I decided to follow a similar format to my earlier pilot study and schedule all courses to begin in the same week across different areas of the county to increase opportunities for staff to attend and to run the courses in the morning. The timing of the course (10am – 12) was set up so that staff did not get caught in the busyness of work prior to attending on that day and so that whatever benefits they gained from the morning could be taken through the day. **Top Tip 5: Consider Course Timings Carefully**

Finding suitable rooms to book for eight weeks in a row in the same location at the same time for three separate courses was my initial challenge and still continues to be so. It was difficult to find meeting or training rooms that were big enough and not next to noisy adjoining offices or busy corridors and then of course parking on Hospital sites was usually difficult. The participant's experience of the mindfulness course can certainly be affected by the location. A correlation was noted between the lower retention rates on courses and the quality of the location that the training was held in. **Top Tip 6: Use Quiet, Spacious Training Spaces**. As one participant noted: "Maybe a different venue! There was quite a lot of distraction and it didn't feel intimate enough".

The initial courses were well received and attended, however, another issue began to surface. Some of the course participants managers had not bought into the importance / relevance of the course and requested that their staff take holidays or time off to attend. I was made aware of this information as the courses progressed and I, therefore, put a question on the next round application paperwork asking staff if it was easy for them to attend the course or get time off work? One participant commented: "Initially I had problems convincing the line manager I could do the course in work time".

When I then found out that some managers were still asking their staff to take holidays to attend, I took this information back to my manager and also asked to meet with the members of the Board and the Executive Team to introduce them to the benefits of mindfulness, but to also get their support for staff to attend without taking holidays. I was supported in my request to allow staff to attend the courses and made this very clear when talking to staff at future introductory sessions and also offered to communicate this message to the participant's manager if needed. **Top Tip 6: Prioritise the Importance of the Intervention**.

PAUSE, CHECK, RE-ADJUST

At this point I took a good look at my own health and well-being and evaluated the impact of working with clients who present with stories of trauma and the impact of this type of work had on me in the long-term. I felt I was becoming de-sensitized to the stories (a protective barrier), but also stressed about dealing with safeguarding issues on a daily basis. I decided to take a complete career change and phase out the private counselling practice and at the very least take a break from this type of work. I was fortunate to be offered more work for the Mindfulness Association (MA) as a Lead Tutor (also teaching on the Studies in Mindfulness MSc) and a member of their Management Team and I also offered to work on the MA Board. I was more than happy to direct my attention to extra work and juggle lots of balls in the air while I found my feet in the world again in this period of transition.

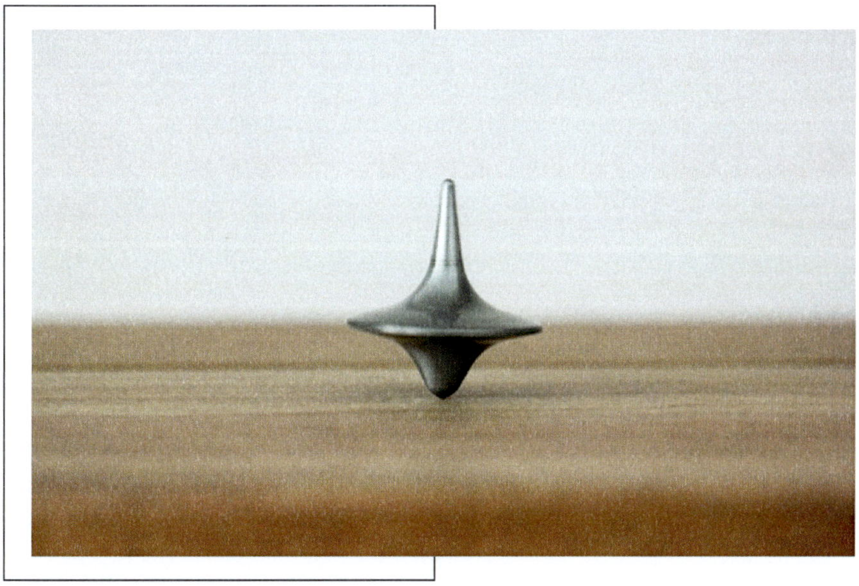

Figure 3: Balance. Photo by Christophe Hautier.

After working in this way for a year or so, I realised that while I was very fortunate, I was also now officially too busy. The frenetic pace was not sustainable. I reflected on needing to walk the talk and stop being so busy multi-tasking myself. I dropped running private community mindfulness courses, phased back my work with the MA and stepped down from the Management Team and Board. This was quite a big step for me, because my style is to take on a lot and I have difficulty saying no to requests. When I watch my mind it just cycles through to do lists and is mainly future focused.

> **Pause and Reflect**
>
> When you watch your own mind, what do you notice?

WORKING WITH AND BEING IN THE BODY

As mentioned earlier, I have been drawn to the benefits of yoga and in recent years I have been immersing myself in a style called Budokon and have found a home in their community of movers. Budokon translates as "the way of the spiritual warrior" and yoga is only one of its avenues of exploration. Budokon requires students to be highly skilled teachers and practitioners of both a Movement Curriculum: Martial arts, Yoga, Mobility, Calisthenics, & Animal Locomotion, and a Mind Curriculum: Intelligence, Emotion, Relationship, Nutrition, & Environment. Budokon has been a huge influence on working with my own edge in all of the above areas and has taken my understanding of movement to a whole new level. This has had a profound effect on valuing the importance of movement and how to introduce it to others.

> **Pause and Reflect**
>
> Go to You Tube and type in Budokon Red Belt Kata for some high-level mindful movement

Movement is becoming a key theme across a number of the chapters in this book. Both John Arnold and Jacqueline Seery, highlight the relevance and importance of mindful movement. The things that now motivate and sustain me are my daily meditation and yoga practices and also sharing this work with others. For once in my life I feel I am living a life that is authentically me and congruent with my beliefs and I love what I do. This must be "following my bliss" as stated by Campbell and discussed by Vin Harris in Chapter 2.

TRENDS

I am collecting data on the effects of the Mindfulness Based Living Course as I go along and at the end of each year, I compare the data against previous years and then make adjustments to the administration and delivery of the courses as needed.

Participants recorded the following annual average scores during 2018: Mindfulness increased by 30%, self-compassion by 26% and perceived stress decreased by 90%. Here's what three participants had to say about their experience:

> I think this course has been the most significant course I have ever undertaken. Its effects have been felt in all aspects of my life. Brilliant!

It has really helped me to focus my attention and improved my ability to leave difficult issues in the past and to stop reliving painful memories. It has helped me in too many ways to mention."

I feel I am more in tune with my emotions and less reactive, which has led to what I feel are better relationships and improved communication.

For details of my research including the quantitative and qualitative instruments used and research findings, you are welcome to read the dissertation I completed for the Studies in Mindfulness MSc (Rigg, 2013) and the continuation of this research (Rigg and McColl, 2017). I also carry out a detailed analysis of the data and document my findings in an end of year annual report.

The following information pertains to the different trends I have noticed over the last three years:

TREND 1) PRE-COURSE DROP-OUT

The courses are well attended and often there are waiting lists, however, an interesting trend began to emerge. Staff book onto the courses quickly, often 3-6 months in advance, however, a percentage of staff drop out of the course prior to attending the first session. They often do this at the last minute and the majority of them cite work pressures as the reason for not attending. Bearing in mind there is often a waiting list, this then has an impact on the number of staff who then attend. I attempted to the balance this pre-course drop-out by accepting 18 - 20 people per course, which appeared to help. I then noticed that there was strong correlation between the staff that did not attend the introductory session and the pre-course drop-out. At the time I accepted staff onto the course who could not make the introductory session. I then changed this to not accept staff onto the course unless they had attended an introductory session. Immediately following the implementation of this rule, the retention rate figures for the courses became the highest I had ever recorded, although the pre-course drop-out continues to be an issue.

TREND 2) PRIORITISING PERSONAL HEALTH AND WELL-BEING

Health care workers are very good at taking care of others and are less likely to put themselves first. While this may be a very bold statement to make, in my experience, from my observations and from the feedback gained from participants, there is evidence to suggest this may be the case. Indeed, a topic of conversation that emerges on every course, is that of participants stating that they feel selfish or a little guilty for taking time out to focus on their own health and well-being for 30 minutes a day throughout the eight weeks. When this emerges, I pause, underline this thought process and have participants reflect. One participant mentioned how they had met and overcame challenges to practice:

> Time, routine, family, friends and perception were all challenges in practices. I overcame most of them by using the tools from the course and allowing time for myself which I have never done before.

Pause and Reflect

Do you feel guilty or selfish when you set time aside for yourself? Drop the story and each day set aside a period of time where you take time to take care of yourself.

TREND 3) TOO BUSY TO PRACTICE

This is the main issue participants struggle with in the first few weeks of an 8-week course. If you have a mindfulness practice you will realise that it requires effort to practice and certain new habits need to be formed to allow oneself the time to sit and practice. When I say to the group that I expect them to set aside 30 minutes a day for practice (I dropped it from 45 minutes to 30 to make it more achievable for the participant), half of the room moves nervously in their chairs. I then ask them to reframe it in their own minds. Don't think of it as an extra burden, think of it as I am going to prioritise my health and well-being every day for eight weeks.

I also make it clear that I am aware that a participant may miss the odd session because of work, illness or holidays etc, however, if they are going to miss more than two of the eight sessions, then they should leave it until they have more time and if they are not prepared to do the home practice, they should also not attend. One participant explained how they overcame this obstacle: "Attending classes due to workload was an issue, which I overcame with better organisation of time and planning".

> **Pause and Reflect**
>
> Are you telling yourself you're too busy to practice? How will you overcome this story?

TREND 4) HELPING, OFFERING ADVICE AND LISTENING OR NOT

I make it very clear at the beginning of the course how we will work together as a group; letting participants know that when listening to each other there is no need to offer advice or attempt to "fix" things. We are actually just being there for the person and really listening to what they are saying in a mindful way and noticing the impulse to jump in and offer advice or to drift off into not listening. I also ask participants to stay content free, meaning that we can talk about our experience of a practice without adding unnecessary content or disclosing personal information. Listening mindfully in this way takes practice as we are accustomed to figuring out the answer ahead of time and formulating a response before the other person has finished and then often delivering this response before they have done so.

Once we practice and allow ourselves to listen mindfully and also drop the story, the common story about how I am right, and you are wrong, then the whole conversation takes on new meaning and can have significantly different results. Upon reflection, I realise that Donal Creedon has had an influence here on getting me to take a different stance on dialogue, inquiry and communication. One participant commented on the power of really listening to another: "Being able to really listen to our clients and demonstrate compassion and kindness more openly".

> **Pause and Reflect**
>
> How many times have you heard people interrupting each other, finishing each other's sentences or observed yourself waiting to jump in without hearing the other person fully?

TREND 5) THE BENEFITS OF CONSISTENT PRACTICE

Around session three and onwards you can really see how the practice is taking effect, as a weight appears lifted from many of the participants shoulders, as they begin prioritising their health and well-being and slowing down, pausing and noticing this one precious life we all have. Week three onwards for me is my favourite time in the course, because this change is evident in the participant's faces, their bodies and their attitudes. I have recently advised participants that if they can't make the first three sessions, then they should also not attend the course, because we are really sowing the seeds in the first few sessions. One participant mentioned the impact that the practices had on them:

> Changing my work style from multi-tasking to one task at a time. Being kinder to myself over perceived underachieving; kinder to team members as all under pressure and all trying to cope. Learning to prioritise my well-being through exercises and breaks and leave work at work.

TREND 6) MOVE MORE

A growing number of us have jobs that are office based and because of this contributes to a more sedentary lifestyle. Part of making the mindfulness-based interventions successful at work, is making them relevant to work and life. When presenting mindful movement and the body scan, I begin by saying to the participants, "Let's do the maths here!" We sit down at our desk for eight hours a day, we drive for two, sit on our couch for four and then lie down and go to sleep with a bit of walking in between. Our bodies are effectively in a contracted posture for most of the day, therefore, it's no wonder we have problems with our backs, shoulders, necks and wrists based on this lifestyle.

In addition to the body scan, we can bring our awareness to the body as we inhabit it at different times during the day and then move it more often. As our lifestyle habits contract the body in, we need to spend more and more time expanding outwards to counteract this. We have already been told about the benefits of exercise all our lives, but how about the joy of moving and stretching in a very simple way on a daily basis. Moving and expressing energy in the body is an undervalued activity that is a key to one's health and well-being and paying attention to the body in this way is also an early indicator of what the body needs and how we should respond. One participant commented on how an increased body awareness had an impact: "Just being in my body and trying to become more aware of the body which carries me around and how to appreciate it, look after it and be there for it. It is amazing!"

Pause and Reflect

Get up and move every hour. Even doing a few simple stretches out of your seat will begin to help.

TREND 7) TAKE A BREAK, DON'T BE SILLY

When I suggested that participants should take regular breaks at work and dare I say it a "lunch break", I received laughs and noticed nervous fidgeting from certain members of the audience on a regular basis. As we explored the outlandish statement I'd made, I began to uncover language that had made its way into the working culture that made people uncomfortable and also conform. "I don't have time for a lunch break!" "If someone leaves the office on time at the end of the day, my colleague says, it must be alright for her eh?" Have you ever met someone who routinely states the following rather loudly in the office: "I haven't had a chance to take a break!" "It's three o-clock and I'm only just having a sandwich now!"

Some of us have bought into this crazy system, based on the routine use of the preceding language in this trend and it needs to be challenged! So I point this one out with a big underline when it comes up (which it does more often than we'd like to admit) and I even say things like "stop being a mug and take a break!" "I think you can safely challenge anyone that objects to you taking a lunch break." "Stop being part of the problem you're complaining about and take a break when you need one." One participant commented on the work-related positive impact of taking a break: "Taking a break actually helps productivity".

On occasion participants would also point out the attitude of their colleagues to the training they were attending. This sometimes manifested as making fun of them for doing that weird mindfulness stuff, to questioning why they got to leave the office to go and do the training when their work should take priority. One participant mentioned the difficulties encountered along the way: "Getting into the habit of regular practice was at first challenging. I needed to make it part of my daily routine. Colleagues attitude to "it" was also an issue".

> **Pause and Reflect**
>
> Are you one of those people that "choose" not to take a break or eats while driving or checking emails? Get a grip! They stopped giving out gold watches for retirement years ago!

CONCLUSION

As I finish writing this (it's August 2018), I have now worked for three years in the role of a Mindfulness Facilitator in the Health Service. To date I have introduced mindfulness to around 300 participants in an organisation that is set to have upwards of 8000 staff; so you could say I have a way to go. I have recently written a developmental plan for mindfulness, which recommends the training of new facilitators and lists our priorities for areas of expansion in the immediate future. I can say that I am well supported by my manager and by an organisation that recognises the inherent benefits of sharing the "boon" of mindfulness with staff. Staff put others first and as a consequence may often put themselves last. It is a humbling experience to "follow my bliss" and to have the opportunity to share it with others (while dodging the limelight and side stepping the hugs). The friends that I asked to proofread this chapter, have suggested that I say more about my own personal practice. It may suffice to say that I still attend around a month's worth of retreat each year with exceptional teachers and I get my bum on the cushion most days. Each day after sitting I expand the body outwards by doing yoga and stretching and I go for a walk a week by myself in the mountains to make a connection with space and nature.

Good luck on your own journey, Ian

FURTHER RESOURCES

Budokon Mixed Movement Arts University at:
www.Budokon.com
Budokon demonstrations found on You Tube:
https://www.youtube.com/watch?v=lwRGC3xTLDE
Melayne Shayne:
https://www.youtube.com/watch?v=m_52T0vhz8U
Tara Rokpa Centre:
www.tararokpacentre.co.za

REFERENCES

BOELLINGHAUS, I., JONES, F.W., and HUTTON, J. 2012. The Role of Mindfulness and Loving-Kindness Meditation in Cultivating Self-Compassion and Other Focused Concern in Health Care Professionals. Mindfulness 5 (2), pp. 1-10.
BUDOKON http://budokon.com
CAMPBELL, J., 2nd Ed, 2008. The Hero With a Thousand Faces. New World Library
DRUPON, RINPOCHE., 2013. Teaching on Meditation. Samye Ling Tibetan Buddhist Centre, Scotland, 26th of July, 2013.
HAUTIER, C (n.d.) Spinning Dream, photo taken by Christophe Hautier and released under Unsplash license. Public Domain Free Photo
https://unsplash.com/photos/902vnYeoWS4
IRVING, J.A., DOBKIN, P.L. and PARK, J., 2009. Cultivating mindfulness in health care professionals: A review of empirical studies of mindfulnesss-based stress reduction (MBSR). Complementary Therapies in Clinical Practice, 15 (2), pp. 61-66.
JUAREZ, J (n.d.) Mindfulness, photo taken by Lesly Juarez and released under Unsplash license. Public Domain Free Photo https://unsplash.com/photos/DFtjXYd5Pto
KORNFRST, B. (n.d.) Jedi Training, Photo by Ben Konfrst and released under Unsplash license. Public Domain Free Photo https://unsplash.com/photos/DfPi82f-pqc
MACKENZIE, C.S., POULIN, P.A. and SEIDMAN-CARLSON, R., 2006. A brief mindfulness-based stress reduction intervention for nurses and nurse aides. Applied Nursing Research, 19 (2), pp. 105-109.
MINDFULNESS ASSOCIATION LTD. Mindfulness Based Living Course 8 Week Programme Course Manual. The University of Aberdeen: Studies in Mindfulness.
NAIRN, R., 1997. Tranquil Mind: An Introduction to Buddhism and Meditation. Kairon Press: South Africa
NISARGADATTA MAHARAJ, S., 1974. I am That: Talks with Sri Nisargadatta Maharaj. Chetana
POULIN, P.A., MACKENZIE, C.S., SOLOWAY, G. and KARAYOLAS, E., 2008. Mindfulness training as an evidenced-based approach to reducing stress and promoting well-being among human services professionals. International Journal of Health Promotion and Education, 46 (2), pp. 72.
RIGG, I., 2013. The Effects of the 8-Week Mindfulness Based Living Course (MBLC) When Delivered to a Mixed Group of Health Care Staff: A Prospective Pilot Study. Thesis (MSc Commendation). University of Aberdeen.
RIGG, I AND MCCOLL, J., 2017. Mindfulness based living: an exploratory study with health care staff. In: Garcia, Irene and Tur-Viñes, Victoria, (eds.) Bilateral dialogues between researchers from Glasgow Caledonian University and University of Alicante (Spain). Spain, University of Alicante Spain, pp. 153-173
WACHOWSKI BROTHERS. The Matrix. Film. Directed by Wachowski Brothers. USA: Warner Brothers, 1999

CHAPTER 11

DOING WHAT NEEDS TO BE DONE: MINDFUL COMPASSION TRAINING FOR NURSES

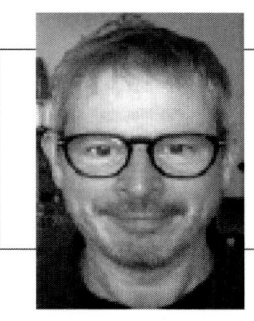

Gavin Cullen

g.cullen2@napier.ac.uk

INTRODUCTION: PROMISES TO KEEP

Mindfulness training taught me to reflect on my intention and motivation for practicing mindfulness. Doing so has become a crucial way to kick-start daily practice. It helps me stay in touch with my reasons for practicing, enriching what could otherwise become a predictable and ultimately dull routine. Here, my intentions are to describe a project that is important to me, that may be of interest to you, and to do so as clearly as I can. My motivation is going to sound a bit rude initially, although what I have to say is borne out of passion.

For me, the current context in which nurses work is like the proverbial "tale, told by an idiot, full of sound and fury, signifying nothing" (Shakespeare, Macbeth, Act 5, Scene 5, 2015, p85).

What I mean is that the backdrop of political, professional and societal posturing, meddling and ever-increasing expectations make the notion of providing consistent, effective nursing care almost impossible. Further, nursing as a profession has done little so far to coherently explain one of the key qualities associated with it: compassion.

I will attempt to explain myself. I worked as a mental health nurse in the National Health Service (NHS) for twenty-five years, before becoming a university lecturer, helping teach pre-registration nurses. In both contexts, I have found it useful to answer this question periodically: am I doing what is needed, for patients, carers, colleagues or myself, or am I doing what I might prefer to be doing? There can be a profound difference between these two positions. To give an extreme example, emergency situations often require nurses to move towards and deal with danger, when every cell in their body naturally screams for retreat. Fires can break out in hospitals; suicides are attempted; and sometimes violence needs to be contained. More subtle instances are more pervasive. These include nurses busying themselves with bureaucratic task after task, often in a 'duty room', rather than spending more time outside that safety zone, being present with, and therefore responsive to, people who are suffering. I am not blaming anyone here, and I recognise my own behaviour in this too; mental health nursing is deeply challenging work.

And there is seemingly no limit to how busy current health and social care can be. There are endless audits, procedures and targets. Such endeavours may have a reasonable starting-point, and might serve to re-assure politicians, NHS senior managers and the public about that inevitable 'bottom' (or 'top') 'line'. For me, however, cumulatively they can overwhelm and distract nurses from their more important function of providing direct care. They can also, arguably, become sticks to punish services with, create climates of fear and unnecessary competition, and in the worst cases contribute to poor standards of care (Ballatt and Campling, 2011).

The busyness is also a consequence of the exponential increase in the volume of referrals to the services nurses work in, which has not been accompanied by a concomitant rise in staffing; an increase in people developing complex health and social care needs; health and social care integration; continually evolving technological advances; and the current recruitment crisis, some of which is arguably related to political uncertainties (Audit Scotland, 2018; Bland et al., 2015; Fahy et al., 2017; and Stephenson, 2018).

One constant in all this is that most people using the NHS are suffering. This is unlikely to change. And, of course, nurses strive to meet that suffering with kindness and compassion. All the nurses I worked with were motivated to do so, and all of us experienced distress at the prospects of leaving needs unmet. However, despite the myth that nurses respond to 'a calling' to enter the profession and are somehow therefore naturally compassionate beings all the time (perhaps even angels), compassion does not happen by magic. Maintaining compassionate motivation can be a struggle, even for the most skilled nurse practitioners.

This chapter describes a project that was designed to introduce mental health nurses to what I called 'Mindful Compassion Training for Nurses' (MCTN). The training took place in a National Health Service (NHS) Child and Adolescent Mental Health Service (CAMHS). The MCTN model, which combines training in mindfulness with compassion meditation techniques, is outlined further below.

I was motivated to do this because I was fed up with the 'idiot's tale' described above, including my ultimate NHS role as a team leader, which often involved becoming embroiled in work distancing me from the heart of nursing practice. But please hear me when I also say I love being a nurse and my time working in the NHS, where a diverse staff group gather on a daily basis to at least try to do something good for other people. The MCTN project was also driven by a wish to give something back, to courageous and inspiring colleagues, and indeed to the people I helped provide care for.

The decision to offer the project to nurses was based mainly on the notion, as my Granny often said, that:
> "Ye cannae pour from an empty cup!"

I was interested in sharing the understanding and techniques I felt I had benefitted from in meditation training. I wanted to do something to check that we were all looking after ourselves well, to open up a dialogue about what compassion 'really' is, and perhaps create a safer context in which it could flourish. To be truly honest, I also wanted what I believe all nurses yearn for, to be of proper use to others, and to offer the hope of something better.

I hesitate to call my part in this project 'heroic'. The term conjures up images from cinema and literature of super-human figures, overcoming insurmountable odds to save the world, using powers which only they possess. As enjoyable as those fantastical tales can be, they are also a bit comical, like the idea of a caped superhero from another planet who wears his underpants over his trousers as he goes about being heroic.

Nonetheless, the stages of the 'Hero's Journey', as described by Vin Harris in Chapter 2, are apt. First, this project was a definite point of departure for me, and, I believe, the nurses who took part in it. I had to suspend being a pushy, controlling nurse leader and manager, and we were going to explore the sometimes messy but rewarding territory of compassion together. Between us, the group who participated in MCTN had over a hundred years' nursing experience. Strange, perhaps ridiculous, that we had not undertaken such a journey before.

And journey we did, together, as Yoda might have said. This is my real problem with the term 'hero' - the implication that it revolves around solo effort and achievement. For me, there is no such thing, as I hope to demonstrate.

Pause and Reflect

What does the word 'compassion' mean to you?
You might want to take a note of any ideas that come to you – and see how they compare to the way compassion is discussed in the rest of this chapter.

When I say that providing compassionate care is the central creed of nursing I may be stating the obvious. Certainly, key stakeholders in nursing, from the nurses' governing body, the Nursing and Midwifery Council (2015), to the Scottish Government (2010 and 2017), expect nurses to deliver on compassionate promises.

The first curiosity, for me, however, is that there is no clear agreement on what compassion in nursing (CIN) is (Goetz et al., 2010). Further, in nursing, ideas like 'sympathy' and 'empathy', the ability to perceive things from another person's perspective, have long been confused with 'compassion'. For me, the former concepts can be helpful places to start, but arguably they are but two items on a longer list of compassionate attributes, which includes: a sensitivity to suffering; the motivation to care; the capacity to tolerate difficult feelings; being non-judgmental; and warmth (Gilbert and Choden, 2013). And while I am here, my working definition of compassion also comes from Gilbert and Choden (2013): an awareness of and engagement with suffering, along with a commitment to intervene and do something about that suffering.

The second, unpleasant, revelation relates to the existence of healthcare scandals which demonstrate or imply sometimes shocking and even fatal deficits in compassionate care. These include the events at Mid-Staffordshire NHS Foundation Trust. Media reports suggest potentially hundreds of people could have died in that Trust as a consequence of poor care standards (Owen and Meikle, 2013). While some commentary suggests that the Trust was under-resourced and caught up in meeting harsh Government targets, this tragedy also led to much soul-searching in nursing and subsequent re-vamping of nurse education and ongoing professional development standards (Ballat and Campling, 2011, and Report of the Willis Commission, 2012). A more recent Scottish example involves allegations of bullying and inappropriate use of physical restraint in NHS Tayside mental health services (British Broadcasting Corporation, 2018). Those allegations are to be the focus of an ongoing Public Inquiry (NHS Tayside, 2018).

I find such scandals upsetting, and I would never condone malpractice. Simultaneously, as already implied, I do not believe that the average practicing nurse has much control over the increasingly challenging conditions they find themselves working in. And yet the expectations of nurses to be compassionate are, if anything, increasing.

A more innocent theme related to compassion in nursing but one which has unintended unhelpful consequences, is the emphasis in nursing on compassion as observable behaviour. In Scotland, for example, the Government requires nurses to deliver 'safe, effective and person-centred' practice, preferably with the concrete supporting evidence of completed checklists, audits or patient/carer testimony (see, for example, NHS Education for Scotland, 2011). It is understandable and appropriate that there is such a focus on compassion-as-action. After all the public purse is being spent on providing nursing care, and we all want to ensure the best standards of care possible are being delivered – and to avoid further scandals. Further, as the nurse participants in this project are testament to, nurses like to be busy; compassion is often seen as something you do.

So, this 'compassion from the outside-in' is a reasonable idea. But for me, there is another, equal, if not more important side to this story: the potential to develop 'compassion from the inside-out' offered by mindfulness and compassion meditation training. There is some evidence to suggest that nurses begin to struggle with maintaining their compassionate motivation quite quickly following registration (Maben et al., 2007). Further, even well-educated mental healthcare professionals can develop negative views of their patients following experience of adverse events like violence or suicidal behaviour (Friedrich et al., 2013). I believe that this is partly because the focus on compassion from the outside-in does not help nurses and their colleagues understand how to reconcile conflicting feelings about their experiences, while simultaneously being able to sustain compassion for patients and indeed themselves. And let's make no bones about it, nursing involves prolonged and often psychologically intimate contact with human suffering.

There are some supportive mechanisms already in existence for nurses, such as 'clinical supervision'. This involves individuals or groups of nurses reflecting on their working practice in supportive ways with more experienced 'mentors' or peers (Butterworth et al., 2008). Supervision is, however, linked with meeting organisational targets and can therefore be perceived by nurses as a management tool used to control their behaviour (Hawkins and Shohet, 2012). Also, from experience, supervision sessions occur infrequently, and its provision is at the mercy of other service demands. Even if nurses get regular supervision, I have long-wondered what they do in the weeks to months between sessions, and what they do day-to-day, and moment-to-moment, to sustain compassion.

Meanwhile, nursing has been slow to pick up on the increasing interest in mindfulness and compassion-based meditation practices, whether they are used to address problems, prevent them arising, or enhance resilience. In the build-up to this project I found one promising research trial offering mindfulness to student nurses and another which included some nurses in a wider multi-disciplinary team (Beddoe and Murphy, 2004, and Brady et al, 2011). I did not find examples of compassion meditation training for nurses.

PROJECT DESIGN: A KIND OF MAGIC

I was skeptical about magical thinking earlier in this chapter. To be honest, however, designing this project and choosing research methods initially felt like being a newly-anointed novice magician, with an inexhaustible, indestructible power source in the form of meditation training and ongoing practice. Having been trained by wise elders, I was now ready to change the world forever. What transpired, of course, was modest, ordinary and hard-won. And thank goodness for that.

There certainly seem to be magical spells cast in the research world. Arguably the most powerful of these relates to 'quantitative' methods and 'randomised controlled trials' (RCT'S) particularly. RCT's involve randomly assigning research 'subject's' to either the intervention/ new thing being tested or what in healthcare is described as 'treatment-as-usual' (TAU) (Burns and Grove, 2010). RCT's are 'quantitative' in that they use numbers to measure how well the new thing worked or did not compared to TAU, for example by asking people to score responses to pre-determined items on 'self-report questionnaires'.

RCT's monopolise healthcare research, including mindfulness trials. They are prized for their objectivity in creating laboratory-like conditions, where as many factors as possible, such as age or gender, are 'controlled for', so that the clearest picture of the new thing's effectiveness emerges (Kendall, 2003, and Edwards et al., 2015). At the time of this project I struggled to see how RCT's could truly represent mindfulness as I experienced it. To me, mindfulness practice is a personal, intuitive process almost impossible to translate into words, never mind numbers. Mindfulness RCT's also tend to focus on individual responses, seemingly ignoring the fact that most mindfulness training has a strong social component, taking place in groups, and in being facilitated by instructors every bit as human as group members.

Bentz and Shapiro's (1994) work gave me a platform to adopt research methods I could believe in more fully. They argue that research is a very human pursuit, involving 'participant's', not 'subjects', who actively choose involvement in projects, or not, and with whom researchers have dynamic relationships. I found similar ideas in Pawson and Tilley's (1994) 'realistic evaluation' (RE) model. RE recognizes that neither researchers nor participants operate in laboratory conditions, but instead exist in multiple, complex, interacting social systems, including those related to their personal and professional lives.

In RE, researchers can still use outcome measures, but the approach is not interested in outcomes alone. It focuses instead on the relationship between outcomes, the context of participants' lives and the study, and the 'underlying mechanisms' or ways in which project activities worked for them, or not. These relationships are referred to as 'Context-Mechanism-Outcome configurations' or CMOc (de Souza, 2013). In other words, RE is not interested solely in whether or not an intervention like mindfulness works, but why, for whom, and in what contexts. This understanding can then help other researchers and project funders decide if and how the intervention could be transferred to a different setting. For me this is a potentially powerful antidote to beliefs that mindfulness is a panacea for all the world's problems and will assuredly benefit everybody.

Another key element of RE research design is that the researcher needs to develop and then test a theory about the research topic in question, in my case compassion in nursing.

I based the Mindful Compassion Training for Nurses (MCTN project) on recruiting and comparing two groups of nurse colleagues. Cohort One would receive eight weeks of MCTN in a group, and Cohort Two would be used as a comparison. I would also ask all participants, in both Cohorts, to complete outcome measures before and after the MCTN group ran. During the second run of asking participants to complete the measures, I also interviewed ten nurses individually, recruited from both Cohorts. Findings from the first set of outcome measures informed my compassion in nursing (CIN) theory development, and the theory itself formed the basis of the participant interviews.

The project involved a 'mixed methods' approach. I set out to obtain quantitative findings via the outcome measures and qualitative findings via verbal feedback related to participants' experiences. Overall, I was more interested in the latter, with quantitative findings playing the supporting role described earlier, because I wanted to engage in a dialogue with colleagues about compassion. Nonetheless, I found the quantitative findings, and even colleagues' reactions to the questionnaires, as fascinating as the verbal feedback. One message I can offer you here is: this research stuff can really work- you can find things out! More on that later.

PROJECT AIMS

The project's central focus was to answer the question: could Mindful Compassion Training for Nurses (MCTN) be useful to nurses in 'real' terms? In order to explore that question there were two key project aims:

1. To identify individual, social, professional and organisational contextual factors which influence MCTN outcomes, and
2. To identify key 'enablers' and 'inhibitors' for participants in those four domains.

> **Pause and Reflect**
>
> Links to the outcome measures used in the project are given below. Copy them to a browser and try them for yourself. You can download them and print them out or just score them on a piece of paper, then score them using the guidance given on the questionnaires. What do the questionnaires tell you about yourself? Are there any surprises?
>
> The Self-Compassion Scale:
> http://self-compassion.org/wptest/wp-content/uploads/Self_Compassion_Scale_for_researchers.pdf
>
> Fears of Compassion Scale:
> https://compassionatemind.co.uk/uploads/files/fears-of-compassion-scale.pdf

Ultimately twenty nurses were recruited, ten for each Cohort. As noted earlier, Cohort One were invited to participate in the Mindful Compassion Training for Nurses (MCTN) group. Cohort Two's important role was to provide a comparison group; they did not participate in MCTN and were asked to carry on with their working lives as usual. If they were interested in MCTN I promised Cohort Two participants I would share the techniques taught in the group with them after the project was finished. Between the Cohorts the ratio of female: male participants was 13:7, and the age range 26 to 53 years. There were 17 registered nurses and 3 nurse support workers. 14 nurses had worked in adult mental health services previously, and all 20 had worked in a psychiatric inpatient unit. The participants length of nursing service varied from 1 to 25 years.

75% of participants had previous meditation practice experience. This was, however, limited and no participant had recently been engaged in meditation practice or had an ongoing practice routine.

THE MINDFUL COMPASSION TRAINING FOR NURSES (MCTN) GROUP

MCTN was a hybrid programme using mindfulness as a foundation to then explore compassion practices and theory. It was derived from a combination of: a) the MSc course training (Nairn et al., 2010a and b; and Nixon et al., 2011); and b) Gilbert and Choden's (2013) 'mindful compassion' training.

The programme comprised of eight weekly, ninety-minute sessions. The eight-week structure is mainly a tradition in secular mindfulness training, and I went with ninety-minute sessions because the group was held during the 'handover' period between an early and late shift for the inpatient unit. This meant that colleagues not in the group had to 'hold the fort' while the group was on, and instinct told me MCTN participants would not want to keep those colleagues, or indeed, CAMHS service users, waiting for longer.

I facilitated each group session, which comprised of a combination of information sharing, experiential guided practice, shared reflection on the practice, and home practice advice and support. The practices included mindful breathing; the body scan; mindful movement; and a range of compassion practices including visualizing a safe place, and the loving kindness practice. If you would like more information about the programme, please contact me.

THE MINDFUL COMPASSION TRAINING FOR NURSES (MCTN) PROJECT IN ACTION: EMBODYING IMPERFECTION

THE EXPERIENCE OF TEACHING

Despite years of personal mindfulness practice and mindfulness teacher training, I was anxious as the first group session started. The participants knew me well, and they knew how much I had invested in mindfulness training, and indeed how much the NHS had invested in me too (mainly the MSc course fees). It also felt like facilitating the MCTN project was akin to coming out of the compassion closet. I would be making a declaration of sorts, one that I would need to stick to. And I just wanted it to work.

I was also excited, and had prepared enough material for a four-hour group, never mind ninety minutes. I had also prepared detailed plans for each subsequent session. Halfway through that first session, I relaxed on realising that the most important thing was to go at the pace of the participants, to work with that sense of an 'open curriculum' that McCown et al. (2010) describe. To do so was itself a form of mindfulness practice, of living in to:

> "Knowing what is happening, while it is happening, without preference".
> (Choden and Regan-Addis, 2018, p9)

That does not mean each session was without structure It means the training quickly settled in to a more spacious routine:

Activity	Approximate time
Settling/ arriving practice	5 minutes
Check-in with participants	10
New theory or practice	25
Guided practice and group reflection/ discussion/ inquiry	45
Closing practice	5

The 'without preference' aspect of mindfulness practice noted above could also be described as a kind, positively curious, warm and accepting stance (Choden and Regan-Addis, 2018). I needed to draw on these qualities in relation to a key personal learning point from the project: just how much nurse participants valued mindful movement.

During my own mindfulness training, I had sometimes felt like the only person at the disco with no rhythm when I practiced mindful movement techniques, even though I tried to live by more of my Granny's more particular advice:

"no need to dance like a block of wood, Gavin – let go!"

And so, I taught the first round of gentle yoga exercises feeling shy and clumsy. These feelings were heightened by the venue for the group: the relatively small 'school room' in the CAMHS concerned, chosen because it was the only room available consistently. Its advantage was that it was in the quietest part of the building, its disadvantage that, with eleven adults in it, it could feel quite intimate. There was certainly no hiding place.

But the participants loved being able to move. In fact, they needed to. They told me, and once or twice showed me, that if you put busy, hardworking people in a room and ask them to be still, they will fall asleep sooner or later. Or worry that they should be off somewhere, being busy again, a theme I will return to later.

Another thing which stood out was a sense in which guiding practices and teaching mindfulness lifted the veil of roles we adopt in life, professional or personal, to reveal our shared, precious humanity. For example, when I led the body scan practice, the participants lying on the floor around me were not colleagues then. They were living, breathing, sometimes snoring, people, sharing a desire for peace and happiness. What I am trying to indicate here is that, although I facilitated the training, the participants were of course in reality teaching themselves, as a group and as individuals. For example, although we discussed whether we should all wear shoes during the group, the group itself developed a ritual of taking their shoes off before coming in to the class room, leaving them in an organic pile outside.

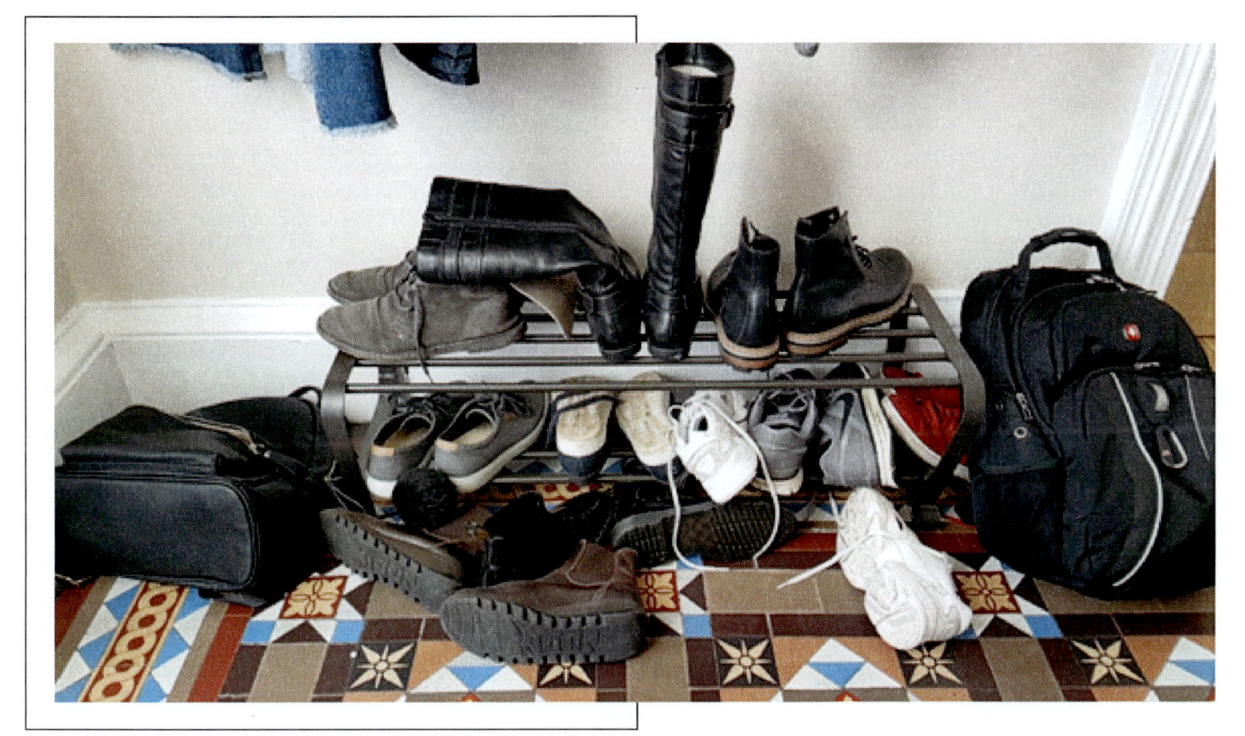

Figure 1: An organic pile of shoes. Photo © Cullen 2019

PROJECT OUTCOMES AND PARTICIPANTS' EXPERIENCES

Project outcomes and participants' experiences

OUTCOME MEASURES

In terms of the Self-Compassion Scale (SCS), Neff's (2003) scoring advice is that overall 'self-compassion' ratings of:

- 1.0 - 2.4 indicate 'low' self-compassion levels;
- 2.4 - 3.5 are 'moderate'; and
- 3.5 and over are 'high'.

Possessing moderate to high levels of self-compassion has been correlated with better psychological health, emotional resilience and quicker recovery from health problems in related research (Neff, 2011; and Neff and Germer, 2013). In this project, 'compassion' scores gathered suggested that both Cohorts' participants already possessed healthy levels of self-compassion and that MCTN was additionally helpful for Cohort One nurses. As Figure 2 (below) shows, the mean 'self-compassion' score for cohort one rose from 3.07 to 3.4, an increase of 9.9 %, while cohort two's score remained the same at 3.11.

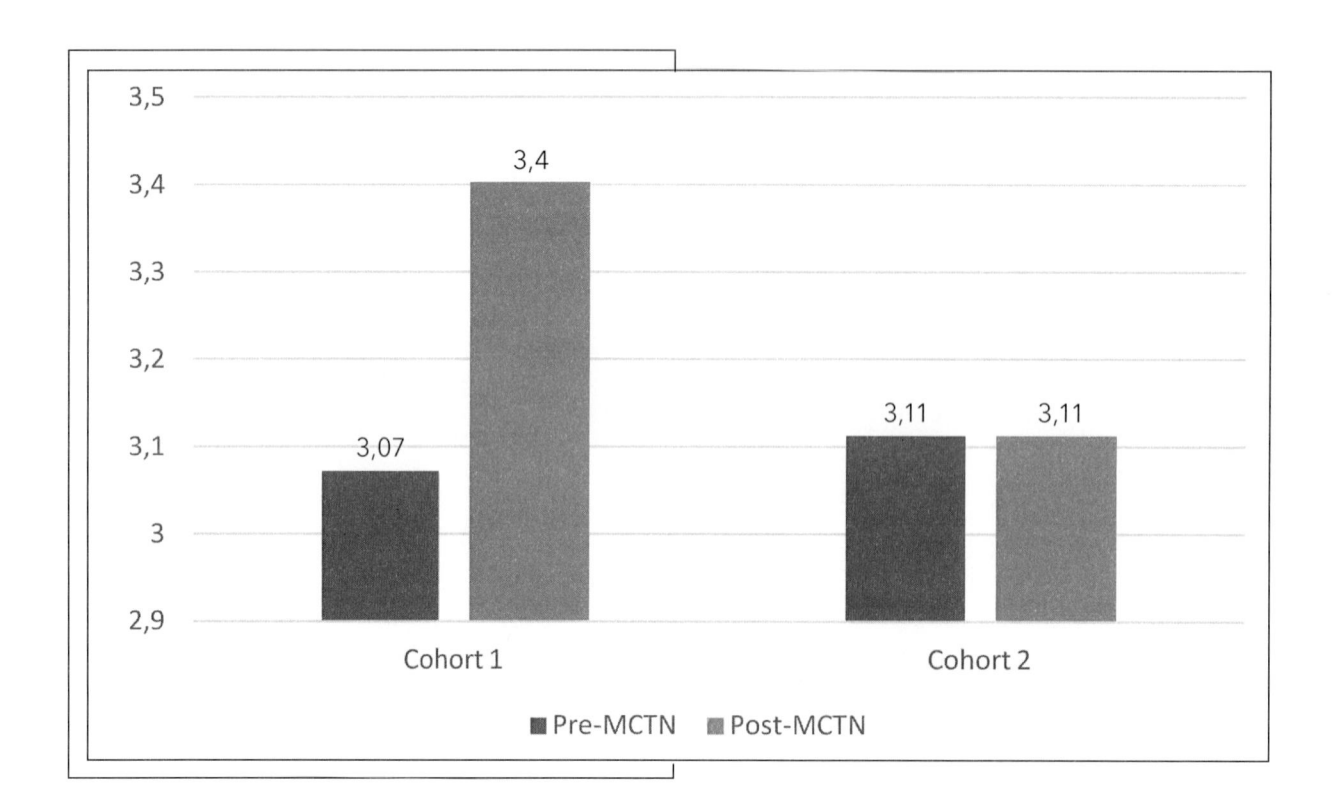

Figure 2: Mean pre and post-MCTN 'self-compassion' scores using the SCS

The findings above are also fairly typical of research involving healthcare clinicians: generally speaking we see ourselves as fairly healthy and resilient (see, for example, Shapiro et al., 2007; and Heffernan et al., 2010). However, a closer look at the six SCS scores reveals that Cohort Two nurses fared worse on two of the negative sub-scales, self-judgement and over-identification with thinking, as shown in Figure 3 below:

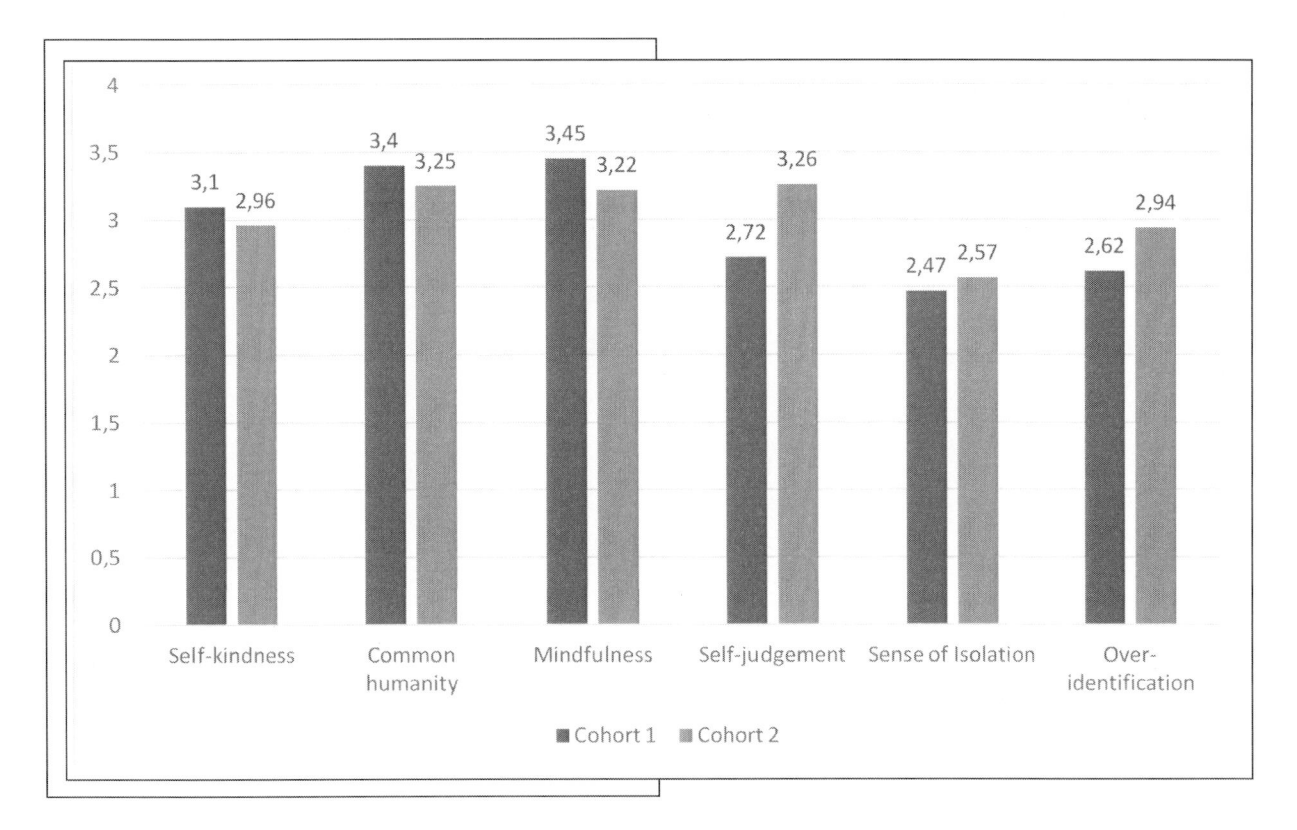

Figure 3: Comparison of mean post-MCTN SCS sub-scale findings

The Fears of Compassion Scales (FCS) results were more striking. In brief, the higher a person's scores on the FCS the greater their reported fears of compassion will be (Gilbert et al., 2010). In this project the main finding was that Cohort One's mean scores on all three scales reduced significantly within the Cohort and compared to Cohort Two, as Figures 4 and 5 demonstrate. In Cohort One, mean fears of expressing compassion for others fell by 23.03 % within the Cohort and were 33.12 % less than Cohort Two's mean results at follow-up; fears of responding to compassion from others fell by 27.89 % within the Cohort and were 51.93% less than Cohort two's at follow-up; and fears of expressing kindness and compassion towards yourself fell by 41.53% within the Cohort and were 52.42 % less than Cohort Two's at follow-up.

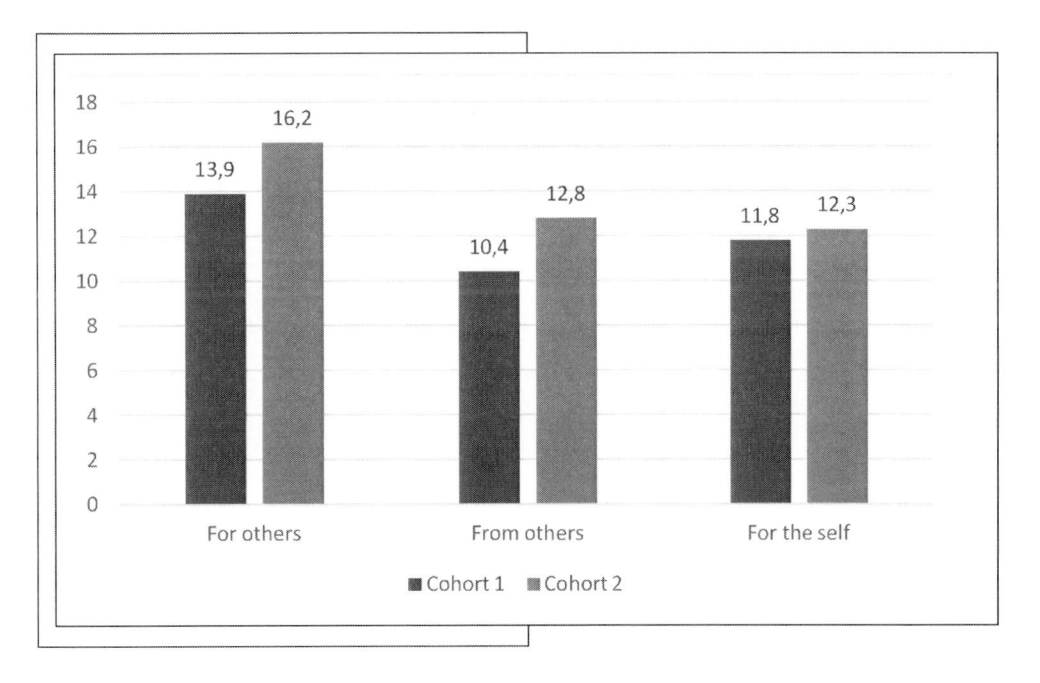

Figure 4: Comparison of pre-MCTN FCS scores

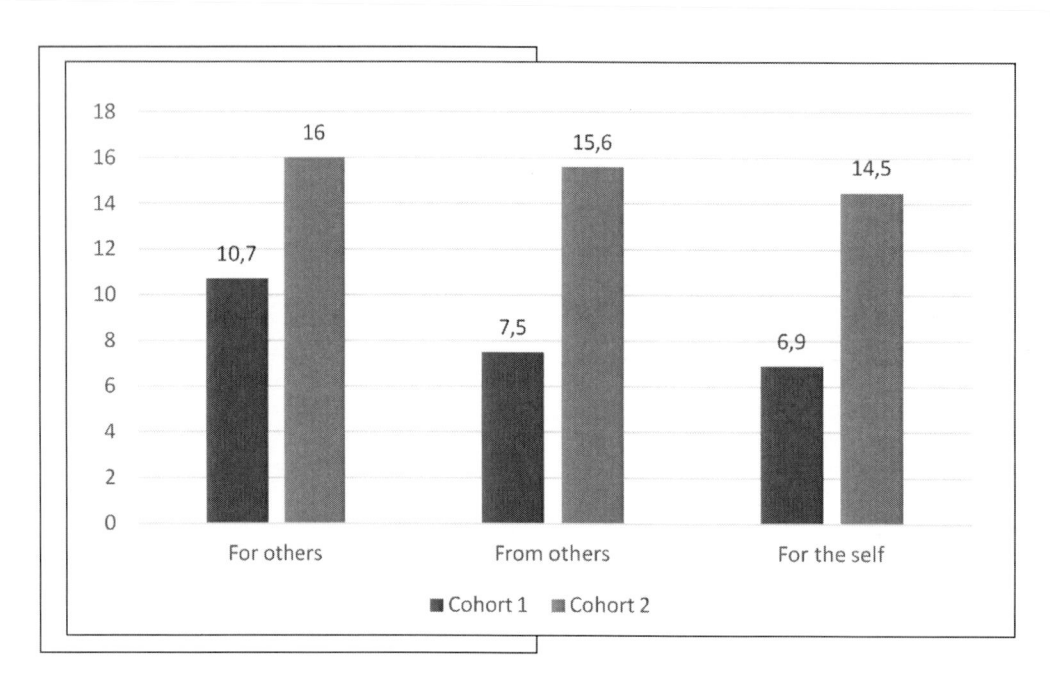

Figure 5: Comparison of post-MCTN FCS scores

INTERVIEW THEMES

The compassion in nursing (CIN) theory noted earlier was a useful springboard for interviewees to explore why fears of compassion can arise and what we might be able to do about that. I have grouped the interview responses below under five theme headings derived from my CIN theory and analysis of nurses' responses to it. All names given are pseudonyms.

Theme 1: compassion in nursing (CIN) is important to nurses
All participants agreed CIN is crucial. As Colin, a charge nurse, put it:

> "I don't think you could do the job without it."

However, some participants also noted that not all nurse colleagues lived up to the compassionate ideal, and all identified significant factors potentially adversely affecting CIN. These included time pressure and organisational targets being prioritised over staff support and development. As Colin also said:

> "The good bits of the job are when you...have time to think about what sort of care are we giving this young person and their family....and being thoughtful about it, but that's not as much as the time we spend thinking: 'have I done the hand hygiene audits'?"

Another interviewee recalled a former role as a child health nurse. In the children's hospital concerned, she said that nurses were expected to carry on with their duties without support even if children on the ward died.

There was also agreement between participants that nurses lacked self-kindness and compassion. As Rachel, a staff nurse, said:

> "we do lack being able to look after ourselves a wee bit."

Theme 2: compassion in nursing (CIN) is linked with nurses' clinical experience
There was unanimous support for linking adverse incidents involving patients with developing 'fears of compassion'. Jemma, who worked in the CAMHS inpatient unit said such fears were a:

"natural reaction to working somewhere like the inpatient unit."

Meanwhile, Anna, another staff nurse, remarked:

"it's difficult to be compassionate towards people you know have been violent towards people you work with."

The year before this project took place, a young person in CAMHS had died by suicide. Norma, a community nurse reflected on that tragedy:

"..of course that affected everybody and how you managed things, and how you lost confidence in what you were doing."

Theme 3: nursing involves more 'doing' than 'being', and nurses equate being compassionate with being busy

For all participants there was a pressure to be busy and for some there was also a need to be seen to be busy. Rachel summarised this idea well:

"there's certainly a…feeling of if you're not seen to be active or doing something physical therefore you're not doing anything beneficial to people".

Further, for some nurses being busy also served a protective function; the activity prevented them from dwelling on distressing experiences or their own psychological issues. One nurse noted that she found it: "very difficult to settle down" after being involved in incidents where a young person was physically restrained to prevent them attacking other people or themselves.

Theme 4: nurses engage in their own individual and social ways to manage their feelings

Participants reported engaging in a range of diverse individual and social coping mechanisms to 'let off steam'. Susan, another Staff Nurse, said she managed by:

"probably just taking time out by myself…and speaking to people."

Andrew, a community nurse, reported he would:

"talk to my wife, do stuff with my kids, go-kartin'."

There were differences in how useful going to the pub was. Some participants valued this as a 'release valve' after a 'bad day' or particularly busy time. Karen, a nursing assistant, however, did not always like pub events or nights out, because she would feel she was just: "surrounded by the same conversations" there. Some nurses, like Andrew, even wondered if there was any way of managing workplace stress:

"is there anything you could actually do to get rid of that in this job? I dunno if there is…there's always something round the corner in this job."

Theme 5: Mindful Compassion Training for Nurses (MCTN) could benefit nurses in managing their feelings and in sustaining compassion in nursing (CIN)

One of my key aims was to harness a sense of camaraderie and safeness in the MCTN group, partly by making the sessions closed and for nurses only. That aim was achieved in the main. As Anna said:

"it helped that it was just nurses, it felt a bit more relaxed and comfortable, because we were all roughly the same level."

Karen too, thought that the group was: "really comfortable…a nice space." Norma shared this sentiment, however only after several sessions had passed:

"did I feel camaraderie? Eventually, yes. It felt a very safe group…it was good to see familiar faces, it was inspiring and positive that way…people were genuinely keen and everyone contributed."

Another key aim was of course to introduce colleagues to mindfulness and compassion meditation techniques. Anne, firstly, stated that engaging in group practices had made her notice that she was: "really tired", and that she could: "fall asleep like that." She also felt that the practice had made her realise that her:

> "mind's busy a lot of the time…I've got, like a narrative all the time."

Further, she described finding herself: "getting upset a few times" during compassion practices, for example when visualising other people who were suffering, and remarked that MCTN has made her aware that she was:

> "not as kind as I thought I was…I've noticed quite a lot, em, I can be quite stern, maybe I need to work on that a bit."

Despite these issues, and a previous brief trial of meditation practice that left Anne believing it might not: "work for me at all", in MCTN Anne:

> "learned that I can do it and that it benefitted me."

She summarised the sessions as: "quite precious."

For Veronica, another charge nurse, the meditation practice challenge included:

> "nurses are very used to keeping busy, so the idea of just stopping and sitting still just to be and hang out…is really strange."

She too felt sleepy during group practices but ascribed that to initially keeping her eyes shut during them. This was something the author subsequently discussed with the whole group. Then, in Veronica's words:

> "the fact that I could actually do the exercises with my eyes open was a revelation to me."

Veronica also appreciated the definition of compassion provided in MCTN, prior to which she had conceived of compassion as an:

> "amorphous, unstructured thing that you can't really get a grip of."

Like her Cohort One peers, Veronica had, for instance, found it helpful to learn of Gilbert's (2010b) three-way flow of compassion:

> "for yourself, from other people to you, and from you to other people."

Despite this, and previously conceiving of herself as: "a visual person", however, she sometimes found the visualisation aspects of compassion exercises challenging and reported an: "exam pressure" to get them right, a feeling others in the group shared. On the other hand, Veronica found that the MCTN programme also:

> "clarified a couple of things about myself and about…my tendencies to…be… worrying about stuff in the past that I can't actually do anything about now, em, or projecting some terribleness into the future."

Norma also criticised herself sometimes during MCTN experiential exercises:

> "my brain kept challenging myself, c'os every time I would sit and say… 'have peace, have love, have com(passion)'… (a) bit of my head…would contradict it. Immediately my head went to a: 'no, you don't mean this'."

The compassion practices nonetheless led Norma to reflect on CIN. She wondered if nurses sometimes lost compassion: "because of the tough boundaries" they imposed on therapeutic relationships with patients. She ended MCTN with a: "broader understanding of it now", even though it was a: "difficult" concept which nurses can be: "scared of". Norma, like Anne and Veronica, also found it challenging to:

> "have a busy schedule to then come in and just switch off."

Her self-assessment in relation to mindfulness practice was that:

> "I need to practice the being able to sit still…
> but the gentle movement is good for me."

Here, Norma was referring to the yoga and mindful walking introduced in the MCTN programme that, as already stated, the whole group valued highly. Although not referred to in the interview, Norma reported in a group session that she practiced mindful walking to and from her car during and immediately after work, and that doing so helped her both relax and pay more attention to her day.

Karen reported that she found some group practices relaxing too, for example during the session where I invited participants to keep their eyes open during them. At that time she felt:

> "drained in a nice way, really relaxed and not wanting to move."

However, Karen also remarked that sometimes when she had finished a group session she was: "ragin'", and this irritability had been noticed by a colleague. Karen ascribed it to getting in touch with issues which had been troubling her. In her words:

> "it might be subconsciously that I was thinking about things that maybe I could be changing, that I was annoyed at myself for."

Indeed in Karen's interview she gave examples of going on to address personal and social problems from this perspective of considering her own role in maintaining them. Those examples cannot be noted here, however, for ethical reasons.

Karen, Norma, Anne and Veronica all stated that they were aspiring to be kinder towards other people, including colleagues. Notably, most Cohort One participants did little, if any, between-session meditation practice, despite my encouragement to do so. I do not see this as a significant problem; this project was an invitation to colleagues to try the various techniques. They did just that, and indeed committed fully to each group they attended. Further, most participants wanted facilitated mindfulness practice to continue. As Norma said:

> "I need to find a protected time…to do it every day, em, but yeah I'd quite like the teaching of it as well to continue on a weekly basis so I could protect it that way as well."

SUMMARY OF PROJECT INTERVIEW FINDINGS

I believe that during this project my colleagues were describing the following vicious cycle: although nurses aspire to be compassionate, distressing clinical experiences can instil fears of being compassionate; pressure on nurses' time and pressure to be busy, whether internally driven or externally imposed, places further strain on nurses' compassionate intentions; and although nurses can describe personal and social coping strategies, their working environment is continually stressful. Programmes like MCTN could help nurses manage stress and gain broader understanding and experience of compassion, including making important links between self-compassion and kindness for others.

DISCUSSION: HOW THE LIGHT GETS IN

This project is of course small in scale and its findings are not therefore generalisable. Nonetheless I believe the project has something valuable to contribute. I do not believe that my colleagues, the participants, had lost their compassionate intentions and motivation for nursing. Some of them had, however, developed fears of being compassionate. I believe that those two potentially conflicting positions, wanting to be compassionate, but being afraid of it, could ultimately cause problems.

As I noted earlier in this chapter, one of the purposes of realistic evaluation is to produce 'context-mechanism-outcome' (CMO) models. For me, this project suggests the following model:

Contexts and Possible Negative Implications

- Nursing practice, in which compassion is expected and nurses themselves aspire to being compassionate
- Distressing clinical experiences
- Pressure on nurses' time and the pressure to be busy
- (Unintentionally) inadequate personal, social and formal organisational support to meet the demands of the nursing role and sustain compassion

⬇

Mechanism:
- Development of a split between 'being' compassionate and fearing being compassionate

⬇

Potential outcomes
- Nurses losing touch with compassionate intentions
- Increased stress
- Decreased job satisfaction

Figure 6: Context-mechanism-outcome model one: Contexts:

Doing nothing about CIN is not an option. Nurses need access to supportive mechanisms which can help them cope with emotionally demanding roles and sustain compassion. In that respect, programmes like MCTN could usefully support traditional options, such as clinical supervision, whilst also having the potential to facilitate enhanced understanding and even experience of compassion.

This, therefore, is my second CMO model to come from the project:

Contexts and Possible Positive Implications:

- Nursing practice continues as described in model one above
- Mindfulness and compassion meditation group training/ practice sessions

⬇

Mechanisms:

- Safeness, supportiveness and inspiration of the shared group experience
- Yoga, mindful movement and mindful walking facilitate a sense of competence in practising mindfulness and function as a 'good fit' for busy nurses
- Nurses given 'permission' and the means to reduce stress
- Nurses experience increased awareness of own thoughts and feelings
- Nurses introduced to a broader understanding of compassion, including the value of self-compassion

⬇

Outcomes:

- Reduced fears of compassion
- Increased or renewed aspirations to be kinder to others and to be self-compassionate
- Increased responsibility for one's own thoughts, feelings and behaviour, for instance in relation to interpersonal conflict
- Increased interest in mindfulness practice

Figure 7: Context-Mechanism-Outcome model two:

I noted earlier that participants did little between-session practice. I believe that was partly related to the MCTN participants viewing the group as an opportunity to reduce stress. Further, my impression is that they preferred mindfulness to compassion training overall and found the mindfulness techniques had a more immediate impact on their stress levels.

For people who have taught or been taught meditation techniques, this might be unsurprising. Compassion meditation training tends to be described by theorists and practitioners alike as a challenging venture, one which can often stir up strong, sometimes conflicting feelings in participants (Gilbert et al., 2010; and Nairn et al., 2011).

I do not regret the decision to include compassion training, however. It did serve an important function in engaging colleagues in necessary debate about CIN. Indeed, ideally, I would like nurses to take charge of the compassion agenda, rather than having other people's views of it imposed on them. Including (ultimately) my own views. And if is a bit messy getting there, or a bit challenging, I do not think that is a bad thing:

"Only the impossible is worth doing."
Choje Akong Tulku Rinpoche (Kagyu Samye Ling, 2017)

> **Pause and Reflect**
>
> Having read this chapter, what (things) do you think it is that is (are) 'impossible'? If you had a say, what would you want to change about the way nurses work?

FURTHER RESOURCES

Nursing:

NHS Education for Scotland (NES) Nursing and Midwifery: https://www.nes.scot.nhs.uk/education-and-training/by-discipline/nursing-and-midwifery.aspx – NES are responsible for the training and ongoing professional development of registered nurses in Scotland. This page takes you to their main initiatives.

Compassion training:

Kristin Neff: https://self-compassion.org – Kristin is one of the founders of the 'Mindful Self-Compassion' programme, and of course developed the 'Self-Compassion Scale' discussed in this chapter. There is some information about her approach to self-compassion on the website and some free resources.

The Compassionate Mind Foundation: https://compassionatemind.co.uk – this website was set up by Paul Gilbert and colleagues to provide information and resources about their 'Compassionate Mind Training' approach.

REFERENCES

AUDIT SCOTLAND (2018). Health and social care integration: update on progress. Edinburgh: Audit Scotland. Available: http://www.auditscotland.gov.uk/uploads/docs/report/2018/nr_181115_health_socialcare_update.pdf [Date accessed: 29/11/2018]
BALLAT, J. and CAMPLING, P., (2011). Intelligent Kindness: Reforming the Culture of Healthcare. London: Royal College of Psychiatrists.
BEDDOE, A. and MURPHY, S., (2004). Does mindfulness decrease stress and foster empathy among nursing students? Journal of Nurse Education, 43 (7), pp. 305-312.
BENTZ, V., and SHAPIRO, J., (1998). Mindful Inquiry in Social Research. London: Sage Publications, Inc.
BLAND, J., KHAN, H., LODER, J., SYMON, T. and WESTLAKE, S. (2015). The NHS in 2030: a vision of a people-powered, knowledge-powered health system. London: Nesta. Available: https://media.nesta.org.uk/documents/the-nhs-in-2030.pdf [Date accessed: 29/112018]
BRADY, S., O'CONNOR, N., BURGERMEISTER, D., and HANSON, P., (2011). The impact of mindfulness meditation in promoting a culture of safety on an acute psychiatric unit. Perspectives in Psychiatric Care, 48 (3), pp. 129-137.
BRITISH BROADCASTING CORPORATION, THE (BBC) (2018). Carseview drug allegations passed to police. BBC. Available: https://www.bbc.co.uk/news/uk-scotland-tayside-central-44778332 [Date accessed: 29/11/2018]
BURNS, N and GROVES, S., (2010). Understanding Nursing Research. 5th edn. Maryland Heights, Missouri: Elsevier Saunders.
BUTTERWORTH, T., BELL, L., JACKSON, C., and PAJNKIHAR, M., (2008). Wicked spell or magic bullet? A review of the clinical supervision literature 2001-2007. Nurse Education Today, 28, pp. 264-272.
KAGYU SAMYE LING (2017). Quotes. Eskdalemuir, Dumfries: Kagyu Samye Ling. Available: http://www.samyeling.org/quotes/ [Accessed 29/11/2018]

CHODEN and REGAN-ADDIS, H. (2018). Mindfulness based living course. Winchester, UK: O-Books.
CRESWELL, J., and PIANO-CLARK, V., (2011). Designing and Conducting Mixed Methods Research. 2nd edn. London: Sage Publications, Inc.
DE SOUZA, D., (2013). Elaborating the context-mechanism-outcome configuration (CMOc) in realist evaluation: a critical realist perspective. Evaluation, 19 (2), pp. 141- 154.
EDWARDS, R., BRYNING, L., and CRANE, R., (2015). Design of economic evaluations of mindfulness-based interventions: ten methodological questions of which to be mindful. Mindfulness, 6 (3), pp. 490-500
FAHY, N., HERVERY, T., GREER, S., JARMAN, H., STUCKLER, D., GLASWORTHY, M. and MCKEE, M. (2017). How will Brexit affect health and health services in the UK? Evaluating three possible scenarios. The Lancet, 390, pp. 2110-2118.
FRIEDRICH, B., EVANS-LACKO, S., LONDON, J., RHYDDERCH, D., HENDERSON, C., and THORNICROFT, G., (2013). Anti-stigma training for medical students: the education not

discrimination project. The British Journal of Psychiatry, 202, pp. 89-94.
GILBERT, P. and CHODEN, (2013). Mindful Compassion: Using the Power of Mindfulness and Compassion to Transform Our Lives. London: Constable & Robinson Ltd.
GILBERT, P., MCEWAN, K., MATOS, M. and RIVIS, A., (2010). Fears of compassion: development of three self-report measures. Psychology and Psychotherapy, Research and Practice, 84 (3), pp. 239-255.
GOETZ, J., KELTNER, D., and SIMON-THOMAS, E., (2010). Compassion: an evolutionary analysis and empirical review. Psychological Bulletin, 136 (3), pp. 351-374.
HAWKINS, P., and SHOHET, R., (2012). Supervision in the Helping Professions: An Individual, Group and Organizational Approach. 4th edn. Milton Keynes: Open University.
HEFFERNAN, M., GRIFFIN, M., MCNULTY, R. and FITZPATRICK, J., (2010). Self-compassion and emotional intelligence in nurses. International Journal of Nursing Practice, 16, pp. 366-373.
KAGYU SAMYE LING (2017). Quotes. Eskdalemuir, Dumfries: Kagyu Samye Ling. Available: http://www.samyeling.org/quotes/ [Accessed 29/11/2018]
KENDALL, J., (2003). Designing a research project: randomised controlled trials and their principles. Emergency Medicine Journal, 20, pp. 164-168.
MABEN, J., LATTER, S., and CLARK, J., (2007). The sustainability of ideals, values and the nursing mandate: evidence from a longitudinal study. Nursing Inquiry, 14 (2), pp. 99-113.
MCCOWN, D., REIBEL, D. and MICOZZI, M., (2010). Teaching Mindfulness: A Practical Guide for Clinicians and Educators. London: Springer.
NAIRN, R., NIXON, G., CHODEN, REGAN-ADDIS, H., MCMURTRY, D., and CRAIG, L., (2010a). Aberdeen University Postgraduate Studies in Mindfulness MSc Mindfulness Weekend One. Mindfulness Association Ltd.
NAIRN, R., NIXON, G., CHODEN, REGAN-ADDIS, H., and NEVEJAN, A., (2010b). Aberdeen University Postgraduate Studies in Mindfulness MSc Mindfulness Weekend Two. Mindfulness Association Ltd.
NAIRN, R., NIXON, G., CHODEN, REGAN-ADDIS, H., and ADAMS, F., (2011). Aberdeen University Postgraduate Studies in Mindfulness MSc Insight Weekend One. Mindfulness Association Ltd.
NATIONAL HEALTH SERVICE EDUCATION FOR SCOTLAND (NHS NES), (2011). Education and developmental framework for Senior Charge Nurses/ Midwives and team leaders in all areas of practice. Edinburgh: NHS NES. Available:
https://www.nes.scot.nhs.uk/media/261811/edanddev-framework-final-version2011.pdf [Date accessed: 29/11/2018].
NATIONAL HEALTH SERVICE (NHS) TAYSIDE (2018). NHS Tayside announces Chair of Independent Inquiry into mental health services. NHS Tayside. Available:
https://www.nhstayside.scot.nhs.uk/News/Article/index.htm?article=PROD_303238 [Date accessed: 29/11/2018]
NEFF, K., (2003). Development and validation of a scale to measure self-compassion. Self and Identity, 2, pp. 223-250.
NEFF, K. and GERMER, C., (2013). A pilot study and randomized controlled trial of the Mindful Self-Compassion Program. Journal of Clinical Psychology, 69 (1), pp 28-44.
NIXON, G., CHODEN, REGAN-ADDIS, H., and NEVEJAN, A., (2011). Aberdeen University Postgraduate Studies in Mindfulness MSc Compassion Weekend Two. Mindfulness Association Ltd.
NURSING AND MIDWIFERY COUNCIL, THE (NMC) (2015). The code: professional standards of behaviour for nurses, midwives and nursing associates. London: NMC. Available:
https://www.nmc.org.uk/globalassets/sitedocuments/nmc-publications/nmc-code.pdf [Date accessed: 29/11/18]

OWENS, P., and MEIKLE, J., (2013). Mid Staffordshire Trust inquiry report published. The Guardian: Guardian News and Media Ltd. Available:
http://www.theguardian.com/society/blog/2013/feb/06/mid-staffordshire-nhs-trust-inquiry-report-published-live [Date accessed: 21st April 2014].
PAWSON, R. and TILLEY, N., (1997). Realistic Evaluation. London: Sage Publications Ltd.
REPORT OF THE WILLIS COMMISSION, (2012). Quality with Compassion: The Future of Nursing Education. London: The Royal College of Nursing. Available:
https://docplayer.net/19476155-Quality-with-compassion-the-future-of-nursing-education.html [Date accessed: 29/11/2018].
SCOTTISH GOVERNMENT, THE, (2010). The Healthcare Quality Strategy for NHS Scotland. The Scottish Government. Available:
http://www.scotland.gov.uk/Resource/Doc/311667/0098354.pdf [Date accessed: 29/11/2018].
SCOTTISH GOVERNMENT, THE, (2017). Nursing 2030 vision: promoting confident, competent and collaborative nursing for Scotland's future. Edinburgh: The Scottish Government. Available:
https://www.gov.scot/publications/nursing-2030-vision-9781788511001/ [Date accessed: 29/11/2018]
SHAKESPEARE, W. (2015). Macbeth. London: Penguin Classics.
SHAPIRO, S., BROWN, K., and BIEGEL, G., (2007). Teaching self-care to caregivers: effects of mindfulness-based stress reduction on the mental health of therapists in training. Training and Education in Professional Psychology, 1 (2), pp. 105-115.
STEPHENSON, J. (2018). Scotland ramps up efforts to recruit nurses from overseas. London: Nursing Times. Available:
https://www.nursingtimes.net/news/workforce/scotland-ramps-up-efforts-to-recruit-nurses-from-overseas/7024955.article [Date accessed: 29/11/2018]
Partial quotes used in section headings
'Promises to keep', used in the introduction heading, is taken from Robert Frost's (1923) poem: "Stopping by woods on a snowy evening".
'How the light gets in', used in the discussion heading, is taken from Leonard Cohen's (1997) song lyric for: "Anthem", on the album: "The Future", released by Sony Music.

CHAPTER 12

INTRODUCTION TO STORIES OF MINDFUL HEROES IN BUSINESS

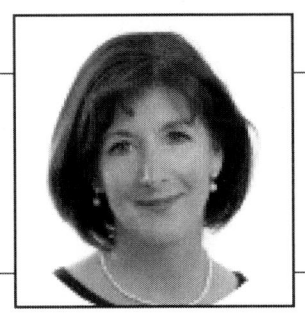

Joanne O'Malley

info@mindfulnessatwork.ie

I set up Mindfulness at Work in 2012 to offer Corporate Mindfulness Programmes that improve both individual and organisational leadership, wellbeing, resilience and relationships. At this stage, I have provided training to thousands of people and feel very privileged to have worked with a great many of the leading organisations in Ireland and internationally.

With continuous advancements in technology, today's workplace is a dynamic, non-stop, information overloaded environment. People spend so much of their time working, and yet for many this is the most stressful and least rewarding part of their lives. The level of personal suffering is often hidden, as people are afraid to admit they are struggling. Paradoxically, success in organisations relies on the very things that disengagement and stress erode: focus, concentration, communication, teamwork, cognitive flexibility and good decision making. Research shows that stressed workers are less engaged, have reduced productivity, high levels of absenteeism and turnover, as well as higher healthcare costs.

The reason I am bringing Mindfulness and Compassion Training to workplace settings, is that these practices have the power to positively transform the way people relate to themselves, their work and even time! I've really enjoyed reading the two business chapters. Both connect closely with my own journey, as well as with the breakthroughs I see in the people I train. The feedback I receive is very similar to the personal accounts included in these chapters.

I admire Tarja's courage in disclosing her 'helplessness' at the outset of her journey forcing her body to be numb and not having any tools to work with her emotions, beliefs and values. She exposes a phenomenon I encounter everyday. Human beings at work struggling with their bodies, minds and hearts; simply not having the awareness and tools to work in a way that is healthy, effective and fulfilling.

The analogy of Boxer from Animal Farm is particularly poignant and resembles a familiar way people deal with the pressure and non-stop demands of work now. Some people are similar to our hero: "beating myself up, being extremely harsh on myself and asking much more from myself than from others." (Tarja, Chapter 14). Tarja recounts how mindfulness led to a shift in her perception, allowing her to start making gradual changes that cultivated mental well-being and enhanced her quality-of-life. She reveals each step of her growing awareness, laying a pathway for you to follow. Each step resonating with my own experience and the experience of many people I have trained. In particular, she stresses how vital self compassion is in enhancing one's relationship with oneself. She explores the courage cultivated by this accepting, compassionate way of relating, breaking free of enslavement to old limiting patterns. Finally, she tells stories of growing new habits that underpin working joyfully and effortlessly.

Boxer never learnt to read (or a better way to work) and he collapsed from overwork. Many working peoples' fate is similar, unless they learn a new literacy: "Mindfulness sheds light into our habitual patterns and reveals our inner drivers... helps to develop the capacity to see more clearly...so that we can make conscious choice" (Tarja, Chapter 14).

The title of Chapter 13: Is there time for Mindfulness in Business? reads like a koan. A koan is a philosophical riddle in Zen practice, used to encourage insight / enlightenment to occur.
Susan admits something that is also true for me and I would imagine many of you...
"to describe time as an illusion felt incredible to me! It challenged a long held unquestioned belief of mine that time is real. But, as my research continued a compelling case to the contrary surfaced" (Susan, chapter 13).

This delusion leads to: 'time famine' and 'sacrifice syndrome', terms used by the author to evoke a sense of the level of suffering that acute time pressure causes. The problematic outcome of this perception is that: "the more you are focused on time, past and future, the more you miss the Now, the most precious thing there is" (Eckhart Tolle, 1997, p.49).

It's baffling because I am old enough to remember a time when we worried about how we could possibly use up all the free time we would have as a result of technology automating and speeding up processes/communication etc. We anticipated a three-day working week.
However, as Susan outlines the impact has been the opposite. People find they are less productive and effective, less able to focus, unable to relax and increasingly stressed and anxious by the very things that were designed to make work easier and more efficient (such as email, computers, mobile phones). In addition, activities that require people to shift their focus between the past and future like strategic planning, goal setting, performance reviewing can be disorientating and result in a lack of presence.

Yet, the truth is: "Any planning as well as working toward achieving a particular goal is done NOW. The enlightened person's main focus of attention is always the Now, but they are still peripherally aware of time..." (Eckhart Tolle, 1997, p.57). In the world of work, learning to 'pay attention' to NOW (mindfulness) is a radically new perspective and a lot of education is still needed. This essential skill has been completely neglected by the educational system. It seems absurd that simple practices like taking a pause and awareness of the breath and body would have the power to change our experience as they do. So, this is not easy to explain coherently and the learning comes experientially.

Susan's exploration of the two states people can be in at work - entanglement and disentanglement is helpful in facilitating understanding. People who practice mindfulness are more aware of where there attention is; so even when involved in thinking, doing, planning, reviewing etc. they benefit from bringing a mindful awareness to it. My own experience and that of my clients supports her findings that this state of awareness allows you see through the illusion of time as something solid and fixed. Instead, of feeling enslaved, you feel empowered which changes your approach to managing time. So though, the skill of mindfulness (like language acquisition), requires time and discipline to gain expertise of this 'new literacy', the result of being mindful at work is more effective use of time.

Unfortunately, this perspective is still new to many people. So, despite the obvious need for mindfulness solutions and the fact that corporate employees are positively disposed to this training, (75% express an openness to attend a course, VHI, 2018), the paradox between trying to cope with a perceived lack of time and creating time for mindfulness practice remains. And there are other significant but not insurmountable workplace barriers.

It's true that workplace culture can either encourage or inhibit a mindful approach to work. Senior management teams play a leading role, as they set the tone for how staffs feel they must behave. Research studies from Harvard University show that when leaders are stressed and anxious, they pass these negative emotions onto the entire organisation.This is a persistent issue.

Traditionally, peoples' humanity and suffering at work was ignored causing dis-engagement statistics to soar. Now, research shows clearly that organisations and businesses do best when they pay attention to the human needs of their workers. Responding compassionately not only improves peoples' performance and loyalty, but also creates an atmosphere that is safe for learning, collaboration, and innovation—which all impact the bottom line.

This is why I advocate Mindful Leadership Training as an essential starting point for companies. Today, leaders need to be enablers; creating the optimum conditions for their employees to be at their best in work. This requires high emotional intelligence; skills that result from Mindfulness Training (Reitz and Chackalson, 2016). As Susan says, leading by example is important and shifting culture requires visible action from senior people in organisations (Susan, Chapter 13).

Finally, it is unlikely that the workplace will slow down, or pressure and distraction will disappear. Yet, our heroes have shown us that when they practiced mindfulness, they changed their perception and experience of work and time. They gained control over their minds and mental/emotional states, and this led to freedom from the automatic reactive and limiting patterns and perceptions in which they were stuck. They could see more clearly what was important and therefore where to invest their energy; they were more effective, compassionate, discerning, relationships improved and lots more…

I hope that the heroes' stories have inspired you to take control of your own mind and heart and develop your ability to work mindfully and joyfully. I'm in agreement with Susan (Chapter 13): "In organisations, presence and being present is where people can offer the greatest level of contribution."

This is your choice. As another hero, Nelson Mandela told us in Long Walk to Freedom: "I realized that they could take everything from me except my mind and my heart. They could not take those things. Those things I still had control over. And I decided not to give them away."

FURTHER RESOURCES

Mindfulness at Work
https://mindfulnessatwork.ie/

REFERENCES

REITZ, M. AND CHACKALSON,M., (2016) How to Bring Mindfulness to Your Company's Leadership. Havard Business Review.
https://hbr.org/2016/12/how-to-bring-mindfulness-to-your-companys-leadership
TOLLE, E. (1997) The Power of Now: A Guide to Spiritual Enlightenment. San Frasico: New World Library
VHI (2018) A Route to Mindfulness: Finding the way to better health in the workplace, Health Insight Report. Dublin : Voluntary Health Insurance.

CHAPTER 13

IS THERE TIME FOR MINDFULNESS IN BUSINESS? MAKING THE CASE FOR A HEALTHIER APPROACH TO TIME.

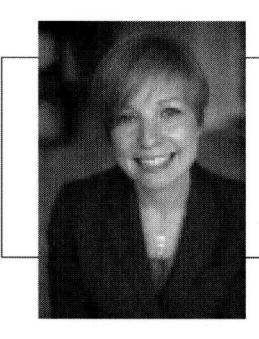

Susan Grandfield

susan@susangrandfield.com

SETTING THE SCENE

PURPOSE AND INTENTION

This chapter reveals both a personal and professional journey into time viewed through a mindful lens. Through my MSc Studies in Mindfulness research and my own experience I have discovered how mindfulness can shift people's experience of time and time pressure. My intention here is to share those discoveries with you. Why? - Because there is a growing trend for people in business to experience acute time pressure on a regular basis leading to time famine and sacrifice syndrome. This trend is having a detrimental effect on people's health, well-being and effectiveness in the workplace and I believe mindfulness could offer a way to reverse that trend. "Right mindfulness recovers for the man the lost pearl of his freedom, snatching it from the jaws of dragon time" (Thera, cited in Taylor, 2008).

MY POINT OF DEPARTURE

My journey began in 2010 when my good friend Laura asked if I'd like to join her on an introductory session for a mindfulness course in Glasgow. Despite being more than a little bit sceptical I said yes, on the proviso that if it felt too "tree-huggy" I wouldn't sign up for the 8-week course. Needless to say, not only did I sign up for the course, I completed it, continued to develop my personal practice for 8 years, completed a master's degree and became a qualified mindfulness teacher!

That introductory session connected with a deep sense that I was missing out on the experience of living by being more concerned with what might happen next than what was actually happening now. I was an ambitious person who had spent 10 years in the corporate world in Human Resources and Learning and Development before stepping out and setting up my own coaching and training business. I recognised that I was on a treadmill - always focused on moving forward, achieving, striving - and that at some point the treadmill would stop and I'd be in a wooden box. A bit of a wake-up call you could say (and I was only 35 years old at the time!). This was the point of departure on my hero's journey.

WHERE PERSONAL AND PROFESSIONAL CONTEXTS COLLIDE

Developing my mindful practice and experiencing how it influenced my life inevitably influenced my work. I felt more present with my clients and noticed that had a positive impact on them, so I gradually started to integrate mindfulness into my client work.

The experience of integrating my practice into my professional context is why I chose to do the masters through the University of Aberdeen. As Graeme Nixon described in Chapter 3, the University's intention is to offer students the opportunity to explore mindfulness in a variety of contexts and to make that exploration and research real and meaningful to them. The idea that I could not only deepen my learning and practice of mindfulness but also contribute to two things I felt very passionate about - mindfulness and personal development in the business world - clinched the deal for me. And so, my journey continued.

A JOURNEY INTO TIME

In my 20 years as a coach and trainer one enduring challenge has kept emerging with my clients - how to manage time. The increasing pace of work and the drive to do more with less have contributed to a feeling of time scarcity, sacrifice and lack of fulfilment. The knock-on effect on people's mental and physical health is staggering. A YouGov poll in 2018 found that 74% of people feel so stressed that they have become overwhelmed and unable to cope.

One solution for organisations is to offer time management training, which they have been doing for decades. Yet, this approach does not seem to have mitigated the crisis we find ourselves in today and, having delivered this type of training myself in the past, I feel that the problem perhaps lies in the misleading message that time is something we can "manage".

MY QUEST

I set out with the aim of exploring how mindfulness influences the way people relate to time in organisations and as a result offers an alternative approach to traditional time management training to enable people to thrive in busy, time pressured workplaces. I was particularly interested in:

- the effect mindfulness has on people's perceptions of time
- how mindfulness influences their relationship with time
- how people bring mindfulness practice into their work and the impact that has

Exploring these questions helped me answer the big question - Is there time for mindfulness in business?

In all of the organisations I've worked with over the years, if an idea, initiative or system did not offer tangible benefits (and usually the quicker the better) then it would not get the same time, money or energy investment that would be given to something which could demonstrate a clear return on that investment. I think the same applies to mindfulness. In an environment where time is scarce the only way to encourage people to explore something which requires an investment of time (like practicing mindfulness) is to be able to demonstrate that it makes a difference to the individual and can therefore make a difference to the performance of a team and the whole organisation. That is where my research aims to make a contribution. Before I set the scene and share the highlights from my research, I'd like to invite you to pause and consider your own relationship with time.

Pause and Reflect

What part does time play in your day?
What is your experience of time pressure?
How does it feel?
What is your current approach to time management?

WHAT OTHERS HAD TO SAY ABOUT MINDFULNESS AND TIME

OUR ENSLAVEMENT WITH TIME

There was a time when time did not exist. That is hard for us to comprehend in our time obsessed world but time, in its present form, is socially constructed. Time has developed a solidity and value that is based on how humans have related to it over centuries. Barbara Adam (2004) offers a comprehensive and complex exploration of the evolution of time and concludes that time is something humans have been on a quest to control ever since we realised that certain events in the flow of life could be predicted (such as the changing seasons and night turning into day). As a result, we developed ways to define, categorise and label this flow of life into the units we now refer to as "time".

Tom Evans (2015) describes the point at which there was a collective awareness of time as the point we also became enslaved by it. He states that much of our suffering at the hands of time comes from the relationship we have with it and the desire to want to control it. So, how did we get here? How did we evolve from a place where life flowed without our intervention, to a place where we are obsessed with "managing time"?

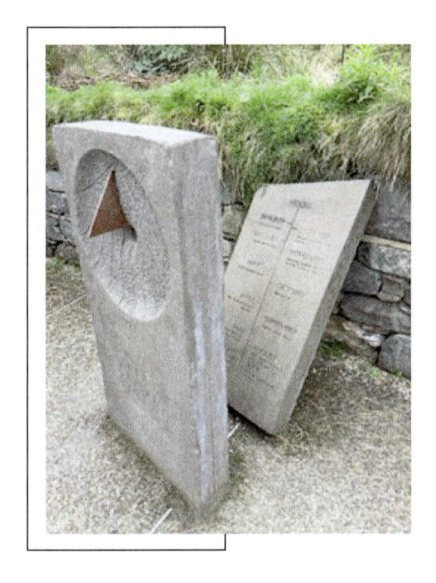

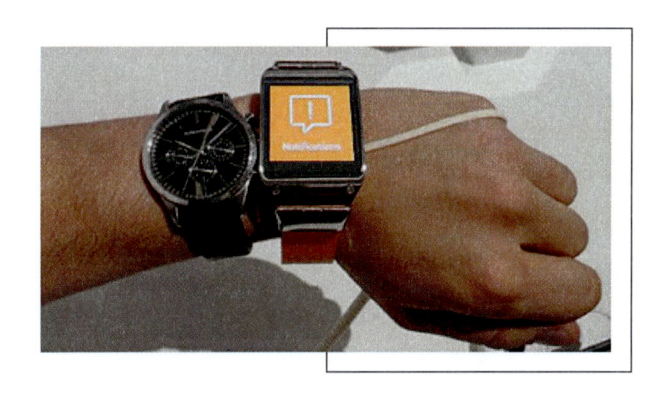

*Figure 1a: Example of early time pieces,
Photo © Susan Grandfield 2017*

*Figure 1b: Current time pieces,
Wikimedia Commons contributors*

As I discovered, there have been some critical points in the evolution of time. These include the advent of clock time in the 14th century and the invention of pocket watches in the 17th century. Being able to measure and mark time became an integral part of how people and communities worked collectively, traded and co-ordinated activities with others. In the 19th century, Fredrick Taylor's time and motion studies demonstrated a growing interest in the management of time as a resource to increase productivity and competitive advantage (Taylor, 2008). Whilst this approach yielded progress in industry and production, the movement towards controlling, compressing, commodifying and colonising time (the 4C's as described by Adam) resulted in some unintended consequences for us today.

Many people now find themselves being less productive and effective, less able to focus, unable to relax and increasingly stressed and anxious by the very things which were designed to make our lives easier and more efficient (such as e-mail, computers, mobile phones). The resulting effect is time famine (Perlow, 1999) and sacrifice syndrome (Boyatiz & McKee, 2013) which are experienced by more and more of us as the pressure to do more with less increases and our ability to switch off decreases. The impact of this is wide reaching in terms of mental and physical health and the subsequent impact on productivity, effectiveness and engagement in the workplace. Yet, if time is something we have constructed, can't we re-create it? This was an interesting question that arose from my initial research. I found myself asking, "has time itself remained unchanged through this evolution and is it simply our relationship with time that has changed?" If so, "do we have the opportunity to re-engage with time in a way which mitigates these negative effects?"

OUR SHIFTING RELATIONSHIP WITH TIME

Time is lived, experienced, known, theorised, created, regulated, solid and controlled. It is contextual and historical, embodied and objectified, abstracted and constructed, represented and commodified (Adam, 2004).

There are many layers and facets to time and the way in which we relate to it. Our sense of time emerges about the same time as our sense of self, around 5 years old. As newborns we are timeless and even as young children time has no meaning for us. As our sense of self develops we begin to see ourselves as separate from others and as having experiences occurring in a linear timeframe - past, present and future (Taylor, 2008).

Past, present and future are concepts we frequently talk about in relation to mindfulness. Being present is at the core of mindfulness practice; recognising when our thoughts have pulled us into the past or drawn us into the future and bringing our attention back to the present moment. However, in business a great deal of energy is directed towards the future and to using the past as a way of defining, forecasting or predicting how the future will look. Strategic planning, goal setting, performance reviewing and so on require people to shift between the past and the future. In my experience, this can often result in a lack of presence. Here is where mindfulness and time start to dance with each other. At this point it is useful to pose the question - what is time? Is it the numbers on a clock? Is it the dates on a calendar? Or is it in fact an illusion of the mind?

WHAT IS TIME?

To describe time as an illusion felt incredible to me! It challenged a long held, unquestioned belief of mine that time is real. But as my research continued a compelling case to the contrary surfaced. If we go back to Greek mythology we discover that they had two words for time - chronos and kairos. Chronos referring to the chronological passing of hours and minutes and kairos referring to an openness to the experience of time, to making the most of it and taking advantage of opportunities as they present themselves (Kairos Momentum, 2011). In the context of this research kairos bears a striking resemblance to mindfulness. Less about a linear, fixed and pre-conceived view of the world; more fluid, open, curious and attentive to each moment.

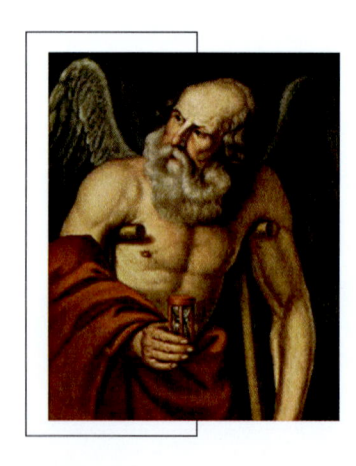

Figure 2a: Chronos by Artus Wolffort (1581-1641) Wikimedia Commons contributors

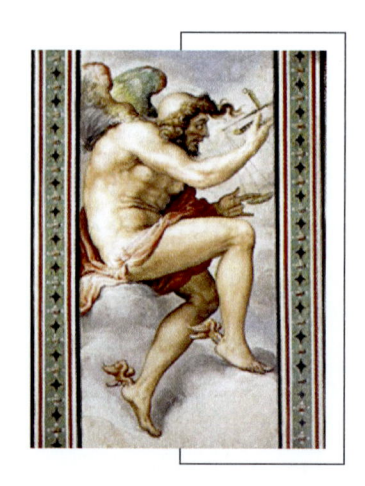

Figure 2b: Kairos by Francesco de'Rossi (2010) Wikimedia Commons contributors

The Greeks were not the only people to offer an alternative view to the one that time is linear or universally experienced. Social scientists and anthropologists through history have offered up the possibility that time is non-linear, is psychological and can be experienced differently by two people at the same time and by one individual in different circumstances. Mihaly Csikszentmihalyi (1980) suggested it is possible to experience timelessness in certain situations when we get into a state of Flow. When we are in Flow time seems to disappear. We become focused, we perform at our best, we can do what we are doing with ease. There is a sense of being totally connected to whatever we are doing. Rudd et al (2012) conducted a study in which they found that when we experience awe we experience a sense of having more time and being less impatient which results in a greater sense of satisfaction. Similarly, Eckhart Tolle (1999) proposed that when we let go of ego (which happens when we are in Flow) our experience of time expands and we are less constrained by past, present and future thinking. So, where does that leave us today?

> **Pause and Reflect**
>
> Take a moment to reflect on your experience of Flow and the impact it has on you:
> Bring to mind a time when you felt in Flow:
> What were you doing?
> How did you feel?
> What did you notice?

HOW WE RELATE TO TIME TODAY

There is an interesting paradox in how we relate to time today. On one hand many of us feel we are too busy, that we don't have enough time to do what we need to do. And yet, we tend to get bored if we find ourselves with time on our hands! We are constantly seeking simulation from smart phones, tablets, iPods etc.

"Each of us gets the same twenty-four hours in a day......we fill those hours with so much doing that we scarcely have time for being" (Kabat-Zinn, cited in Good et al, 2016). Our everyday lives are guided by chronos, linear time. We organise our day into chunks of time which are defined by the numbers on a clock. We co-ordinate with other people using the common language of time. We are often at the mercy of other people's time frames e.g. bus or train timetables, shift working patterns, retail opening hours. Despite this enslavement to an externally defined time structure (which we seek to fill up with activity) there is a growing recognition of the value and benefit of the kairos, non-linear way of relating to time, of slowing down and being less concerned with filling our time.

The Slow Movement is one example of that. It began in 1986 when Carolo Petrini set up the slow food movement in protest against the opening of a McDonalds in one of the famous Piazza's in Rome (Honore, 2005). The slow movement has been described as a cultural revolution against the notion that faster is always better. Now the movement is entering a host of different areas of life including travel, gardening and parenting. It seems that people are recognising that the fast pace at which they live their lives is neither sustainable nor healthy and so they are looking for a way to re-balance and re-connect. However, is this compatible with business? Some believe it is not, that you can't stay competitive if you slow down. On the other hand, there are an increasing number of people and organisations who are recognising the value that the clarity and awareness that comes from slowing down can bring; shifting from a mind-filled state to a mindful state (Nakai & Schultz, 2000).

THE DANCE BETWEEN ENTANGLEMENT AND DISENTANGLEMENT

Let's look into the question of whether it is desirable or even possible to be mindful in a busy, target driven business environment. Some research suggests that mindfulness is incompatible with certain work environments or jobs. My concern is that this may be holding organisations back from embracing a more mindful way of working. But what if it is not a case of either/or? What if it's not a case of being busy and future focused at the expense of mindfulness or that being mindful comes at the expense of achieving goals and getting tasks done?

Lyddy and Good (2017) describe two states people can be in at work - entanglement and disentanglement. As you might imagine, entanglement is when we are in "doing" mode, we have our head down, getting on with tasks and caught up in our thinking. I'm sure you know how that feels and recognise that some days you get into this mode without being aware that it's happened. You'll also know how it feels to be disentangled. That is when the mind is quieter, there is a feeling of spaciousness, we have lifted our head up and can see more clearly. We become more aware of "being". We dance between these two modes throughout our day but unless we are aware it's happening and are able to make the shift consciously, our environment, other people or our habits determine which mode we find ourselves in. Similarly, to Lyddy and Good, I discovered that people who practice mindfulness notice when they have shifted between modes and are able to activate the state of disentanglement for longer which results in a continuity of mindfulness. That means even when they are involved in thinking, doing, planning, reviewing and so on, they benefit from bringing a mindful awareness to it. The implications of this for time management are that if we are able to disentangle ourselves from our thoughts and habitual "doing" we will be able to see more clearly where to place our attention and energy; resulting in a more effective use of time.

VIEWING TIME THROUGH A MINDFUL LENS

Two factors stood out from the research as I began to look at time through a mindful lens - clarity and intention. In Geoff McKeown's book "essentialism" (2014) he highlights the importance of becoming very clear of our intention and focusing our energy and attention in that direction as a way to transform our productivity, effectiveness and wellness. Lyddy & Good's study suggests that mindfulness practice enables people to be aware of deadlines and priorities but not be controlled by them in the same way. It seems mindfulness helps people have the headspace in which to make more effective decisions about what to do, when to do it and how.

Studies in the field of neuroscience offer substance to these claims with research pointing towards the positive impact mindfulness can have on how the brain deals with challenges such as mind wandering, attention, overloaded working memory and stress. Brewer et al (2011) found that experienced meditators showed reduced activation in the neural networks associated with mind wandering. Cahn & Polich (2009) concluded from their research that the attentional control developed through mindfulness results in practitioners using less mental processing unnecessarily and therefore being more efficient with their attention. I'd like to add to this debate by sharing with you what I discovered as I explored the experience of mindfulness practitioners in the business world.

WHAT I DISCOVERED

A MAP OF MY JOURNEY

As research was a new discipline for me I approached it with a mindful attitude of curiosity, non-judgement and patience. I chose to use a qualitative methodology, in part because numbers are not my thing(!) but more seriously because I felt I'd gain more insight and understanding of how mindfulness has an impact on our relationship with time and to do that I felt I needed to have conversations with people about their lived experience.

I carried out in-depth interviews with 4 participants all of whom were recruited from my professional network. I conducted 2 interviews with each participant between 5-8 weeks apart. The first interviews were semi-structured and as I moved into the second interviews I chose to go with an unstructured approach. From the 8 interviews I extracted themes about their experience of time in the workplace and of practicing mindfulness. The participants came from a variety of business backgrounds and all had some level of experience of mindfulness ranging from; starting an on-line 8-week course to 20+ years of mindfulness practice.

THE 3 A'S - A MODEL FOR A MINDFUL APPROACH TO TIME IN BUSINESS

The most striking theme that emerged from my research was how people relate to time now compared to how they related to it before they began practicing mindfulness. Where previously time was seen as a resource to be managed, planned and programmed, now they were able to experience time as a flowing, moving element of their day. This improved the quality of their work, the quality of their experience and their ability to get things done. There seemed to be 3 factors which contributed to this shift which I've defined as the 3 A's: Attitude, Attention and Action.

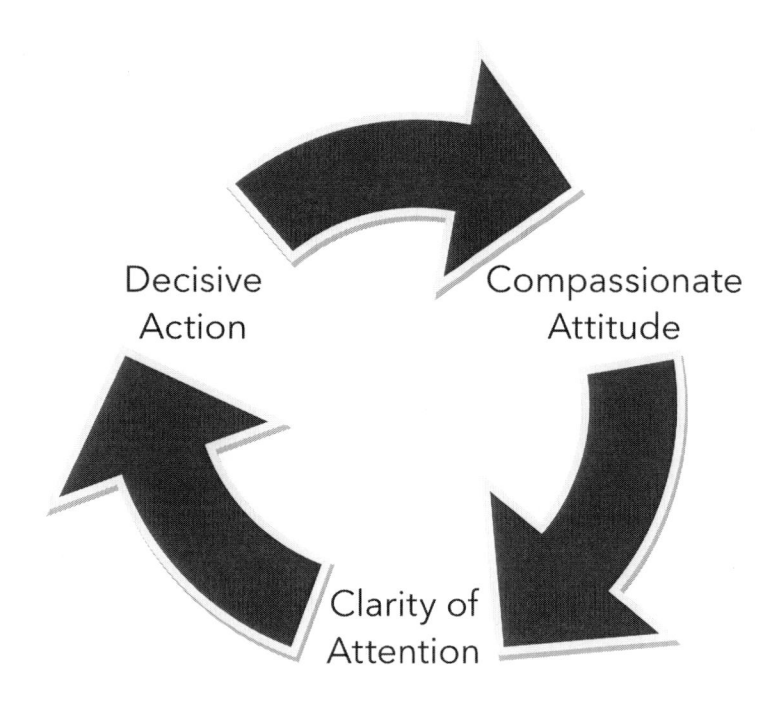

Figure 3: The 3A's - A Model for a Mindful Approach to Time in Business

COMPASSIONATE ATTITUDE

The attitude participants displayed was of openness, curiosity and compassion. They described how they felt less constrained by time and more empowered, as if they had more choice about how to use their time. They found themselves choosing quality of experience over quantity. This was not just in terms of the tasks they faced each day but also in terms of the interactions they had with other people. They became curious and open to finding more effective ways to achieve what they needed to achieve both in work and outside of work. They described stepping out of their old routines, being willing to slow down and take time to work out what to do next rather than rushing on to the next task simply to get it finished. It was like they were bringing a beginner's mind to their to-do list.

A sense of compassion came through in how they described approaching their working day. They were less hard on themselves if they didn't manage to achieve everything they wanted to in a given time period, recognising that often they set their expectations too high to be achievable in the first place. They were also less hard on other people and described a compassionate attitude towards colleagues, their boss or staff members who they could see where struggling to deal with time pressure.

CLARITY OF ATTENTION

Where and how they focused their attention also changed. It emerged that through formal and informal mindfulness practice they were able to see more clearly what was important and therefore where to invest their energy. All the participants described the importance of making the most of their time and as such checked in with themselves regularly to notice what they were doing and whether that was the right thing to be doing in that moment.

Having a clear sense of intention and purpose seemed to act as a reference point from which participants could make moment by moment choices about how to spend their time. Knowing what was needed from them (by others) or what they wanted to achieve each day enabled them to prioritise their activities. Sometimes this meant they recognised an imbalance in how they were spending their time (e.g. between work and home or between completing a task and engaging with their team) and felt more confident about taking action to address it. Focusing their attention on a clear intention and purpose also helped them to manage distractions. When they felt drawn to engage in a distraction such as an email or a ringing phone, it was easier to ignore or put off until later if they had a clear purpose or sense of commitment to what they were doing at that moment. Saying "no" was also made easier by this clarity of focus enabling them to manage their workload and daily to-to list more effectively.

DECISIVE ACTION

The shift in attitude and attention positively impacted on the action participants then took. All of the participants, to some extent, explained how their approach to managing their time had shifted as a result of practicing mindfulness. They described the paradox between structure and fluidity and how striking a balance between the two was critical to effectively (and mindfully) managing their time. They described using useful practices such as; prioritising, writing to-do lists, using a diary and having a notebook to record tasks and activities. It was interesting that instead of applying structure and process rigidly they recognised the importance of being more flexible in their approach to time and allowing fluidity to emerge.

The image this created in my mind was of stepping stones across a flowing river. The stones being the priorities which form the structure for the day and the space around the stones where the water flows representing the fluidity. Traditional time management practices of prioritising and planning are important and useful but what is more useful is the ability to allow space in one's day for the natural flow of life to occur and in which to respond to the unexpected. (Because life doesn't always fit neatly into a four-box model!).

IS THERE TIME FOR MINDFULNESS IN BUSINESS?

Taking all of the above into account, the answer to the big question I was asking is simply....."Yes". We should be creating more time for mindfulness in business because it offers a way of being which has many positive implications.

According to the participants in my study, the impact of their shift in attitude, attention and action was:

- improved quality of work
- greater sense of achievement and getting things done
- less time wasted
- improved quality of time with others (e.g. family, customers)
- less multi-tasking and more focus

I didn't ask participants to quantify these (which would be worth exploring further) however there are clearly financial, productivity and efficiency benefits to be gained from people delivering higher quality work, being more focused, wasting less time and connecting with others more effectively.

Whilst the aim of this research was to explore time and mindfulness, what emerged from all participants was the wider impact of mindfulness on their work and their lives. In different ways, each participant volunteered the broader benefits they have experienced which include health, well-being, energy management, ability to take different perspectives and clarity of mind. Clearly there are reasons beyond time management which support mindfulness in business. An important question to address, however, is how to make time for mindfulness practice when people feel they have a lack of time to do what is already on their to-do list.

ADDRESSING THE PARADOX

It was clear that participants noticed a difference in their day when they practiced mindfulness. They experienced value from clarity, focus and awareness. Three participants talked about how they have integrated formal and/or informal practice into their day and how it frequently feels effortless to be mindful. The participant who was the least experienced mindfulness practitioner did not report the same level of insight and ability to manage their time mindfully as the other participants did. This reinforced the point that the more we practice mindfulness the more benefit we experience.

Another participant highlighted the time investment required to practice mindfulness stating that it shouldn't be underestimated. I agree and feel it is important to address the paradox between trying to cope with a perceived lack of time and creating time for mindfulness. When faced with a decision between taking 10 minutes to meditate or 10 minutes to finish an important report for your boss, it is easy to see why many people may fall at the first hurdle of establishing a mindfulness practice. It is the classic chicken and egg scenario....."if I had more time I'd practice mindfulness but if I don't practice mindfulness I don't feel I have the time". How do we break out of this cycle? What bearing does the culture of the organisation have on whether people feel they can make the time for mindfulness?

RE-DEFINING OUR RELATIONSHIP WITH TIME IN BUSINESS

Exploring organisational culture was not in the initial plan for my research but it emerged as a challenge participants faced. They described how other people had an impact on how they were able to bring a mindful approach to work. At a micro level, the demands and energy of colleagues or customers could disrupt their flow and at the macro level, the culture of the organisation could inhibit or prevent a mindful approach to work.

There needs to be a more sincere recognition of time as a driver of people's behaviour, an acceptance of the negative impact that has and a willingness to explore new ways of working which support the stepping stone approach to time management. It isn't enough to offer people time management training or mindfulness training because neither, in themselves, will change the organisational landscape people are working in. There is, therefore, both an individual and an organisational responsibility to confront this situation and re-define our relationship with time in work.

THE RETURN

Exploring time made me, as well as the research participants, think about it in a way which we had not done before. We looked at it from different angles, we viewed ourselves interacting with it and we stood back and considered how our mindfulness journeys have influenced our approach to time. Just as Joseph Campbell describes in the hero's journey (take a look at Chapter 2 for more on this), I was changed by my experience of researching this topic. I'd like to share the insights I have gained from my experience of this process and to offer those of you in the business world a new approach to time management and those of you in the mindfulness community a new perspective on mindfulness.

FREEING OURSELVES FROM OUR ENSLAVEMENT WITH TIME

I set out to explore if mindfulness could offer an alternative approach to traditional time management training to enable people to thrive in busy, time pressurised workplaces. My journey revealed that mindfulness practice creates a shift in how people think about and relate to time which changes their approach to managing time. Instead of feeling constrained by time they feel freer and more empowered. It is not that mindfulness creates more time but that how we relate to time and the choices we make about how and what we do is influenced by the practices and attitudes that mindfulness cultivates.

The mindfulness practitioners I spoke to experience time as more than simply clock time. They each described how important quality of time is for them and the conscious and considered way in which they now engage with activities. They find themselves less and less enslaved by or entangled in time. It appears to me that simply pausing to reflect on our relationship with time begins the process of changing our relationship with it. I hope that this chapter has begun to serve you in that way.

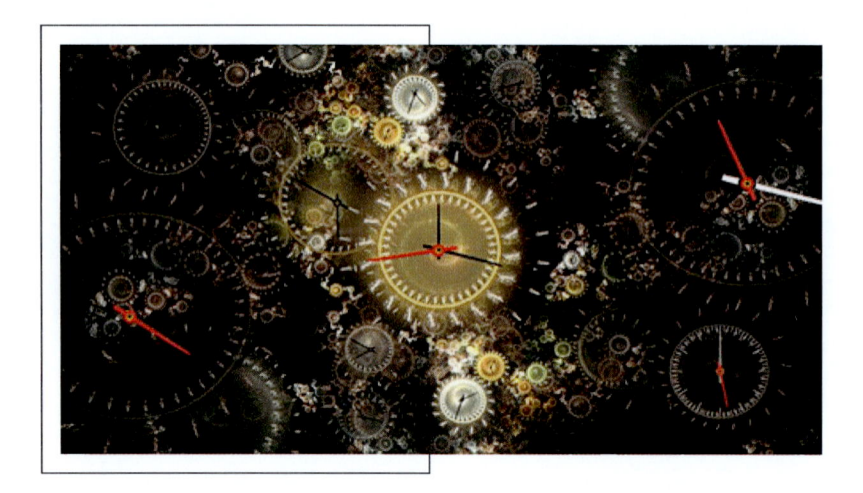

Figure 4: Reflections on time, Mobilos 2013 Wikimedia Commons contributors

Pause and Reflect

What has resonated with you on this journey into time so far?
What does this tell you about your relationship with time?

WHAT IT MEANS FOR BUSINESS

If you recognise the effects time pressure is having on your staff or are considering how mindfulness could benefit your organisation, I have 3 recommendations for you:

1. Stop running time management training courses

The main finding in my research was that people benefit most from being able to balance structure with fluidity. This is something which can't be taught to people in a single intervention like a training course. Striking that balance requires practice and the ability to adapt to moment by moment changes. It is hard to bring the reality of everyday life into a training room and so I'd suggest that there is an opportunity to replace skills-based time management training with a more blended approach.

The reality is that life throws us curve balls all the time. Our ability to manage our attention is tested constantly in a busy work environment and, as was discussed earlier in the chapter, other people can also impact on our good intentions when it comes to managing our time. So, we need to support people to recognise when they are in a state of entanglement (or caught up in their thinking) and to develop the ability to transition into disentanglement. This requires people to become more consciously aware of what is going on as it happens rather than trying to recall it as they sit in a training room. Encouraging people to begin to explore their relationship with time by looking at key elements such as managing distractions, developing clarity and focus, working with purpose and managing energy levels is important. Through short facilitated sessions people can begin to explore the ways in which they can build structure into their day (stepping stones) whilst also becoming aware of the need to allow fluidity and space (space for the water to flow).

Being comfortable with allowing space to be more flexible with time is where my 3A's Model for a Mindful Approach to Time in Business comes in. Developing the compassionate attitude, clarity of attention and decisive action that results in a healthier approach to time management takes time and comes with practice. One training session won't be enough. Giving people the opportunity to check in with themselves regularly in small groups, to share experiences, explore ways to support each other and identify opportunities to improve how they approach work would add value.

2. Take a broader view

Don't consider time management in isolation. The causes of time pressure are not just down to people's inability to plan and prioritise. It is important to think about the wider system in which individuals are operating. Workload, team dynamics, leadership, systems and processes and technology are all factors which regularly eat into people's time and sap their energy. If poor time management appears to be the cause of stress, missed deadlines, poor standard of work and so on, I'd encourage you to step back and take a broader view. There may be a different reason.

There is a cultural aspect to how people relate to time. In many of the organisations I have worked with it is common for people to have back to back meetings taking up their whole day, to take work home regularly to meet deadlines and to spend hours of their day just answering emails. Working in this kind of environment will make it very difficult for even the most mindful of people to maintain balance. In fact, in my experience the most mindful people would choose not to work in such an environment.

By becoming aware of the common practices in your organisation you may recognise that a broader review of how people use their time could be of value. This is where engaging your leaders will be crucial to success. To create a shift in culture (e.g. stopping endless meetings or excessive emails) will require some visible action from senior people in the organisation. If people see them relating differently to time it will send a strong message about what is accepted and expected.

3. Advocate "the pause"

In my research, much of the benefit participants experienced came from pausing at various points in their day: stepping back from engaging in activity and allowing themselves to shift out of autopilot and into mindful awareness. It benefits decision making, creative thinking, communication, stress management (to name but a few!). Taking time away to meditate at work can feel like a big step and it is far easier for people to see the possibility of pausing in the midst of a busy day for a few minutes. Advocating regular pauses doesn't mean scheduling them at specific times of the day or even defining when and how people pause (introduced this way it simply becomes another thing to do). Instead make it clear that taking a few moments to step back and become present are encouraged. Leading by example is important and if leaders began meetings with a short pause, perhaps a breathing space, that would send a signal that the organisation sees the value in slowing down and investing a moment to be present. Pressing pause allows people the space to become more present. In organisations, and in life, presence and being present is where people can offer the greatest level of contribution.

WHAT IT MEANS FOR THE MINDFULNESS COMMUNITY

For those of you who are mindfulness practitioners/teachers working with people in organisations the first thing to say is that there is a huge opportunity for you to help individuals and whole organisations tackle this perennial problem of time and at the same time help them improve productivity and effectiveness, reduce stress and enhance performance. The point above about taking a broader view applies here as well. You need to be aware of the impact that the culture of an organisation has on people's ability to be mindful at work. What are the norms, accepted (and expected) practices and behaviours which will support or detract from a more mindful approach to time?

When engaging with an organisation a key first step is to get a sense of whether mindfulness is being seen as a "quick fix" or whether there is a wider context in which the organisations sees mindfulness playing a part. It can be very tempting to deliver taster session and lunch and learn sessions (which are very useful and I'm not suggesting you stop running them), but too often what they do is dangle the carrot of possibility in front of people and when they leave the meeting room they get sucked back into the organisational system and revert to habits.

How we introduce mindfulness plays a big part in whether it continues to have an impact beyond the introductory session. As my study shows, even novice practitioners can be motivated and inspired to approach what they do differently through an awareness of mindfulness and some basic mindfulness practices. The sustainable benefits such as ability to focus, manage distractions and be purposeful were more pronounced in those who had received mindfulness training, who had a regular practice and had regular contact with other mindfulness practitioners. This suggests that creating more opportunities for people to easily access regular mindfulness practice sessions is important.

Seeing mindfulness through the lens of time management may have opened up a new avenue for you to explore. Whether you work with individuals or groups, in organisations or in your community there is a pretty good chance that time comes up in your discussions (even if only in relation to how to find the time to practice). The fundamental message is that time is not as solid and fixed as we think. Acknowledging the way in which we have been conditioned to relate to time and opening up to the possibility that we can relate differently to it, serves to give us more options about how and when we allocate time to our practice.

A few quotes from my participants are worth sharing as a way of reminding ourselves of the value in investing time to practice mindfulness:

> I'm slowing down and it's actually giving me more time

> How I work with time and my experience of delivering my job has been improved [through mindfulness] there's no doubt

> I think what mindfulness does for me is it gives me a greater clarity about what matters in the first place

FINAL REFLECTIONS

We are living in a time where time has become ingrained in our everyday life and work. It is unlikely that we are going to dispense with all of the clocks, timetables and calendars as a way to free ourselves from the constraints and pressures of time. But we are also living in a time where time is still evolving. The 24-hour culture means we have access to many goods and services whenever we want them. Technology has enabled us to be able to work whenever and wherever we need to and to do so more efficiently. No longer do we need worry if we miss our favourite TV programme because they are available on-demand whenever we are ready to watch them. This all points to the fact that time has already become more fluid for us.

So, how we relate to time is still evolving. Mindfulness can support this evolution by enabling us to make more conscious, healthy decisions about that relationship. The experience of exploring this topic has had a profound impact on me how I respond to time pressure. I am also noticing when I talk to people about my research there is a shift in awareness that happens for them too. It seems that just turning our attention towards time and pausing to recognise our own habits and behaviours opens up the potential for change.

I see the findings from my research as an opportunity to open up new conversations with people in organisations about how to shift perspectives of time and the controlling influence it has on us and to create a movement towards a new, more balanced approach to how we get things done. It is not about getting rid of the structure that time gives us but there is a middle way which combines it with a greater sense of empowerment and fluidity.

Final pause

Before rushing on to the next chapter or your next activity, allow yourself a moment or two to absorb what you have read here.

How are you feeling?
What are you thinking?
How has your perspective on time shifted as you read this chapter?
What adjustments can you make to ease any time pressure you feel in your life or work?

FURTHER RESOURCES

Copies of:

- "Pressing Pause: a practical guide to mindfulness in everyday life"
- "Pressing Pause: developing a healthier approach to time"
  can be downloaded from my website - http://www.sgdevelopmentsolutions.com

REFERENCES

ADAM, B., (2004). Time. Cambridge. Polity.
ALLEN, D., (2002). Getting things Done: The Art of Stress-free Productivity. Piatkus.
BABAUTA, L., (2012). Zen to Done: The Ultimate Simple Productivity System. Phatbits LLC
BENTZ, V.M. and SHAPIRO, J.J., (1998). Mindful inquiry in social research. Sage Publications.
BOYATZIS, R. and MCKEE, A., (2013). Resonant Leadership: Renewing Yourself and Connecting with Others Through Mindfulness, Hope and Compassion. Harvard Business Press.
BREWER, J.A., WORHUNSKY, P.D., GRAY, J.R., TANG, Y.Y., WEBER, J. and KOBER, H., (2011). Meditation experience is associated with differences in default mode network activity and connectivity. Proceedings of the National Academy of Sciences of the United States of America, 108(50), pp. 20254-20259.
CAHN, B.R. and POLICH, J., (2009). Meditation (Vipassana) and the P3a event-related brain potential. International Journal of Psychophysiology, 72(1), pp. 51-60.
CSIKSZENTMIHALYI, M., (1990). Flow and the psychology of discovery and invention. New York: Harper Collins.
EVANS, T., (2015) Managing Time Mindfully: A Mindful Approach to Time Management. Tmesis.
HONORE, C., (2005). In Praise of Slowness. HarperCollins.
KABAT-ZINN, J., (2009). Full Catastrophe Living, Revised Edition: How to cope with stress, pain and illness using mindfulness meditation. Hachette UK.
KAIROS MOMENTUM (2011). cited on http://www.kairosmomentum.com/ [date accessed: 9th August 2017].
KVALE, S. and BRINKMANN, S., (2009). Interviews: Learning the craft of qualitative research interviewing. Sage.
LYDDY, C.J. and GOOD, D.J., (2017). Being While Doing: An Inductive Model of Mindfulness at Work. Frontiers in Psychology 7:2060. doi: 10.3389/fpsyg.2016.02060
McKEOWN, G., (2014). essentialism; The disciplined pursuit of less. Random House.
NAKAI, P. and SCHULTZ, R., (2000). The mindful corporation: Liberating the human spirit at work. Leadership Press (Long Beach, CA).
PERLOW, L.A., (1999). The time famine: Toward a sociology of work time. Administrative Science Quarterly, 44(1), pp. 57-81.
RUDD, M., VOHS, K.D. and AAKER, J., (2012). Awe expands people's perception of time, alters decision making, and enhances well-being. Psychological science, 23(10), pp.1130-1136.
TAYLOR, S., (2008). Making Time. Icon Books
TOLLE, E., (1999). The Power of Now. Hatchette.
YouGov poll cited on https://www.mentalhealth.org.uk/statistics/mental-health-statistics-stress [accessed 23/05/18]
WIKIMEDIA COMMONS CONTRIBUTORS, Hi-tech@Mail.Ru Commons, the free media repository, https://commons.wikimedia.org/wiki/File:Samsung_Galaxy_Gear_Comparison.jpg [accessed 02/11/18]
WIKIMEDIA COMMONS CONTRIBUTORS, 'File:Artus Wolffort - Chronos.jpg', Wikimedia Commons, the free media repository, https://commons.wikimedia.org/w/index.php?title=File:Artus_Wolffort_-_Chronos.jpg&oldid=314906759 [accessed 17/08/18]
WIKIMEDIA COMMONS CONTRIBUTORS, 'File: Francesco salviati, storie di furio camillo, 1543-45, kairos 02.JPG', Wikimedia Commons, the free media repository, https://commons.wikimedia.org/w/index.php?title=File:Francesco_salviati,_storie_di_furio_camillo,_1543-45,_kairos_02.JPG&oldid=312981985 [accessed 1/08/18]
WIKIMEDIA COMMONS CONTRIBUTORS, 'File:Fractal clock.jpg', Wikimedia Commons, the free media repository, https://commons.wikimedia.org/w/index.php?title=File:Fractal_clock.jpg&oldid=222022751 [accessed 17/08/18]

CHAPTER 14

LOST IN WORK: MY STORY OF RECOVERY

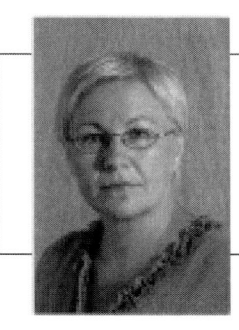

Tarja Gordienko

tarja.gordienko@gmail.com.

INTRODUCTION

My name is Tarja and I used to be a workaholic.

To realise that I have been an addict is a huge thing, a shock to me. To say it out loud feels like coming out of a closet. And to recover by creating a new life has been – and still is – a long and painful process. As a groundbreaking experience it has been like learning to walk again. My understanding of my work addiction has made me totally change my way to be and live with my work: how to start the day, how to act during the working day, how to eat my lunch, how to end the working day, how to be when I am not working.

How did I manage to do it? This chapter is my hero's journey – the journey of a recovering work addict.

A RESPECTABLE ADDICT

My story is connected with a phenomenon which has been titled "the addiction of the 21st century" (Griffiths, 2011, p. 740.). Work addiction - a phenomenon with negative consequences both to mental health, physical health and to interpersonal relationships. The problem is not marginal in today's working life. It has been estimated that ten per cent of people living in the western countries are suffering from work addiction (Van Gordon, Shonin, et al., 2014b) and younger adults are more likely to be affected (Andreassen, et al., 2014). People even die because of extreme working. In Japanese language there is a special word for this: karoshi, defined by Japanese scientists to describe sudden death from overwork (Li, 2016).

There are many factors that speed up obsessive work orientation in the modern lifestyle. Advanced technology makes it possible to access the internet and email accounts on computers, mobile phones or tablets anywhere, even at the dinner table. Effectiveness rules, and everything is measured. People try to reach deadlines, meet incentives and beat competition. Still there are only 24 hours in a day. This makes multi-tasking a highly valued skill. Instead of concentrating on one task at a time, people handle many things at the same time, for example, check e-mails during a meeting or plan next week's projects during the weekend. A substantial investment in work is also a cultural thing. According to the old Calvinistic philosophy and work ethic, working hard and putting in long hours has been a desirable way to live. Already within early Christian teachings sloth was one of the seven deadly sins.

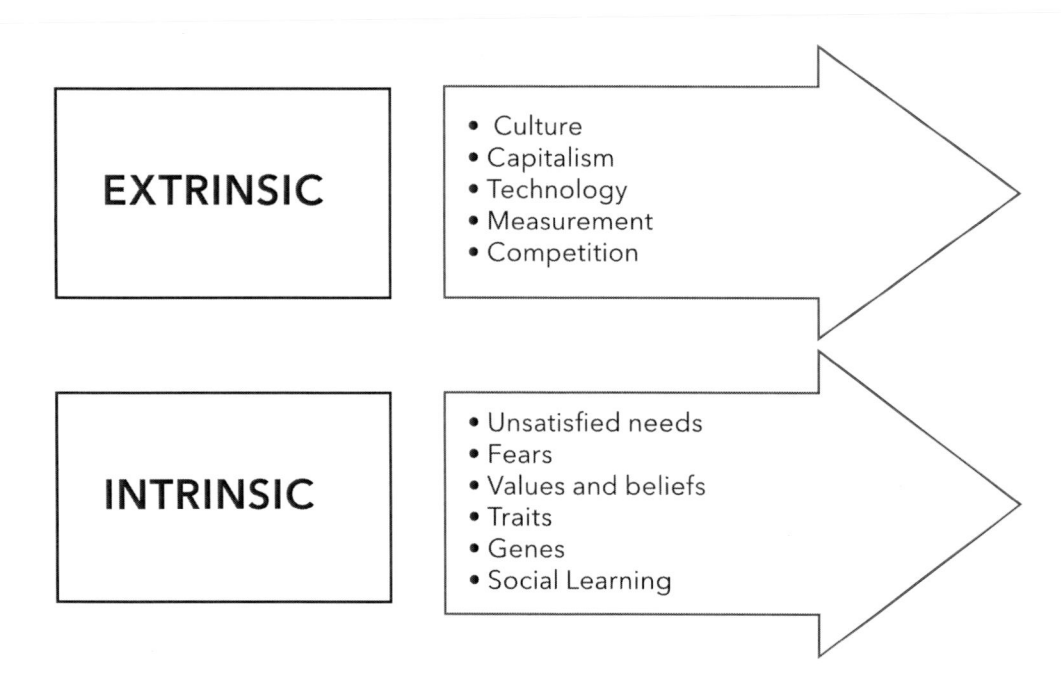

Figure 1: The Extrinsic and Intrinsic Factors of Work Addiction

One may easily mix work addiction with work engagement and strong work ethic, which are positive and desirable features at work. Because of its apparent benefits to employers and in building a career, work addiction is socially more accepted than other addictions (Griffiths, 2005a). Workaholics have been called "the respectable addicts" (Killinger, 1991). It is more challenging to set boundaries to work addiction than it is to fight addictions like gambling or smoking, because we need to work in order to make a living. Work is also highly interrelated with other important areas of life such as family, leisure, religion and community. This makes work addiction hard to handle.

In order to face problems like work addiction and to establish a new pattern of behavior, one needs to do more than just quit. One must take care of the emotional state underlying maladaptive behavior or avoidance. As Graeme Nixon says in Chapter 3 of this book:" … to be human is to be a creative, autonomous, freethinking being. However, to be made thus is also to be capable of anxiety, misperception, rumination and shame." Mindfulness sheds light into our habitual patterns and reveals our inner drivers. It opens up a wide perspective on life and helps to develop the capacity to see more clearly the things we are attached to. The hidden areas of resistance, e.g. negative emotions, rejected hopes or past experiences, can be noted and examined so that we can make the conscious choice to reject them. This gives a possibility to explore emerging emotions, thoughts, beliefs and physical sensations, and noting habitual patterns, openly and without judgement (Germer, 2009; Kabat-Zinn, 2013; Mindfulness Association, 2014).

EXPLORING MYSELF BY WRITING

On my hero's journey, I combined work addiction and mindfulness, using self-reflection as a tool to explore my condition. I asked myself: How might practising mindfulness and compassion influence a person like me, suffering from work addiction? My exploratory window was autoethnographic. Autoethnography is a form of qualitative research in which an author uses self-reflection and writing to explore one's personal experience and to connect one's story to wider cultural and social understanding. As Carolyn Ellis describes: "…I start with my personal life. I pay attention to my physical feelings, thoughts, and emotions. I use what I call systematic sociological introspection and emotional recall to try to understand an experience I have lived through. Then I write my experience as a story" (Ellis 1999, p. 671).

The method is especially useful when handling sensitive topics and emotions. In my case, I explored myself by writing, interviewing myself, and studying my practice diaries, and generating understanding from recurring themes and patterns. I have included some of my texts into this chapter.

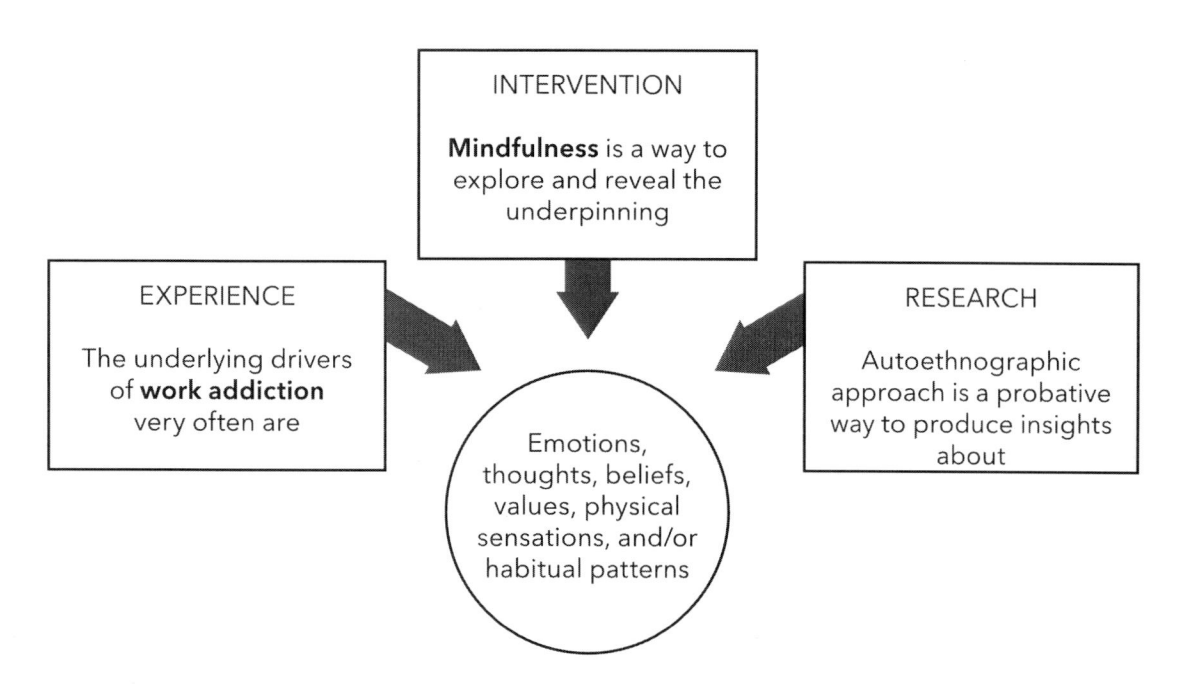

Figure 2: *Combining the Experience in Work Addiction, Mindfulness and Autoethnographic Approach*

FEELING FLOW – OR IS IT AN ADDICTION?

Addiction in the narrow sense entails the use of substances like alcohol or drugs to create an altered state of consciousness, in a way that is compulsive and destructive. The intention is to avoid pain and increase pleasure, enhancing a positive experience (Bien, 2009). However, behavioral addictions which do not involve a substance misuse, such as sex addiction, eating disorders, gambling or work addiction, can be just as serious as substance addictions.

Many signs and effects of behavioral addiction are parallel to the symptoms and consequences of substance addiction. The reason for this is that addictions are the state of enslavement to a habit or practice of something that is psychologically or physically habit-forming (Griffiths, 2012). In behavioral addiction, it is the psychological dependence that creates the addiction and related compulsive behaviors, but the mechanism of getting "high" is in fact quite similar to the analogous experience of drug or alcohol addiction (Griffiths, 2011).

Not everybody working hard is a work addict. So what does work addiction really mean? How does work addiction differ from work engagement or flow experience which are related to excellent job performance and generally seen as positive and desirable personal qualities of a worker? Work addiction has been known as a phenomenon since the 70's and defined in many different ways. Nowadays it is usually viewed as an addiction characterised by excessive work causing harmful consequences. For example, being overly concerned about work, being driven by an uncontrollable work motivation, and spending so much energy and effort on work that it impairs private relationships, spare-time activities and/or health (Andreassen et al., 2012).

Therefore, excessive working itself does not necessarily mean that a person is addicted to work. The real issue is to determine to what extent excessive working negatively impacts the other areas of the person's life, since an addiction always brings negative consequences. Work engagement is a positive condition characterised by energy, dedication and experiencing flow. A work addict, on the other hand, thinks that work is important but does not enjoy it. Instead, he or she is driven by his/her inner obsession (Schaufeli and Bakker, 2004).

> **Pause and Practice**
>
> What kind of personal values do you connect with your work?
> Does your work give you inspiration and happiness?

GETTING LOST

In order to clarify my own learning process, I will describe, in narrative description, how work addiction has affected my life and how practising mindfulness and compassion has changed my experience. With this, I hope to give voice to something very personal in order to describe a wider psychological and sociological phenomenon.

I have always been a hard-working person. I am from a poor, protestant farming family. My home was safe and loving, but my parents had to drudge to get their living. Of course, they wanted us children to be more successful and financially secure than they had been in their youth, so they taught us to work. The untouchable family value of being hardworking and diligent was tattooed on me already in my childhood. However, I think my relationship with work was still within normal limits when I was a child, a schoolgirl and a student. The habit of working hard did not turn into an unhealthy obsession until I was in my 30's, when I was a young mother having my first permanent job as a journalist. Recalling those years, I now notice some changes in my working habits:

> I am sitting by my desk and trying to make the world complete. But I can't get any satisfaction because my incoming mail box is never empty.

I invested more and more time in working, sweating sometimes from dusk till dawn to meet deadlines, starting to make excuses to get to work and hiding the time spent at work from my family. At first I was in a constant flow and loved my job. My work place was full of interesting challenges and people. I got a lot of good feedback for being so committed and was promoted to a team leader. This added fuel to my fire, but in a few years, this hype turned into a monster. I remember a summer vacation when I started by crying exhaustedly because I had taken myself far beyond my limits at work. My family and my friends complained that I was always at work. I was always tired and put on weight. Finally, my addiction took me to the threshold of a burnout and I spent a few weeks on sick leave:

> I think about my work constantly. I am always at work – even in those moments when I am not at the office but at home. When I play with my child, I am absent. I feel I am a bad mother but I cannot help it.

It took me more than ten years to understand, that there was something exceptional in my attitude towards work. The sick leave because of exhaustion was a crux for me. I knew I needed to change my life and work less. After that my life was a continuous struggle to solve the problem of excessive working. My obsession dominated my life and I spent a lot time and energy seeking help from friends, colleagues and superiors and making rules and regulations to control myself and work less. My efforts were not successful. Gradually, I started to realise that I was a work addict but only on the level of reason, in my thoughts. Reasoning did not help me since I had no tools to manage my addiction:

> I feel I have been crawling deep in a dark tunnel, doing my work like a deaf, blind and emotionless animal. I realised it's late, my son must be waiting for me at home, I am really tired, I could eat an antelope, I desperately need to pee. And I feel like shit.

Work addiction influenced deeply on my life at the level of emotions, thoughts, values and beliefs, physical condition, habitual patterns and social wellbeing. I felt ashamed, guilty and worthless because of my compulsive behavior. Moreover, excessive working and poor work-life balance caused me permanent stress with several negative side-effects. In my thoughts I was constantly afraid of failing to meet the expectations of my parents and my employer. On the other hand, I was always anticipating losing my job, so my survival strategy was to be always at work – either in person or at least in my thoughts:

> I usually work nine to ten hours or even more. My body has got used to that, and it feels fed only after a really long work day. I must feel beaten up, hungry and totally exhausted before I am satisfied and let myself walk out of the office.

Constant working caused me serious physical problems which included tension and sleeping problems. I ignored most of my physical needs, such as suffering from aches and pains and putting on weight, and worked even when I was ill. My obsessive habitual pattern to complete every task made it difficult for me to finish my working day. I invested more and more time in working, and as an addict also needed to work constantly more to feel satisfaction. Work centrality in my life made me neglect many things in my social life, including family, friends, hobbies and my own leisure time:

> I understand that I work too much. My family, my friends, my colleagues and even my superior says the same. What have I lost during all these years, working like a lunatic? It makes me dizzy to think about this. I need to change. I need help. So I do everything to change - to kill my addiction.

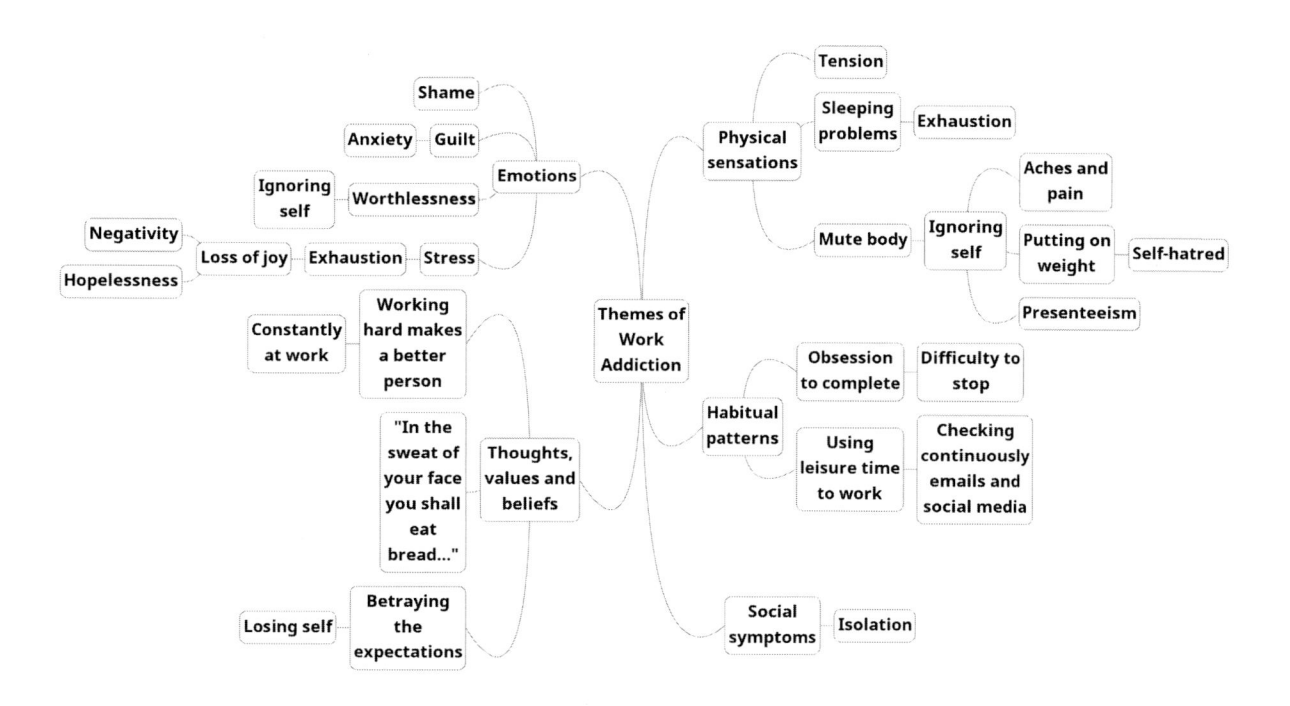

Figure 3: Themes of My Work Addiction

Components of addiction	Accounts in My Story (Gordienko, 2017)	Accounts in the Interview (Gordienko, 2018)
Salience	"I think about my work constantly. I am always at work – even in those moments when I am not at the working place but at home."	"Work is hoovering over all my ideas and thoughts and I don't have energy or time to do anything else. It kind of fills all the space so that there's no room for anything else."
Mood modification	"I feel more and more satisfaction and fulfilment at work and I'm in a constant flow with my important projects."	"I got good feedback and loved it but the most important thing was my inner craving to accomplish, to get a lot of things done, to get forward to the next task."
Withdrawal symptoms	"I cannot relax anyway, so why not do something useful? Otherwise I get anxious."	"I am often really nervous because of my work, feeling terrible stress even when I am at home. I kind of never get rid of those work thoughts."
Increased tolerance	"I must feel beaten up, hungry and totally exhausted before I am satisfied and let myself walk out of the office."	"I find it very difficult to stop working. The others seem to have that enough-feeling after 8 hours but I need to work at least 10 hours to feel the same."
Conflict	"Sometimes I even lie to my husband to get to my work. I know it is not ok to lie but I must get going."	"At some point I asked my colleagues to tell me when I needed to leave from work. When they did, I got really irritated. I just wanted to shout them to fuck off and let me work."
Relapse	"I make no progress with my efforts and always fall back into the cycle. And I am more and more disappointed with myself, accusing and beating myself up."	"As a recovering work addict I really need to separate my work and leisure time, otherwise I'll easily slip back into my old pattern."
Health and/or other problem	"All the new things combined with my obsession get me down and I need to take a sick leave."	"In some point I had bad problems with sleeping, awakening in the middle of the night, extreme tiredness, pain and stiffness in my shoulders – but the worst thing was having heart fluttering when working too much."

Figure 4: Seven Elements of Addiction according to the Bergen Work Addiction Scale and the Matching Qualitative Statements Extracted from my Personal Documents

---

Pause and Practice

What effect does your work have on the way you live?

Have a look at your working habits and take this as a challenge to be really honest with yourself. Have you ever neglected hobbies, leisure activities, exercise or time with your loved ones because of your work?

FINDING A MINDFUL WAY

I started my studies in mindfulness practically without any experience of regular meditation. I had expectations that mindfulness would be a soothing and calming method and believed it would diminish my stress. But I never expected it to have any major impact on my attitude to work. Within my MSc studies in Mindfulness at the University of Aberdeen I created personal, regular meditation routines. I started to meditate several times a week following the practices of Mindfulness Based Living Course and Compassion Based Living Course from the Mindfulness Association. The model of these studies and the way of training have been described by Vin Harris in Chapter 2 of this book. Hand in hand with mindfulness and compassion practices, I also included informal practices in my working days.

In my case the slow, gradual but significant change started with my daily practices. I understood that my working self had grown enormous, all the other parts of me serving it. I realised how important it was to recreate and nurture the other roles I have - as a mother, as a family member, as a friend, as a person who loves life and so on. Later I realised that in addition to continuous overload and stress, it was actually work addiction that made me suffer. To sum up, I could finally see my addiction.

There are four key themes reflecting the changes in my work addictive personality after starting my practices of mindfulness and compassion:

Body Does Not Lie. Having been a work addict for almost half of my life and neglecting most of my needs, I used to totally ignore my body. Among my first mindfulness practices was the body scan, which turned out to be my key to recovery. At first my body did not react during the practice at all, it seemed to be mute. However, the awakening of the body started gradually:

> I noticed how aching my muscles are and how little time I take to myself.

Remapping the Brain. What I saw earlier was that I was a hardworking person, that I was suffering from serious, chronic stress, and that this could not be changed. What I see now is that I was a work addict and that there were certain reasons for my addiction:

> The old Me would have acted that way but the new Me does not want to act like that anymore. Through these practices I have learned to listen to myself and to set boundaries.

Finding self-compassion. Self-compassion overthrew my earlier emotions of shame and worthlessness, and gave me permission to love myself and respect my needs:

> What about self-compassion and kindness, I've always been really hard on myself. Especially when this concerns work. I wouldn't ask anybody for more than I ask from myself.

From Avoidance to Acceptance. Seeing and accepting my work addiction and experiencing self-compassion helped me to start my journey towards a new nonaddictive life. Growing mindful awareness cultivated mental wellbeing and enhanced my quality of life. As a result, I was feeling empowered and less stressed, enjoying my life outside work more and more, and setting boundaries to protect my leisure time:

> It shocks me how many barriers I've made for myself. I am really independent and free person and I have made almost all the barriers by myself.

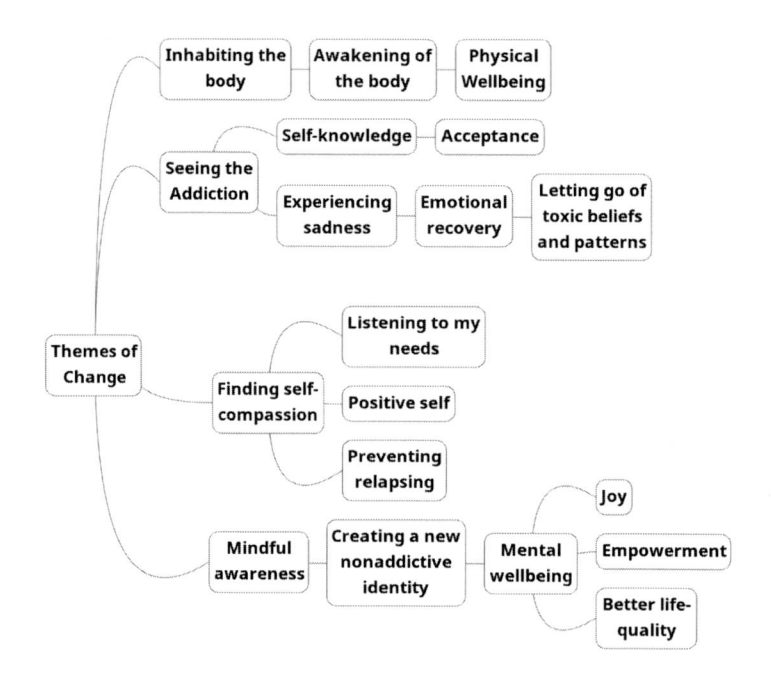

Figure 5: Themes of Change When Practising Mindfulness and Compassion

Components of addiction	Opposing Themes of Change	Accounts according to Personal Documents
Salience	Seeing the addiction, emotional recovery, listening to my needs	"Until now I have been crying three times today, because I listen to myself and have time to feel my feelings." (Practice Diary, 14th February, 2015)
Mood modification	Mindful awareness, self-knowledge, emotional recovery	"At work did some deep breathing and tried to analyze my feelings when noticing that my anxiousness and frustration were rising." (Practice Diary, 20th October, 2014)
Withdrawal symptoms	Awakening of the body, physical well-being	"I started a RAIN practice somehow automatically and concentrated first at my breathing. It calmed me down rather quickly." (Practice Diary, 2nd March, 2015)
Increased tolerance	Awakening of the body, seeing the addiction, letting go of toxic patterns	"I cannot go on like this, working so much. I must change my life and my habit to work too much." (Practice Diary, 18th February, 2015)
Conflict	Creating a new nonaddictive identity	"Thankful today. Early returning home, cooking dinner for my son." (Practice Diary, 14th October, 2015)
Relapse	Finding self-compassion	"It still sometimes happens that I promise to do too much and get into troubles but somehow I feel I find the balance more easily." (Interview, 2018)
Health and/or other problem	Awakening of the body, physical well-being	"I felt pressure in my chest and felt stressed and unstable. I then started a RAIN practice somehow automatically and concentrated first at my breathing. -- In a few minutes the difficulty was over." (Practice Diary, 2nd March, 2015)

Figure 6: Seven Elements of Addiction according to the Bergen Work Addiction Scale and the Opposing Themes of Change with Matching Qualitative Statements Extracted from my Personal Documents

Practising mindfulness and compassion helped me to stop, observe my actions, revise my life and dig the roots of my addiction into sight. Practices assisted me to re-evaluate the role of work in my life and find practical solutions to how to cope with my working day. Finally, accepting my addiction and finding self-compassion helped me to prevent relapsing and to create a new nonaddictive identity with better work-life balance.

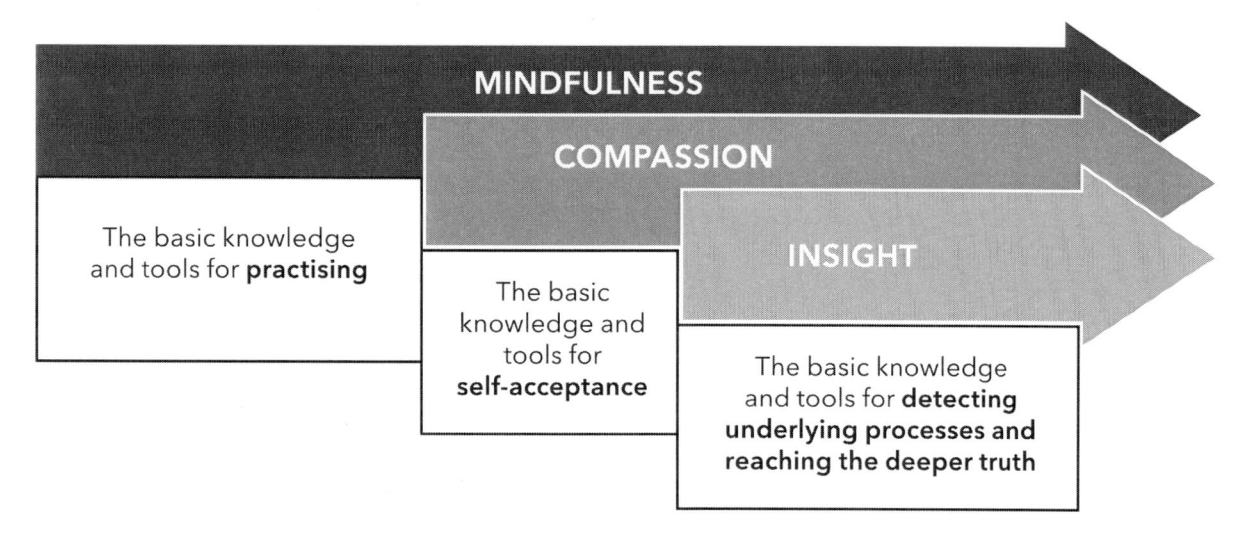

Figure 7: The Core of Mindfulness, Compassion and Insight Practices

CREATING A NEW NONADDICTIVE IDENTITY

Practising compassion and self-compassion balanced my life and supported me breaking away from the work-oriented life. Responding to suffering as a call for action (Gilbert & Choden, 2014) led me to let go of striving and change my daily routines in various simple yet enjoyable ways, for example:

- Changing my breakfast schedule: Instead of reading the newspaper or social media, I started reading poems or just sitting
- Giving myself breaks more often at work
- Enjoying lunch more often in silence
- Allowing myself sometimes to just sit on the sofa, doing nothing
- Doing things more slowly, allowing myself to think before acting
- Reading literature more often, not work papers
- Stopping more often to observe trees, animals and the weather, my own condition, the course of the day…
- Looking out the window observing
- Planning and rejoicing about how to spend my leisure time
- Reflecting on my attitude to work which finally led me having a few months study leave

Self-compassionate people have high self-esteem, but their self-esteem is not particularly dependent on how others evaluate them. They don't need to become grandiose to feel good about themselves. Therefore, self-compassionate people are less afraid of failure and rejection. (Germer, 2009; Neff 2011). My journey with self-compassion was a shift in my physical and emotional being. It helped me to:

- More often reflect on how my actual deeds meet my values
- Understand the importance of saving energy for my own needs
- Feel easier to respect and love my body
- Feel easier to be considerate in everyday situations
- Think more closely about what would be a good and ethical way to act in different situations
- Catch unique moments that would otherwise vanish without noticing
- Enjoy life more

There is a well-known phrase "once an addict, always an addict". This means that once an individual has been addicted, there will always be a risk of relapsing. Based on my brief personal experience, I find this true. Sometimes I still find it easy to fall into my old habitual patterns, especially when I am meditating less regularly. However, I feel I do not have a work addict's identity anymore, and that my mindfulness toolbox helps me to notice when my addiction is starting to re-emerge. As Germer notes - and this is also my experience - self-compassion is a stable way to regulate emotions and a healthy way to respond to lapses (Germer, 2009).

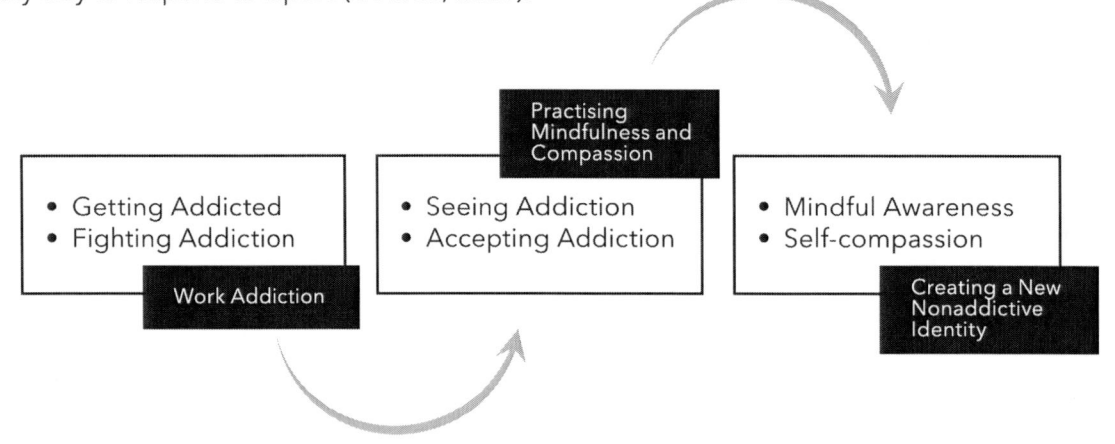

Figure 8: My Journey from Work Addiction to a New Nonaddictive Identity

HOW TO BE MINDFUL AT WORK

Within my studies I created personal, regular meditation routines according to the practices of Mindfulness Association. In my case, the self-reflection with the help of practices and journaling led to self-transformation through self-understanding (Chang, 2008). However, according to my experience and also according to the Thich Nhat Hanh's excellent book "Work" (2012), it is crucial to bring mindfulness training into the midst of working days - to lead one's work and working ability mindfully and to step off the daily treadmill. This may be possible by having short formal or various informal practices during the day, for example taking purposeful pauses, using transitions mindfully, nourishing oneself by eating mindfully, walking between meetings, avoiding social media or for example just taking some mindful breaths every now and then and cherishing self-compassion. There are many mini practices one can do in the middle of the day. Even one breath or a stop for a few seconds may constitute as meaningful, efficient practice.

The most common treatment approaches to work addiction are positive psychology, motivational interviewing, cognitive behavioural therapy, career councelling, and the 12-step program of Workaholics Anonymous (Andreassen 2014). Compared to these, mindfulness and compassion may be - and often are - practiced independently, by oneself, even in the workplace. Mindfulness and compassion practices can be done anywhere and at any time, also in hectic and stressful situations, in meetings and by the desktop. This makes mindfulness and compassion effective and cost-effective ways to make interventions since one may practice them anywhere, even in the middle of an ordinary working day. Work addiction is a multifaceted and ambiguous phenomenon and the reasons for it are always individual (Andreassen 2014). When planning interventions, one must take into account not just biological and genetic predispositions but also the psychological, psychosocial and social environment in which the work takes place in (Griffiths 2011). When it comes to the functionality of mindfulness and compassion practices, every person has an individual path according to the issues essential to him or her. This makes it challenging to give any suggestions or recommendations of the practices which would tackle the work addiction in question the best.

Nevertheless, in my experience it would be important to have both formal and informal practices included in any mindfulness based work addiction intervention. Regular formal practicing is the underpinning for the nonaddictive life and prevents relapsing. Equally important is to bring mindfulness training to work, to the epicentre of the problem of a work addict. In my case, the

Bodyscan and the Settling, Grounding and Resting Practice formed the basis of my formal practicing. Bodyscan is a practice where we give attention to the sensations in each part of our body in turn starting with our toes and ending with the tops of our heads.

> **Pause and Practice**
>
> Settling Grounding and Resting Practice
>
> http://www.mindfulnessassociation.net/wp-content/uploads/2018/03/rob-talk-13-guided-settling-grounding-and-resting.mp3

When it comes to practicing at work, a 3-minute Breathing Space, Self-compassion Break, Loving Kindness and RAIN Practice were easy to implement into the working day. RAIN is a four step practice. Firstly, recognise what is happening in the body, emotionally and what thoughts are arising. Secondly allow the present experience to be just as it is. Thirdly, investigate with gentle curiousity. Fourthly, nurthure with self-compassion.

> **Pause and Practice**
>
> RAIN practice guided by Tara Brach
>
> https://www.tarabrach.com/rain/

I also found Compassionate Bodyscan and Compassion for Self-Critic personally functional at work.

> **Pause and Practice**
>
> Spend a moment to reflect how you might bring mindfulness into the midst of your working days - to be more mindful and to feel better at work.

JOYFULLY, EFFORTLESSLY

For years I had been helpless with my work addiction. I had forced my body to be numb, and I did not have any tools to work with my emotions, beliefs and values. Therefore, I did not understand the reasons for my addiction. For me, mindfulness provided a way to understand the basic reasons for my compulsive working and brought my obsession for work radically and utterly visible. As Kabat-Zinn says: "To avoid workaholism, a person must bring awareness to his life, dare to let go and change ways to respond to things. This is when mindfulness could help" (Kabat-Zinn, 2013, pp. 499-501).

My journey supports Kabat-Zinn's idea that practicing mindfulness can have a positive impact on one's work addiction. In my case, the MBLC and CBLC practices formed a functional union to explore and observe myself and my way to work. In addition, my story bolsters the idea that it is essential for a work addict to bring mindfulness and compassion to a work place in informal ways. Mindfulness and compassion practices do not require any equipment or special space, are highly adaptable, and may be executed even along with work.

In George Orwell's world famous novel "Animal Farm" there is a character called Boxer, a loyal, kind, dedicated, extremely strong, hardworking and respectable cart-horse who believes that any problem can be solved by working harder. His maxim is "I will work harder". Unfortunately, the fate of Boxer is sad: he never learns to read, and when he collapses from overwork, pigs sell him to a local knacker to buy themselves whisky (Orwell, 1993). Orwell's book has strong political connotations but it can be read as a story of a working community where a loyal, kind and hardworking person may well wear himself out.

After my mindfulness journey, I understand that I have been Boxer in my own life, beating myself up, being extremely harsh on myself and asking much more from myself than from the others. The difference is that I have learnt to read. Mindfulness is my new literacy, and I myself am the literature that I am now able to read. This gives me hope to explore and understand my life in a new way, setting myself healthy boundaries and in that way escaping Boxer's destiny.

Carolyn Ellis (2009) says that effective autoethnographies are not victim tales; on the contrary, writing autoethnography well produces survivor tales for the writer and for those who read them. They open up a moral and ethical conversation about the possibilities of living life well. I hope this resonates with you.

In the mandala garden of a distant Scottish island, on Holy Isle, there is a signpost that says: "Work and Practice Joyfully, Effortlessly". These words will also be my sign for the future - for my work, practice and life.

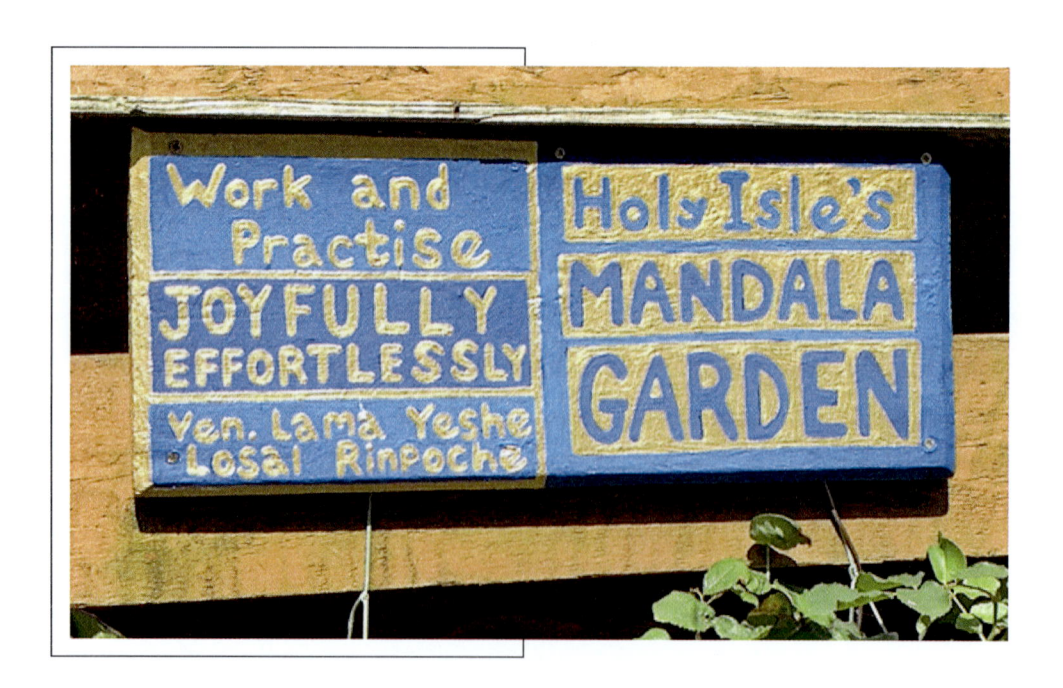

Figure 9: Work and Practice Joyfully, Effortlessly. Photo: © Tarja Gordienko 2018

FURTHER RESOURCES

Thich Nhat Hanh: Work. How to Find Joy and Meaning in Each Hour of the Day. Parallax Press, Berkeley, California (2012).
Blog by Dr. Mark D. Griffiths, an English psychologist focusing in the field of behavioral addictions. See the blog topic category "work": https://drmarkgriffiths.wordpress.com.
The Bergen Work Addiction Scale. See the article "Development of a work addiction scale" by Cecilie Schou Andreassen et al. in Scandinavian Journal of Psychology, 53, pp. 265-272. Issue published: April 10, 2012.
Carolyn Ellis: Heartful Autoethnography, Qualitative Health Research, 9 (5), pp. 669-683. Issue published: September 1, 1999.

REFERENCES

ANDREASSEN, C. S., (2014). Workaholism: An overview and current status of the research. Journal of Behavioral Addictions 3(1), pp. 1-11 [Available from: DOI: 10.1556/JBA.2.2013.017].
ANDREASSEN, C. S., GRIFFITHS, M. D., HETLAND, J. and PALLESEN, S. (2012). Development of a work addiction scale. Scandinavian Journal of Psychology, 53: 265-272. [Available from: DOI: 10.1111/j.1467-9450.2012.00947.x].
ANDREASSEN, C. S., GRIFFITHS, M. D., HETLAND, J., KRAVINA L., JENSEN F., et al. (2014). The Prevalence of Workaholism: A Survey Study in a Nationally Representative Sample of Norwegian Employees. PLoS ONE 9(8): e102446. [Available from: DOI: 10.1371/journal.pone.0102446].
BIEN, T., (2009). Paradise Lost: Mindfulness and Addictive Behavior. In: F. DIDONNA, ed., Clinical Handbook of Mindfulness. New York: Springer. pp. 289-297.
CHANG, H., (2008). Autoethnography as Method. Left Coast press, Inc.
ELLIS, C. (1999). Heartful Autoethnography, Qualitative Health Research, 9 (5), pp. 669-683. Issue published: September 1, 1999. [Available from: DOI: 10.1177/104973299129122153].
ELLIS, C., (2009). Revision. Autoethnographic Reflections on Life and Work. Walnut Creek: Left Coast Press.
GERMER, C., (2009). The Mindful path to self-compassion: freeing yourself from destructive thoughts and emotions. New York: The Guilford Press.
GILBERT, P. and CHODEN, (2014). Mindful Compassion. How the science of compassion can help you understand your emotions, live in the present and connect deeply with others. New Harbinger Publications.
GRIFFITHS, M., (2005a). Workaholism is still a useful construct. Addiction Research and Theory, 13, pp. 97-100. [Available from: DOI: 10.1080/16066350500057290].
GRIFFITHS, M., (2011). Workaholism: A 21st century addiction. The Psychologist: Bulletin of the British Psychological Society, 24 (10), pp. 740-744.
GRIFFITHS, M., (2012). Workaholism: Healthy enthusiasm or an addiction? Blog post. 6th January. Available: https://drmarkgriffiths.wordpress.com/2012/01/06/workaholism-healthy-enthusiasm-or-an-addiction/
HANH, T.N., (2012). Work. How to Find Joy and Meaning in Each Hour of the Day. Parallax Press, Berkeley, California.
KABAT-ZINN, J., (2013). Full Catastrophe Living. How to cope with stress, pain and illness using mindfulness meditation. London: Piatkus.
KILLINGER, B. (1991). Workaholics: the respectable addicts. New York: Simon & Schuster.
LI, J. (2016). Karoshi: An international work-related hazard? International journal of cardiology, ISSN: 1874-1754, Vol: 206, Page: 139-40. [Available from: DOI: 10.1016/j.ijcard.2016.01.092].
MINDFULNESS ASSOCIATION (2011). Mindfulness Based Living Course, 8 Week Programme Course Material. Mindfulness Association Ltd, July 2011.
MINDFULNESS ASSOCIATION (2014). Mindfulness Module Weekend One Manual. Mindfulness Association Ltd.
MINDFULNESS ASSOCIATION (2015a). Compassion Module Weekend One Manual. Theory Section. Mindfulness Association Ltd.
MINDFULNESS ASSOCIATION (2015b). Compassion Module Weekend One Manual. Practice Section. Mindfulness Association Ltd.
MINDFULNESS ASSOCIATION (2016). Compassion Based Living Course, 8 Week Compassion Course Curriculum. Mindfulness Association Ltd, February 2016.

NEFF, K., (2011). Self Compassion. Stop Beating Yourself Up and Leave Insecurity Behind. London: Hodder & Stoughton.
ORWELL, G., (1993). Animal Farm. London: David Campbell (First publ. 1945).
SCHAUFELI, W. and BAKKER, A., (2004). Job demands, job resources, and their relationship with burnout and engagement: a multi-sample study. Journal of Organizational Behavior, 25, pp. 293–315. Published online in Wiley InterScience (www.interscience.wiley.com). [Available from: DOI 10.1002/job.248].
VAN GORDON, W., SHONIN, E., ZANGENEH, M. and GRIFFITHS, M., (2014b). Work-related Mental Health and Job Performance: Can Mindfulness Help? International Journal of Mental Health and Addiction, 'Online First' Published 13th February 2014. [Available from: DOI 10.1007/s11469-014-9484-3].

CHAPTER 15

AN INTRODUCTION TO STORIES OF MINDFUL HEROES IN SPORTS SETTINGS

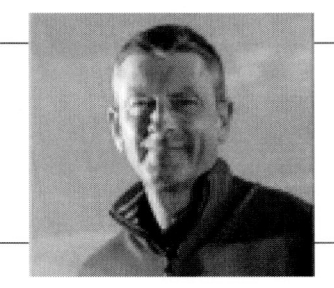

Karl Morris

karl@themindfactor.com

I have been fortunate to be involved in performance coaching for the last thirty years or so. Mainly in the world of golf but in that time, I have also worked with Ashes winning captains in cricket, Premiership and International footballers, title winning Super League Rugby teams and world-renowned snooker players. So it has been a wonderful experience to review the three examples of the practical application of mindfulness techniques in the real world of sport.

I felt an instant connection with the words of Misha Botting in the way he described such an incredible coaching journey with the Olympic Curling Team and his own journey through various approaches to peak performance. I have been fortunate to know Vin Harris for many years and the way he looks at the game of golf is refreshingly honest and forthright. You feel like you are almost on the Ski slope itself as John Arnold describes the sense of being really in tune with your body as a way of improving your skiing technique.

So often we are given great theories and research in the world of performance coaching and psychology yet for me there is nothing better than to be able to connect and learn from people who have actually applied the techniques in a real-life situation. I call it working at the 'coal face'. I have been at that very coal face myself for the past thirty years both as a player and as a performance coach. On this long and meandering journey, I have been promised many solutions from many different approaches. Sadly, most of these techniques lack substance when pitted against the incredibly varied and dynamic landscape of human beings trying to achieve excellence in sport.

Misha points out his own challenges with the standardised approach in much of psychology with Cognitive Behavioural Therapy (CBT). I often get asked in my own work: Do you try to get people to think positive? When I then try to explain to the unsuspecting enquirer this is perhaps one of the most limited and fruitless of approaches, I am mostly met with a quizzical look and the conversation then drifts elsewhere to something less challenging. For many people it would seem thinking positive would be so much better than thinking negatively and to a degree it is, but it wasn't until I myself began to look deeper into mindfulness concepts that I began to understand just how limited this approach can be. Trying to 'think positive' is at its most obvious level a recipe to create an extremely busy mind. You are also in effect trying to convince yourself of something you really deep down don't believe. In golf it would be: "This putt is going in, it is really going in, I am sure it is going in". Then, reality takes over and the ball goes past the hole. What do you do then? Try to think even more positive thoughts? This is what most players will do and then inevitably when the world isn't bending to their whims and wishes they flip to the other side of the coin and drown in self-imposed negative stories of 'I can't do this' or 'I am useless at golf'. Again more and more thinking.

John Arnold makes a great case for the value of acceptance in sport. I could not agree more. To be able to accept the outcome of your actions and move on is at the very heart of mental resilience. Yet as John points out brilliantly, acceptance is not resignation. Acceptance of this particular outcome with a willingness to keep exploring the possibility of the next opportunity. With all of the players

I work with, and I have been fortunate in golf to work with six major champions, I always ask each player this simple question: "When you have been at your very best, when you have won such and such a tournament if you could describe your state of mind at the time with only one word what would that word be?". In all of this time I have never ever heard one single player describe their state of mind as positive. Ever.

The word over the years I have heard time and time again with elite golfers describing their peak moments is CALM. I felt very calm. My mind was very calm. It allowed me to just hit the shots and get the job done. What I have come to understand is we are not in sport looking for a positive mind but a calm mind that allows the wisdom of the body to take over. One of my proudest moments has been publishing my golf book Attention!! The Secret to You Playing Great Golf (Morris, 2014). I often say the mental game in golf can be either incredibly complex or disarmingly simple. You can get lost in all of the technical jargon about the pre-frontal cortex and the effect of the amygdala or you can suggest to yourself that excellence in sport is down to one word. One simple word. That one word being ATTENTION. And my own simple principle is when you play your sport your attention will always be in one of two places for the task at hand. You will either have your attention on something useful or useless. It really is as simple as that. A very simple theory requiring a lifetime of practice.

We think nothing of training our bodies day in day out but what about training our attention? For me this is THE fundamental skill and the tip of a metaphorical iceberg we are only just beginning to understand. That is why mindfulness is such a practical approach to not only health and well-being but a gateway to improved performance on the court, track or course. The game of golf as Vin Harris so wonderfully describes is a very long walk with only intermittent activity over four hours or so. There is a lot of golf that is not golf. Just you and your mind exposed to a huge cascade of emotions and reactions. Nobody to blame but yourself (although many golfers try very hard to find other things to blame!). In this walking time you can get lost in the regret of poor shots you have hit or the anxiety that comes from a mind hell bent on predicting a potential future success. Many golfers never even consider this 90% of non-golf may paradoxically be the key to the other 10% of actual golf.

In this time the principle of 'walking meditation' is such a wonderful place to park your troubled mind. To just 'be' with the walk. To pay attention to the rise and fall of your breath or the feeling of your feet as they come into contact and lose contact with the ground. At all levels this simple mindfulness technique has at the very least a wonderful experiential quality to it as you simply come back to this unique moment in time. John Kabat-Zinn (1990, p.3) has a beautifully descriptive phrase "you only have moments to live'". This phrase really grabs your attention but how many of those moments do we actually pay attention to?

In sport we tend to fall into the trap of what I call 'playing this for that' in the sense that if I play well today it will win me some money in the future or I will qualify for such and such a tour. In the amateur game it tends to be along the lines of if I play well today it will bring me a lower handicap tomorrow. It is fine to have these directions to move towards, but we must be so careful we are not always 'striving yet never arriving'. It is so easy to miss what we have today when all we think about is where we are going to be in the future. As Vin Harris said in his chapter perhaps the most important question we can ask is 'why do I play golf?' or whatever your sport is.

When you really connect with the real reasons you play your sport so many answers are paradoxically available right away. To be close to nature, to feel the freedom in my body, to enjoy the company and camaraderie of others. We can have these elements here and now today if we focus our attention on them and don't get dragged too far into distant outcome thinking. I heard Tony Robbins say many years ago at a seminar in London 'the quality of your life will be determined by the quality of your questions' and at the time I just had no idea how profound a statement that is. Why so important? Well if I asked you now as you are reading this page 'what can you hear in the background?' I am sure your attention has now been pulled elsewhere. The value of questions is because questions focus our attention. One of the key questions I get many of the players I work with to ask before they play is simply 'What am I committed to today?' Such a simple question but by asking it before you play you really increase the chances of having your attention in a place you as a unique individual deem useful. A question I would ask everyone reading this wonderful book is simply 'what are you going to do with this information?'

For me there are two kinds of knowledge. Knowledge we can talk about and discuss and knowledge we can do. Both are important but in sport it is the knowledge that you do on a daily basis that will determine your ongoing experience. To embrace these mindfulness concepts and truly live them on a daily basis will open up endless possibilities. I would encourage you to explore those very possibilities.

FURTHER RESOURCES

The Mind Factor
Train Your Golf Brain
www.themindfactor.com

REFERENCES

KABAT-ZINN, J. (1990) Full Catastrophe Living. London: Little Brown Books.
MORRIS, K. (2014) Attention!! The Secret to You Playing Great Golf. London: The London Press.

CHAPTER 16

MINDFUL LEARNING AND COACHING IN ALPINE SKIING

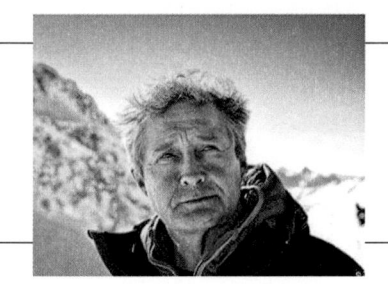

John Arnold

<john@mindfulmountains.co.uk>

INTRODUCTION - THE MYSTERY OF MASTERY

From a young age I became curious about the acquisition of physical skills. I wondered what it was that caused the body to be able to perform some tasks and not others. How some technical skills were easily picked up and 'grooved' whilst others remained elusive? Most people who participate in sports will have memories of their early learning and here's one of mine which remains vivid:

> I failed on the first attempts and was frustrated at this especially as I had taken the beginning step by step breaking down the game of foot hoopla hoop into manageable parts, gradually and painstakingly connecting them into a resemblance of the whole skill. But success eluded me and I left the hoopla hoop motionless on the ground turning away dejected. Later on, I was leaving that place and was thinking about very little, instead I was savouring the cool breeze and sounds of birds in the trees which lined the pathway to the ski centre. Without thinking and with no expectations I stepped into the hoop which had been discarded earlier, flicked the edge up to my ankle and swinging my foot and lower leg in a large circular motion. I felt the air brush over my leg, the pressure of the hoop on my ankle. The balance achieved from the standing leg, I moved surely bringing the leg wide and swinging in towards the standing leg which I confidently hopped enabling the hoop to pass under me. I repeated the cycle each time with perfect balance and timing.

> **Pause and Reflect**
>
> Everyone has had learning breakthroughs. Reflect on some of yours.
> What do you feel was at play in my example here?

In sporting circles, the term 'belief' is common parlance. What is less usual is talk of 'belief in what?' Believing in one's self is a frequent mantra in positive psychology and invariably falls short in eradicating limiting beliefs and performance inhibitors because it points you to look in the wrong direction. Instead, look into the dream itself and feel what it's like to experience it, become mindfully aware of the experience of achieving the goal. Learning and performance is enhanced when we 'can get ourselves out of the way'. The mindfulness faculty thrives in a context of equanimity - it's not the absence of emotions and thoughts which is our goal, it's our relationship with them which matters. Getting yourself out of the way limits the damage which we can exert on ourselves, dissolves learning blocks and clears the way for learning mindfully.

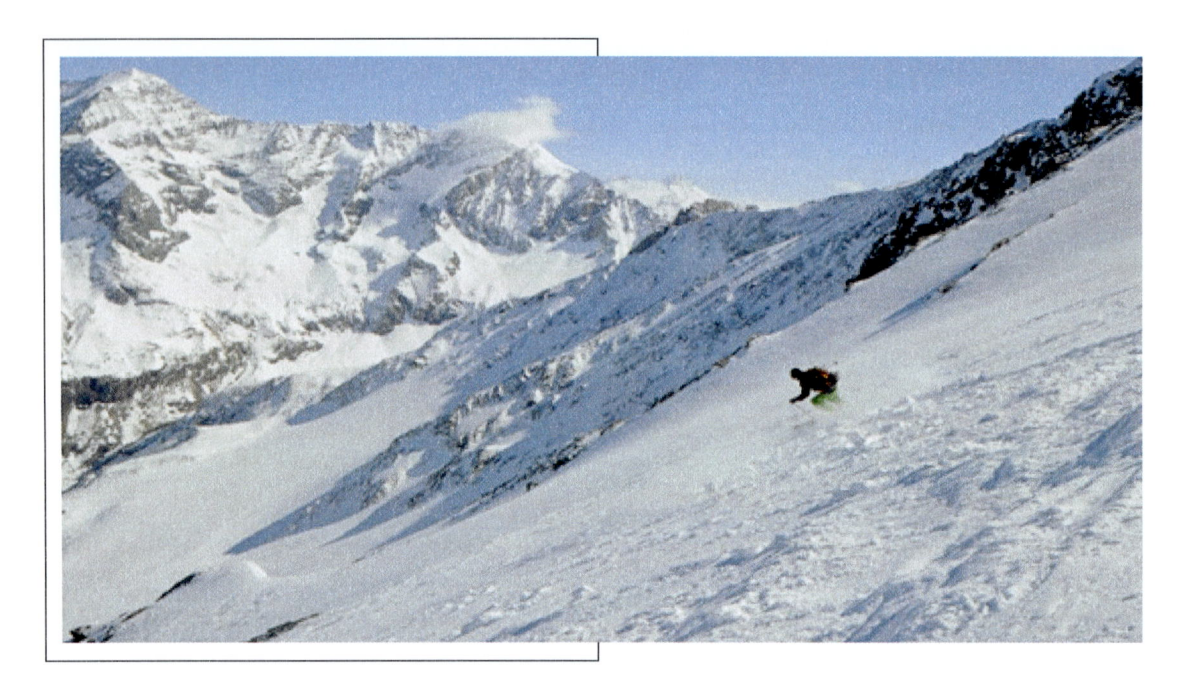

Figure1: Mastery or Madness. Photo © John Arnold 2014

MY JOURNEY

As a coach, teacher and mentor, mindfulness has re-energised my work in sports, life coaching and personal development. It has driven me to change my perspective on learning and developing performance both in sports and the workplace. From a personal viewpoint a daily meditation practice and everyday mindfulness has helped me to cope with stress, loss and improved the way I relate with others.

The majority of my time during the first fifteen years of my career was spent coaching club, regional and national squad ski racers. This work was carried out in Scotland, New Zealand, America and the European Alps, I travelled extensively and was influenced by coaches of various nationalities with different perspectives. For many years I was a ski coach educator running training courses in Scotland and in the Alps. Whilst I was driven by my love of skiing and the mountains, I noticed my curiosity moved more towards the person, athlete and coach, how they learnt and improved performance. With this interest I trained as a life coach and began work in this area as well as ski coaching.

The journey into formal mindfulness studies was an obvious one for me, I had been visiting Samye Ling Monastery on a casual basis for a number of years. The Buddhist teachings and framework for a happier and less suffering life, the advancement of potential and discipline of mental training all appealed to me on a personal and professional level. I continue to deepen my understanding of mindful learning and coaching through coaching skiers in the winter, organising hiking, biking and yoga holidays in the summer and spiritual mountain retreats in the autumn.

POTENTIALITY AND PATHOLOGY

In the early days of my career as a coach and performer my focus was realising athletic capabilities. It was all about realising potential, improving performance and achieving increasing higher levels of personal bests. The context was technical prowess and advancement was measured in the time it took to descend snow covered slopes. As a performer I aspired to higher levels of technical precision following set predetermined rules of the game. I watched, listened and learned from the experts of the time, aspiring to becoming 'better'. I have learned that inherent in the pursuit of better-ness there is often a sense of not being good enough. This self-perception is prevalent in participants of sports at all levels and manifests itself in the learner as striving to be something different from what they are in the present. This 'performance dissonance' as I call it sometimes becomes a block to improving, the learner is just too full of self-limiting beliefs, unable to appreciate their present strengths and capabilities.

As my coaching career became measured in decades rather than years, I noticed a marked shift in the ways I thought about human potential, my scope broadened from the technical, tactical, mental and physical components of sport to the emotional, perceptual and relational. In the snow-covered mountains the only constant is change and I saw how this was reflected in the inner landscape of those I was coaching. I've seen some bizarre behaviours from students on the mountain as they are emotionally challenged and I began to recognise the parallels to everyday life; in my everyday life, I was seeing my pathology obscuring my own potential and the conflict between both was in full view to me, I needed to be a warrior. I needed to get myself out of my own way.

The MSc Studies in Mindfulness, a blend of personal practice, academic study and professional enquiry was perfect. As a coach aspiring to create mindful learning experiences for my students its essential that I am mindful myself and have a depth of personal meditation practice and underpinning knowledge from which to draw. Embodiment of mindfulness in the professional context will only be possible when one's personal practice is disciplined, regular and on-going. Embodiment leads us to getting ourselves out of the way.

Pause and Reflect

What does embodiment mean for you?
Is it a feeling, an emotion and / or mental state?
How do you recognise embodiment in yourself?

MINDFUL LEARNING

To understand mindful learning, we have to look into the whole picture, a holistic view of the learning dynamic. One of the key issues in mindful learning, which is often overlooked, is the learner's motivation for learning. This will shape the learner's readiness for mindful learning so understanding the learner's motivation and needs is crucial. Secondly is the environment, what is the playground and is it suitable for the learners needs? In Alpine Skiing, an open skill, we are fortunate to have whole mountains, the terrain and snow conditions and weather as variables which can be exploited for the learner's benefit. Thirdly is the coach's skill set and expertise in both the specific sport and in mindfulness. A deep understanding of the sport's technical principles, bio-mechanics, physiology and equipment is essential and in combination with the coaches accurate understanding of mindfulness will make creating mindful learning experiences more possible. What I am saying here is that we always begin with the learner – begin from where the learner is, rather than for example, the coach's own agenda or a teaching strategy. In this sense beginning where the learner is in the present moment, rather than where they want to be in the future, is similar to when we are teaching mindfulness or guiding meditations.

ACTIONS FLOW FROM ENERGY

The starting point then is for the coach to understand what motivates the learner to learn? What have been the sequence of events, choices and decisions which brings the learner to seek out and sustain learning? Where is their energy for learning? One of the questions I ask my students on meeting them is why are you here? The responses are fascinating and provide me with valuable information to decide on approach, content, environment, pacing and many other elements of the coaching and learning process.

Some skiers come to coaching sessions for entirely extrinsic reasons, partner pressure being a favourite and occasionally they don't even like the idea of being on a slippery mountain slope in the cold. My approach with these skiers is quite different to skiers who, for example, are there because they find skiing exhilarating, exciting and they love the winter mountain environment. I find out where their energy is in their body. Frequently their energy is in their head, intellectualising the game of skiing and trying to figure out techniques. These are the heady skiers and most are far from being connected with their bodies and what their body is experiencing, something which of course is essential in mindful learning.

In broad terms learner's motivation is both intrinsic and extrinsic, its rarely one or the other. It would be natural to say the learners with intrinsic motivation progress more quickly and enjoy the experiences more so than extrinsic motivated learners, but I don't believe this to necessarily be the case. The power of wanting to please another can be strong in some people and see them through many hardships. With learners like this I believe mindful learning can bring the learner into their body and if the environment is well suited, the learner begins to feel the joy of sliding. As competence increases their ability to manoeuvre themselves down the mountain provides a sense of control and this, for learners in skiing, is a hugely motivating factor, largely because it generates a sense of comfort, confidence and competence.

I have noticed learner motivations often match one or more of the following:

- Pleasing a significant other or others.
- Attaining a skiing grade.
- Performing the perfect technique.
- Feeling the experience of skiing and of being in the environment.

I am not placing a value on any of the four sources of motivation as whatever brings people to the wonderful experience of skiing is welcomed. I have noticed though that where motivation is related to feeling the experience, learners enjoy themselves more, are open to learning mindfully and often less critical of themselves, that is, more self-compassionate. Where learners have more extrinsic motivations, as in the first three above, learning mindfully can help them to enjoy the learning journey by focussing on their experiences rather than external moderators and performance criteria

---

Pause and Reflect

How do you recognise your motivations for learning?
Are they different depending on the subject?
Which have you found to be the most effective?

THERE'S ALWAYS A BIGGER PICTURE

I have noticed that learners in mindful learning have a very different experience to those being taught through more traditional learning methods. I coach in many different styles and approaches and I am able to do this because of my mindfulness practice and my knowledge of a broad range of coaching styles. In mindful learning learners are more able to assimilate their learning experiences and they seem to have deeper meaning, one which impacts them as a human being rather than only in improving performance. I often wonder why this is. According to Langer (2000) mindfulness in the learning arena could be defined as the process of making novel distinctions where attentional capabilities, greater sensitivity to one's environment, and the creation of new categories for structuring perception come to the fore and are developed. This process brings the learner closer to and in tune with their own experiences, their physical and emotional being as they are performing. The resulting openness to knowing themselves deeper during performance heightens the learner's state of present moment 'wakefulness' and naturally spills over into knowing themselves deeper. The learner is observing themselves much closer than in traditional learning methods where the learner is striving to replicate movements and techniques.

I have found that learning mindfully takes the learner into subjective experiences in such a way that present moment body and mind functions and feelings are illuminated. With this awareness the learner can more easily discern between self-reactive impulses, for example, upper body leaning into the mountain (not preferred) and making modification to performance on purpose, for example, leaning away from the mountain (preferred). As the learner becomes more aware of self-reaction and of self-purpose, they experience a greater sense of control of their speed and direction which increases comfort and confidence levels, thereby making their experience a more enjoyable one.

Underpinning mindful learning is how the conscious mind perceives and processes experience and how mindfulness promotes less reactivity to events that can provoke emotional distress and more efficient regulation of that distress when it occurs (Brown, 2009). Within the learning journey, individuals experience varying degrees of stress often increased by their perceptions of their learning and of their environment (a big one in skiing) and when the object of stress is the learning journey itself, mindfulness seems to be able to play a role in helping individuals notice their distress, cope with it and engage more fully. In these moments of stress, I guide learners through a similar process as when guiding meditations and teaching some of the fundamentals of mindfulness. That is essentially comprehending the bigger picture of their own experience by creating internal safe space where the symptoms of stress can be witnessed and held in neutrality, in the absence of engagement with them. I have found that this procedure is more readily accepted on the mountain by those who are daily meditators and this comes as no surprise as they have already learnt on the cushion to recognise their internal landscape and to let it exist in compassion.

> **Pause and Reflect**
>
> How much do you recognise the reflective learner in yourself?
> What is your capacity to see the bigger internal picture when stress is present?

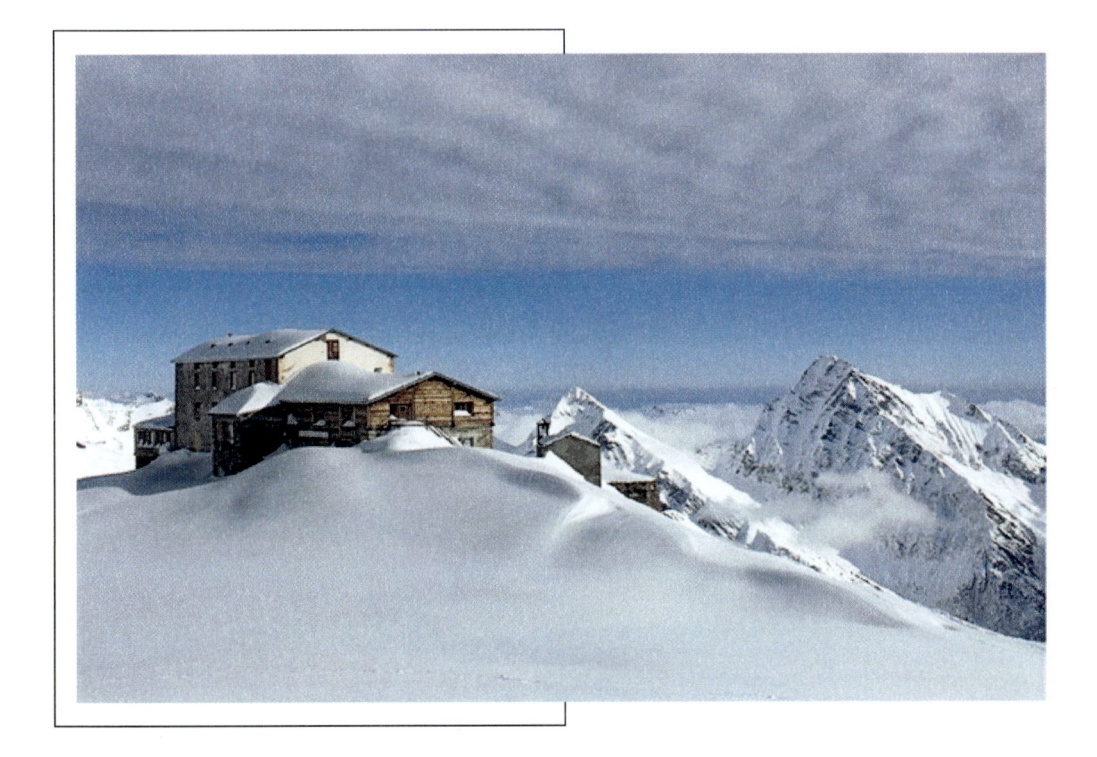

Figure 2: The bigger picture. Photo © John Arnold 2018

ATTITUDE AT ALTITUDE

This is where the rubber meets the tarmac, where the skis meet the snow. In mindful learning there are characteristics which must be evident, if they're not then it's not learning mindfully. Attitudes shape behaviour and this is so true in the learning dynamic of mindfulness. There are certain characteristics inherent in mindfulness, Kabat-Zinn's 'Attitudinal Foundations' of mindfulness (1991) and Ellen Langer's 'six themes of mindfulness' (1989) are examples. With these in mind and from my own coaching experiences and research, my view is that mindful learning must have some or all of the following characteristics.

Awareness: Gaining a deepening awareness of self and present moment experience is the beginning of playing sport with purpose. As it is a precursor to living life with purpose. With awareness of body and emotions the learner more easily perceives self-reactive impulses, their emotions, mindset, the environment and how they are relating to it. The learner understands what is happening as it happens and has the potential to modify techniques and change tactics as they are performing, thereby increasing likelihood of control.

Curiosity: In mindful learning we encourage learners to become curious about their experiences. How they feel physically, emotionally, psychologically and relationally and what present moment sensations they are experiencing. Delving further into what is happening when it's happening. Good coaches achieve this through creating a safe environment (inside and out), effective questioning, reflective episodes and peer sharing.

Novelty: A recurring theme in mindful learning is reference to the notions of novelty-seeking and novelty-producing (Langer 2000; Kee & Wang, 2008; Bain, 1995). The learner's openness to experiences is characteristic in mindful-learning, as is the sense of inquiry, acceptance, flexibility, engagement and non-judgmental experience of performance.

Acceptance: This doesn't mean resignation, rather it's about acknowledging present moment experience, rather than denying it. Acceptance first, change comes later, through exercising non-attachment. We don't need to try and hold on to pleasant experiences any more than pushing away unpleasant ones.

Perspective: This is about perceiving more than one view, creating new categories and welcoming new information simultaneously. The resulting openness to new information and awareness of creative problem-solving brings a subjective 'feel' to the learning dynamic, one where there is a heightened state of present moment 'wakefulness' to the possibilities inherent in learning. The process of peers sharing experiences about their performances encourages seeing things in different ways; recognition that one's way of doing something or seeing it from a particular view, is not the only way. As the learner reflects further, realisations of how and why performance is happening occurs, thereby creating new categories.

Context: When the learner realises and appreciates the value of the performance context much irrelevant information is filtered and the learner is able to focus on what influences their current performance. Context awareness is developed through a realisation of the changing nature of the environment and how technical, physical, tactical and mental components need to align to produce optimal performance. In Alpine Skiing, through the open mountain environment, which is constantly changing, realising the performance context is invaluable and therefore we spend time noting the snow conditions, changing light and varying terrain.

Non-valuing: This sits in what Kabat-Zinn refers to as non-judging, observing whatever you are experiencing in the absence of classifying it into good or bad, like or dislike, that is, not placing it into a value context. If subjective knowledge is to have an impact on the quality of learning experience then the learner will benefit from having the capabilities to bring awareness into current moment experience in the absence of evaluative judgments, elements which are inherent in mindfulness, thus making mindfulness a meaningful approach to subjective knowledge (Bain, 1995).

Non-striving: How do we not strive during learning? Surely the learning process is about developing performance? Well yes and no. Having detailed performance outcomes often causes striving, to be something that one is currently not. I'm an advocate of having the destination in mind whilst being flexible with how one gets there. The main benefit of knowing the destination is that when you arrive it's recognised. What many learners do when setting outcome goals is mistake them for the journey and therefore focus on the wrong things. Non-striving is achieved by having a gentle notion of the destination and then almost forgetting it, thus enabling the learning experience to be fully realised.

> **Pause and Reflect**
>
> Which of these attitudes resonate with you?
> Are you more inclined to some and not others?
> Which ones hold more of a challenge for you?

THE MINDFUL COACH

When teaching mindfully, but not teaching 'mindfulness', the challenge is to teach from a mindful teaching framework and be grounded in the underpinning principles of mindfulness. Mindful coaches prepare their 'being' from which their 'doing' arises. The practitioner's personal mindfulness practice and the embodiment of mindfulness are identified as the foundation for mindful professional practice (Siegel, 2010). Qualities and skills in mindfulness are placed with equal weighting alongside the body of knowledge relating to sports specific performance and teaching / coaching skills. When coaching mindful skiing I frequently pause (chairlift rides are a good time for this) and consider the teaching framework I operate from when teaching mindfulness and guiding mediations and attempt to use this framework to guide me in my coaching approach with skiers.

The coach often uses a broad range of teaching styles, each designed to elicit specific learning experiences and outcomes, in order to create the learning experience. A teaching strategy model which I have found a helpful is Mosston's Spectrum of Teaching Styles. The process highlights the direct relationship, cause and effect, between the teacher behaviour and learner experience. According to the model the teacher consciously decides who (teacher or learner) makes what decisions and when (before, during or after the session). When the teaching-learning process is viewed as a spectrum of decision making where every teaching action is considered in the context of, by whom and when a decision is made, the teacher's behaviour can be matched accordingly to the learner's behaviour and in doing so the learning style can be shaped (Mosston, 2001).

The skillful application of teaching styles, a deep understanding of mindfulness and a personal mindfulness practice are all essential for the mindful coach. They have equal weighting with the sport's specific technical skills and underpinning knowledge. From the mindfulness perspective I keep four things in mind when coaching mindful skiing, Embodiment, Mind-Sight, Equanimity and Compassion.

Embodiment: The commitment to a personal practice of mindfulness is crucial. Daniel Siegel remarks, 'As they say at the beginning of a flight, we need to put our own oxygen mask on first before we can help those around us' (Siegel, 2010, p.xv). The embodiment of mindfulness is nurtured by, amongst other things, the coach engaging in daily mindful meditation practice and on-going mindfulness practices in daily life. These are described in the Good Practice Guidance for Teaching Mindfulness-Based Courses, UK Network of Mindfulness-Based Teacher Trainers (January 2010) where the embodiment of mindfulness is identified as one of the six domains of competence.

The coaches internal frame of being is sustained through levels of awareness which support the present moment recognition of sensing, observing, conceptualising and knowing, in self, others and within the interpersonal relationship between teacher and learner. The state of flow in the coaching / learning process which I experience is more frequent on those occasions when I have prepared myself for the coaching sessions. In my early morning sitting I clear the decks, let go of my coaching agenda and bring to mind my students, their needs, fears and perspectives. Deepening embodiment helps me to, 'get myself out of the way' and as a result I am more present and available for my students.

Mind-Sight - Being with ourselves: Mind-Sight refers to a 'knowing' of one's deeper internal subliminal prejudices at base consciousness, which influence one's surface thinking and behaviour. To be in this place effectively the coach is fully aware of their own internal dialogue as is the case when the coach is working from a mindful embodiment. Mind-sight involves not only sensing the present, but deeply knowing the past so that we are not imprisoned by the unexamined elements of our experience that restrict us in the future (Siegel, 2010).

Equanimity: The mindful coach will see the learner as an equal partner in the coaching / learning transaction. Being with the learner and operating from what the leaner needs is paramount. The coach will not see themselves as the fountain of all knowledge but instead skilled in creating the conditions whereby the learner self-realises - the mindful coach may even aim to make themselves redundant. This process is gained through maintaining a coach / learner relationship where mutual trust, tolerance, empathy, understanding, and appreciation flourishes. Coaching is likely to arise from 'who' the coach is being, rather than 'what' the coach knows. The coach is able to separate the learner from the learner's performance and has an understanding of the challenges and stressors which the learner is experiencing.

Compassion: Manifests in so many varied forms within the learning / teaching dynamic. Compassion in this context is so powerful and worth investigating fully. Where both the learner and coach exercise self-compassion the learning journey will be changed for ever. From my experience the challenge for the mindful coach is to instil in the learner self-compassion, or as Hassed & Chambers (2014) point out, adhering to the golden rule of treating others as we would ourselves. However, in the learning dynamic it seems to be about treating ourselves as we would others. I spend much time with skiers helping them to be kinder to themselves in analysis of their performance. This is not about positivity, instead it's about how we relate to our own performance with kindness and generosity.

Pause and Reflect

How would you describe your style of coaching?
What are your underpinning beliefs about you as a coach?

THE RESEARCH - WHY MINDFUL LEARNING?

Through my early experiences of learning to ski, ski racing and studying sports coaching I realised there was a whole range of types of learning and coaching that were very different to the methods often used in sport at that time (early 1980's). In my coaching throughout the 1990's and 2000's I used various approaches and undertook many forms of coach training, not only in sports but also in life coaching. At this time, I also became interested in Buddhism, particularly the mind training and as I learnt more, I realised the potential benefits of applying some of the Buddhist teachings to learning and developing performance in sport.

It was ten years later when I had the opportunity to formally explore further, during the pilot study which preambles the larger MSc research piece. I eventually had a scenario and resources with which I could carry out some meaningful experimentation. The pilot study, for me, was a significant professional milestone in my MSc Studies in Mindfulness.

I had the unending support of Andrew Maile from Edinburgh University Sports Department to whom I am very grateful. He and his colleagues welcomed me to the Universities Outdoor Centre, Woodlands, at Kingussie in the Spey Valley, Scotland. A very familiar place, having worked there on University ski programmes many times before. With the Physical Education students as the learners and Andy's mentoring, I explored the application of mindfulness principles to the coaching / learning dynamic in Alpine Skiing.

The underpinning reason why I choose mindful learning for my research topic was really very simple – I had believed for a long time that there were other valid ways of coaching and learning than the traditional methods. Having explored many learning theories and coaching methods in my career I always had a feeling that these models and processes could get closer to the learner. I was often left thinking about where the learner is in the process. Mindfulness seemed to answer this not just in concepts but also in action. In mindfulness 'we begin from where we are' and one of the teacher's roles is to help the learner realise where they are now. I had the need to see if this would work in learning sports, namely Alpine Skiing, because that's the sport I know well.

Traditional methods of learning sports have been predominated with teacher centred approaches where the learner attempts to copy what is shown and practices whilst feedback is provided by the coach. The methods are characterised by command, teacher-led and with a focus on the exchange of knowledge from teacher to learner.

In this teaching-learning model, known as EDICT (explain, demonstrate, imitate, correct, test / trial) there is an underpinning assumption that the teacher knows everything and all performance development will originate from them. Learning is characterised by replicating the model performance of the coach, a reliance on external feedback, fault analysis and correction, from the coach. In Mindfulness I found what I consider to be some interesting alternatives to the traditional model, one which essentially shifts the teaching / learning dynamic to the opposite end of the continuum to traditional methods. It moves the learning from command to self-exploration and from replication to reflection and learner creation.

> **Pause and Reflect**
>
> In your own coaching which approach is predominant, command or guided discovery? Perhaps there is a blend depending on the learner.

BEYOND COMMAND

Away from command towards self-exploration learners are guided into deeper levels of self-awareness through body scanning techniques, breathing exercises, experimentation and problem solving. In these approaches the learner constructs their own performance guided by the coach. They value the past experiences of the learner and recognise their current levels of competence. Learners are part of the knowledge production process enabling them to formulate questions and make decisions about their own performance. These approaches are student-centred and lead to the production of performance rather than replication, and in doing so raise the levels of responsibility for their own learning significantly:

> In physical education, constructivist approaches invite students to begin the learning experience with their previous learning experiences intact. They are encouraged to engage with content intellectually and kinaesthetically and to actively participate in solving problems, discovering solutions, and experimenting with techniques and tactics (Singleton, 2009, p. 332).

I begin most sessions with a period of practice, questioning and collaboration, rather than formal performance analysis and fault detection, which often feels like a test to the learner. I encourage learners to interact with each other and to use their current performance and prior knowledge as the primary source of reference for future performances (rather than a 'fault' in performance being the starting place). When I am coaching mindful skiing, I am continuously gathering information and guiding learners towards self-knowledge and not necessarily directing them to predetermined ends. My aim in applying constructivist approaches to the research in mindful learning is in the back drop it creates for developing awareness, enabling inquiry and to hold all the other characteristics of mindful learning. Through my research I needed to understand the constructivist strategy and spent time deciding which coaching behaviour has integrity to this approach.

I also looked at how standard models of education compared with reflective models as the latter sits with mindful learning comfortably. I used the Reflective Paradigm model as put forward by Lipman (1991) and Schon (1991) who discern the move to more person-centred, dialogic and democratic educational approaches, where education is seen as inquiry. Lipman (1991, pp.13-14) draws a comparison between these two paradigms of educational practice which I found helpful:

Standard Paradigm	Reflective Paradigm
1. Education = transmission of knowledge to those who don't know from those who do.	1. Education = outcome of participation in a teacher guided community of inquiry where the goal is good judgement.
2. Our knowledge of the world is unambiguous, un-mysterious and unequivocal.	2. Students are stirred to think about the world when it is revealed that our knowledge of it is ambiguous and mysterious.
3. Knowledge is spread over non-overlapping subjects.	3. Subjects/disciplines overlap and are not exhaustive.
4. The teacher has an authoritative role.	4. The teacher is fallible.
5. An educated mind is a well-stocked mind.	5. The goal is not acquisition of information but to grasp the relationships between subjects.

Figure 3: Lipman's Standard and Reflective Paradigms

The Reflective Paradigm and Constructivist Approach provided me with a framework which lends itself to integrating mindfulness into the learning / coaching dynamic. I hope by sharing this here, albeit briefly, you gain a sense of my perspective on learning which opens the potential to apply mindfulness practices and principles to learning.

CASE STUDY

With the Research completed (Arnold, MSc Research, Mindful Learning in Sport, 2013) and after many hours of shifting through the participant responses to questionnaires and focus group interviews, the participants learning experiences emerged into words. I'll share some of the quotes with you and describe the main three themes which came through very clearly. I begin with a participant quote given in response to the broad, open ended question I put to participants asking them to describe the coaching and learning:

> I was finding out things about my performance from and for myself by recognising what was noticed through feeling bodily sensations as I was performing, I was discovering what my own performance felt like. The coaching approach meant that my learning was totally an internal process with no external / outcome goal whatsoever. I was focused on the experience of my own performance, the focus was not on 'how to' but rather on 'what's happening' during performance, feeling it during the how, so that the 'how' became known to me – we noticed it ourselves.

THE THEMES

I like this quote because it points towards three of the themes which emerged from the study:

1. An increase in self-awareness – not only of the limb movements and muscle tensions but also of the forces generated through skiing which the body feels.
2. An increase in understanding – making sense of sensory information is crucial if the raised self-awareness is to be put to good use. Knowing the cause and the effect within performance.
3. An increase in the ability to modify and adjust the performance at the time it is happening – this points to a higher state of self-regulation during performance, which is a quality of all top performers in any sport.

Participants also reported a heightened awareness of their mental states, mind-set, emotions and how they were feeling about themselves within the learning context. This was really interesting for me because I believe performance is greatly influenced by our being and far too much sports instruction focuses on the doing. It became clear to me that most, if not all, participants experienced some level of heightened awareness of what was happening in terms of body movements (technique), muscular exertion (physical) and emotional state (psychological). They were able to identify what it was, they were feeling and what was happening with their performance as it was happening. Here's some more quotes along these lines:

> Enlightening, it has helped me focus more on my own skiing and how it 'feels' and not to rely on feedback from outside me on what it looks like. I have incorporated this into my own teaching.

> I was finding out things about my performance from and for myself. Through feeling bodily sensations as I was performing, I was discovering what my own performance felt like.

One of the things participants valued most was the time spent on practicing in an atmosphere of unconditional, non-judgement from the coach, peers and themselves. The later of those three was very reassuring to hear as it pointed towards my ability to create a compassionate flavour to the learning, self-compassion being manifested through the absence of self-critical judgement. Another thing which struck me was that participants felt that they could think outside the box, they had permission to create, experiment and explore without fear of the coach telling them it was right or wrong. Many said that time for reflection was very valuable as it gave them opportunity to see and feel deeper into their performance.

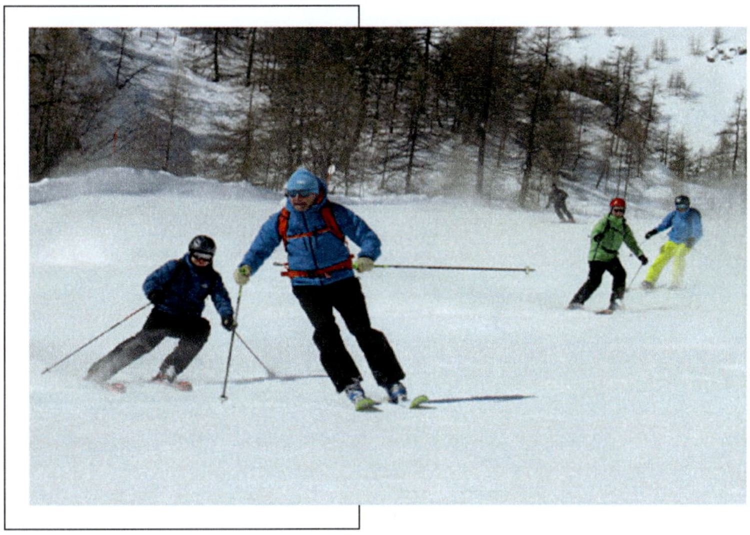

Figure 4: Hear, Feel and See. Photo © Deepak 2018

In a sport such as Alpine Skiing the use of the senses is something good coaches encourage. Clearly the kinaesthetic, tactic knowing of where the body is at any point in time and the muscular effort being applied is something that many sports people can identify with. In Alpine Skiing we guide skiers to hear the sound of the skis over the snow and learn from that information by distinguishing what the action of the skis is against the snow. I often analyse performance from the sound of the skis as they make very different noises depending on what the skis are doing and from this, I know what the body must be doing. Here's some quotes which mention the non-judgemental flavour of the learning:

> Very empowering process; focused my attention inwardly; raised my consciousness of my own performance; did not compare my performance with my peers because through the coaching approach it was not comparable, all working on our own inner stuff.

Connections were being made between the performance itself and the ways in which the performance was being achieved. This is pointing towards context, which in skiing is influenced greatly by the environment, that is, the terrain, snow conditions, weather, equipment. As I've mentioned before Alpine Skiing in the mountains (rather than an indoor snow slope) is a highly open skill, which means there are many variables. On the learning, in which participants immersed themselves, many recognised the collaborative, reflective and self-inquiring nature of the learning and liked it:

> I found the coaching approaches very human, it was very different, quiet, relaxed and sociable; quite unlike my rugby coaching experiences where the coach would become exasperated if you weren't doing what they wanted.

> Coaching felt like guidance rather than teaching; focused on enabling my self-awareness of what was happening to me, rather than thinking about technique and watching a demonstration and trying to figure out what to do.

> It was a new concept to me as I have always applied thought and logic to my learning experiences; I am a thinker; to become aware of feelings of performance was a very different approach for me and very positive and a faster means to learning and improving for me than other more traditional methods.

THE CHALLENGES

Some participants revelled in the learning journey absorbed in practice and gaining a sense of freedom through the absence of value judgments and being encouraged to let go of self-criticism:

> How subtle it was; how the use of self-observation influenced and allowed development; how relaxed and intuitive the learning experience was.

There were challenges for some. The fact that most feedback on performance is intrinsic led some learners to believe they were not being taught. Furthermore the coaches questioning, prompting deeper reflections on their own performance, was met with scepticism particularly by those who are used to 'command' coaches. Those learners were trying to figure out the 'correct' answer. Underpinning all of this perhaps, is the principle of responsibility for one's own learning. Over prescriptive learning can develop the sense that improvements in performance are something which is done to the learner, rather than change coming from within.

Two quotes provide a clue about the ways in which some participants expressed the challenges:

> Initially frustrating then enjoyed the freedom to experiment within the given boundaries.

> Very enjoyable, a bit unsettling psychologically.

Interestingly there are some similarities between the perceived challenges and, 'The Triple Tensions of Mindful Teaching' (Macdonald & Shirley, 2009) which provide purpose, direction and cohesion to mindful teaching as a set of pedagogical principles and practices:

> The first tension of mindful teaching is the tension between contemplation and action. To be mindful, one must take time to become attuned to and reflective about what is transpiring (Macdonald & Shirley, 2009, p. 68).

The challenge to some learners was spending time reflecting and sharing compared to time spent on doing the performance and practicing. Although the time spent on doing and practicing was far more, the periods of self-inquiry and reviewing were an unwelcome distraction for some.

As the sessions progressed, there was 12 hours of coaching in total for each participant, most readjusted their learning expectations. They became to realise how an increase in self-awareness led to an increase in skill and also how the overall process was more enjoyable and empowering. The final quote here is one of my favourites as it expresses a feeling about the learning journey and performances along the way:

> Highly enjoyable and liberating; I started to quieten my own judging mind and experienced improvements in my performance as a consequence; it was fun and felt like a journey and I didn't know where it would end which was great because there was improvement.

CONCLUSIONS

What I have discussed is how learners experience mindful learning and how coaching through mindful methods can be achieved. What you take from this chapter and how much you apply to your own coaching and learning is, of course, your choice. You may be motivated to look into this topic in more detail, follow up on the references and read more widely. If this is the case with just one reader then my job here will be done.

The wonder for me of mindful learning is how these methods of learning increase enjoyment and make participation more fulfilling and joyful. Whether they offer a fast track to higher levels of performance is not important to me. My aim in coaching and leading people in outdoor natural environments is that their happiness increases and suffering decreases. Helping people to put their learning in perspective, particularly learning sports, is a quest of mine, as is having people not take themselves so seriously as learners. This lightness helps people to relax into their learning causing mind and body to be more at ease and in this state, performance will flow more naturally.

For coaches, mindfulness has much to offer, improving how they relate with their students / athletes and more able to attend to their learners needs without interference from their own agenda. I know many coaches are driven by the need to help others and I think mindfulness leads coaches to realise they cannot help others, only help others, to help themselves.

FURTHER RESOURCES

My research can be viewed in full and downloaded from the Mindful Mountains web site. I welcome hearing from any coaches or educators who are interested in learning mindfully, skiing and mindfulness and the place for mindfulness in sport generally. Please contact me through the web site contact page where you can also view and download the full MSc Research Thesis, Mindful Learning in Sport 2013, John Arnold, http://www.mindfulmountains.com
Further information on Muska Mosston's work see here: https://www.spectrumofteachingstyles.org/

REFERENCES

ARNOLD, J. (2013) MSc Research Thesis, MSc Studies in Mindfulness, unpublished research study, Aberdeen University.
BROWN, K.W. CORDON, S. (2009) Towards a Phenomenology of Mindfulness – Subjective Experience and Emotional Correlates, Clinical Handbook of Mindfulness, 2, 59-81.
BAIN, L. (1995) Mindfulness and Subjective Knowledge, Quest, 47 (2) 238 – 253.
HASSED, C. CHAMBERS, R. (2014) Mindful Learning, Shambhala Publications.
KABAT-ZINN, J (1991) Full Catastrophe Living 2nd Edition, Dell Publishing America.
KEE, H. WANG, J. (2008) Relationships between mindfulness, flow dispositions and mental skills adoption: A cluster analytic approach. Psychology of Sport and Exercise 9, 393-411.
LANGER, E. (1989) Mindfulness. Perseus Books USA.
LANGER, E. (2000) Mindful Learning, Current Directions in Psychological Science, Volume 9, Issue 6, 220-223.
LANGER, E. (2000) The Construct of Mindfulness. Journal of Social Issues, Vol. 56, No.1.
LIPMAN, M. (1991) Thinking in Education, Cambridge: Cambridge University Press.
MACDONALD, E. SHIRLEY, D. (2009) The Mindful Teacher, Teachers College Press, London.
MOSSTON, M. (2001) Teaching Physical Education – The Spectrum of Teaching Styles: From command to discovery, 5th edition, Wadsworth Publishing.
SCHON, D. (1991) The Reflective Practitioner, Ashgate Arena, London.
SIEGEL, D. (2010) The Mindful Therapist, W.W. Norton & Company USA.
SINGLETON, E. (2009) From Command to Constructivism Canadian Secondary School Physical Education Curriculum and Teaching Games for Understanding, University of Western Ontario London. Curriculum Inquiry 39:2 Wiley Periodicals, Inc.
UK Network of Mindfulness-Based Teacher Trainers (January 2010) Good Practice Guidance for Teaching Mindfulness-Based Courses.

CHAPTER 17

IT'S GOLF....BUT NOT AS WE KNOW IT: GOLF AS A MINDFULNESS PRACTICE AND A METAPHOR FOR LIFE.

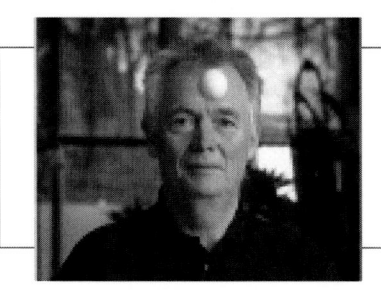

Vin Harris

vinharris.hkt@gmail.com

MINDFULNESS AND GOLF?

Can you imagine an alien spaceship orbiting planet Earth, observing how we busy humans spend our precious free time? What would they think of the thousands of golfers who renounce the concerns of the everyday world and dedicate their lives to hitting a small white ball into holes in the ground? Strutting and fretting for hours out on the course for no obvious purpose. With their strange clothing and mysterious implements, surely they must be taking part in some bizarre religious ritual?

What would these same visitors from another galaxy think as they watch an ever-increasing number of people joining mindfulness clubs: walking very slowly with no particular destination, sitting motionless in silence for extended periods of time, ostensibly doing nothing, watching their own minds (have you ever wondered how is that even possible?). Is this some new kind of lunatic sport without judges or referees where there are no winners or losers?

"Lord, what fools these mortals be!" (Shakespeare, 1605, A Midsummer Night's Dream, 3.ii). Apart from being confusing to aliens, what else do you think golf and mindfulness might have in common? Is there something those who devote their time to these popular forms of human folly could possibly learn from one another? Before trying to answer these questions, I would like to tell you a story which might help to explain how I became fascinated by golf, mindfulness and the mystery of being human.

GOLF - THE FINAL FRONTIER

I was almost forty years old when I took a decision which meant that my life would never be the same again. Driving home from an appointment with my doctor, I was reflecting on the advice she had given me about my health. It was one of those moments when everything falls into place and you just know what needs to be done. The time had come: I was ready to be a golfer.

When I am about to disappear for a few hours (or sometimes for a few days) to play golf, I often remind my wife how grateful I am to her for pointing out that, although I was to all intents and purposes in good health, I ought to take a more active interest in my physical well-being and visit the doctor for a mid-life checkup. After carrying out various tests and asking questions about my lifestyle, the doctor was impressed. She confirmed I was healthy and less stressed out than the average small business owner. I hadn't heard of mindfulness at that time, but I had been a Buddhist practitioner since my early twenties. Maybe I was living proof that meditation actually works. As my business was growing I was spending more time sitting in the office or in the car, less time actively working as a joiner, my doctor suggested I did need to take more exercise. This consultation and my "road to Damascus" experience on the way home was my call to adventure.

Golf was about to bring an unexpected new dimension to what had already been a journey full of variety and wonder. I am a practicing Tibetan Buddhist with a degree in English and European Literature, a craftsman who helped to build a Tibetan Buddhist monastery, an entrepreneur with an MBA, a hippy who has made pilgrimages to holy places in India, Nepal and Tibet. Standing on the first tee, crossing the threshold into another new world I was curious to see what would happen next.

> **Pause and Reflect – Beginner's Mind**
>
> Can you remember a time when you entered an unfamiliar world
> or started out on a new adventure?
> What was it like, how did you feel?
> Could you bring an attitude of "beginner's mind" to the familiar
> reality of your everyday life?

THE SECRET LIFE OF GOLFERS

Golf in Scotland is special. There are the internationally famous Championship links but also many towns and villages throughout Scotland have a golf club and a golf course, that in many cases have been looked after by the local community for more than a hundred years. It is hardly surprising that my approach to golf was unconventional, but nobody seemed to mind; they were probably too busy playing golf to notice. Anyway, it must have been obvious that I loved and respected the ancient game and I received a warm welcome in Moffat Golf Club. During these past twenty-five years I have played golf there in South West Scotland as a member and had the honour of serving as Captain and President.

In a parallel universe my inner journey continues, and it has always seemed pretty obvious to me that golf is a metaphor for the game of life. If you have never played golf you might well wonder why anyone would be interested in this apparently pointless game that many people refer to as "a good walk spoiled" but I prefer my friend Andrew Grieg's view that "a walk is a missed opportunity for golf" (Greig, 2006, p.134). When playing golf there is time and space to feel my body, to notice my mind, to be with nature, to be fully present. But there's more to it than that. Golf shows me my limitations and my potential.

I want to share with you some of the insights into mindfulness and life that I would surely have missed if I had just gone for a good walk. Later in this chapter, as we explore together the inner game of golf, we will understand just how much is going on beneath the surface of golf; or any other form of human folly. But I expect you are wondering what golf has to do with the Hero's Journey.

TO BOLDLY GO

Stories of the deeds of heroes captivate the imagination of people all over the world. A story becomes truly compelling when we identify with the hero or heroine of the adventure and picture ourselves living through the triumphs and disasters they encounter. There are endless permutations but there is a common theme running through the history of storytelling from the plays of the ancient Greeks to the latest science fiction films. Heroes represent courage in the face of adversity and the altruistic qualities we aspire to. The villains they encounter manifest weakness and the selfish tendencies that we wish to overcome. Is this so different from the way in which we relate to our sporting heroes?

We live in a strange world where it is possible to become a multi-millionaire simply on the basis of an ability to run fast or to have a special talent for throwing, hitting or kicking a ball. It doesn't seem to matter that the feats of sporting heroes are in themselves meaningless, as long as our heroes compete in a spirit of integrity. We identify with them and so it does matter to us when, against all the odds, they triumph over adversity and accomplish something that once seemed impossible.

Rejoicing in their greatness we celebrate our own latent qualities. Perhaps this is why billions of people choose to spend so much time and money watching sport.

WE CAN BE HEROES

Sport has become a huge business, an incredibly effective means of extracting cash from the masses. In spite of this can it still be a gateway to a lost spiritual dimension? The Ancient Greeks considered athletic competition as "a concrete demonstration of spirit over matter" (Jackson & Csikszentmihalyi (1999, p. 4). At the summit of their art, Zen archers enter a radically different way of being: "Don't think of what you have to do…. the shot will only go smoothly when it takes the archer himself by surprise" (Herrigel, 2004, p.44). Murphy and White (1995) document many examples of playing in the Zone, an elusive transcendent state sometimes experienced in sport, where athletes find themselves amazed by their own performance. Sincere commitment to physical action can take athletes beyond the mundane into the realms of spiritual experience. In the words of the runner Eric Liddell quoted in the film Chariots of Fire (1981): "I believe God made me for a purpose, but he also made me fast. And when I run I feel His pleasure".

To be a hero is to grow beyond the limits of our own expectations. We all have this capacity. Shivas Irons, the hero of Golf in the Kingdom says of golf:

> …as ye grow in gowf, ye come to see the things ye learn there in every other place…. Ye'll come back from the links with a new hold on life, that is certain if ye play the game with all your heart (Murphy, 1997, p.67).

Setting out to play a round of golf feels like going forth on a hero's quest, leaving behind the everyday world, meeting challenges, returning home to the place I left behind for a few hours, having learnt something of value as a result of losing and finding myself in the game.

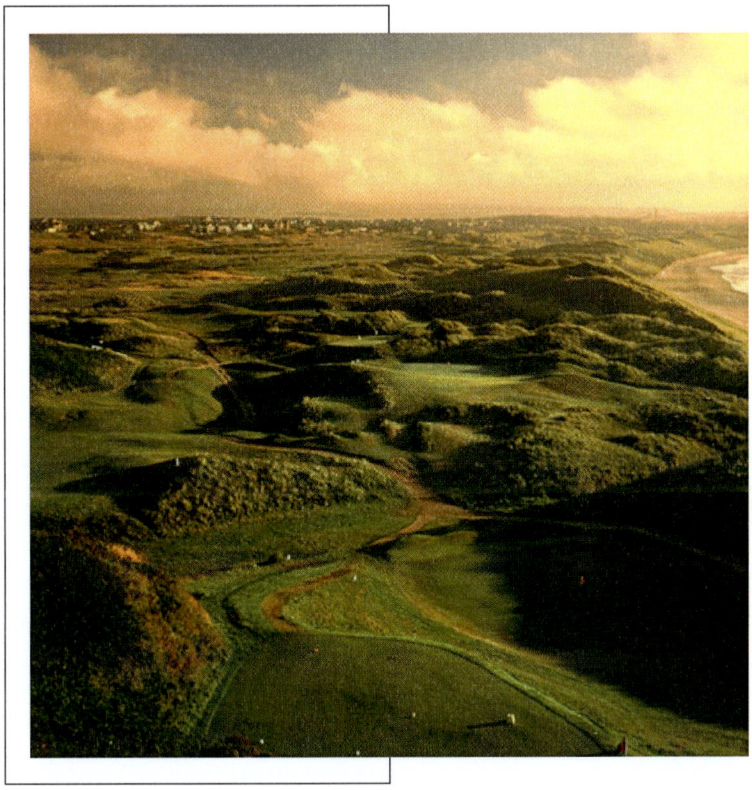

Figure 1: Golf links a field of play where adventures await. Photo © David Whyte, Linksland 2008

FOR THE LOVE OF THE GAME

For amateur golfers, the challenges and rewards are different from those that our sporting heroes can expect; their livelihood and reputation depend on their performance. In the true meaning of the word amateur, we play for the love of the game. Having said that, even when there is not actually very much at stake, golfers of all abilities still tend to get obsessed about how well they play. In his golf novel The Legend of Bagger Vance, Steven Pressfield reflects on the power of golf to cast a spell, to draw us in and lead us on:

> What hooks us about the game is that it gives us glimpses. Glimpses of our Authentic Swing…We feel with absolute certainty that if we could only swing like that all the time, we would be our best selves, our true selves, our Authentic Selves (Pressfield 1996, p. 70).

The enigmatic golfer Moe Norman simply described the experience he loved when hitting golf shots as "the feeling of greatness" (O'Connor, 1995). Most golfers know how it feels to play like this sometimes. When it happens we remember how easy golf can be. But these glimpses don't happen as often as we might wish.

I sometimes find myself in beautiful surroundings, in the company of good friends, away from the complex demands of everyday life and still somehow contrive to not enjoy playing golf. This is not only my experience. Golf is famous for being an exceptionally frustrating game. Success on the course may reveal potential but golf can be a particularly ruthless teacher when it comes to dealing with failure:

> I attribute the insane arrogance of the later Roman emperors almost entirely to the fact that, never having played golf, they never know that strange chastening humility which is engendered by a topped chip-shot. If Cleopatra had been outed in the first round of the Ladies' Singles, we should have heard far less of her proud imperiousness (Wodehouse, 1999, p.228).

Why does it matter so much when results don't conform to my expectations? Why do I play my best golf sometimes, but not all of the time? In essence, I want to understand how I create suffering out of nothing and I want to know what I can do, or refrain from doing, in order to allow my potential to manifest more often. These issues affect us all. I would now like to introduce you to some of the friends, guides and mentors who have helped me navigate the inner world of golf. Whether you are a golfer, a mindfulness practitioner, a curious human or perhaps all three, I trust that their wisdom will hold true when you return to your own world.

EXPLORING THE INNER WORLD OF GOLF

A METAPHOR FOR LIFE

When I first looked beneath the surface of golf I thought I might be the only one who saw golf as a metaphor for life. But I have been lucky to share this journey with so many friends who felt the same way. We have had so much fun exploring the field together. In his book "Preferred Lies", Andrew Greig describes my friend Dave Hares and I as "not so much golfing gurus as golfing guerrillas, here to bring some liberation and light to those oppressed by golf" (Greig, 2006, p.85). I can live with that.

I first met Andrew through a golf workshop called Fairway to Heaven. For the past twenty one years Fairway to Heaven has enticed golfers from around the world to make a pilgrimage to Scotland the Home of Golf. Our purpose is to discover a more rewarding game whilst playing on some of the most wonderful golf courses on planet Earth. The idea for Fairway to Heaven was conceived by my friends Joan Shafer and John Talbot. Taking time out from their regular work as members of the Findhorn Community, they would head for the golf course at Forres to engage in their "special spiritual practice".

Please don't think I underestimate the importance of learning technical golfing skills. However, when we facilitate these programmes, Joan, John and I don't teach participants that aspect of the game. I feel our role is to encourage people who join us for a week of Fairway to Heaven to give themselves a break from playing the game they think they should be playing and play the game they would play if nobody was watching. How do we do this? We provide a space where participants can notice how their hopes and fears play out in their golf games and in their lives. Through meditation, yoga, reflection and discussions we explore the insights that happen through playing golf in a spirit of friendship and curiosity.

Maybe the true value of regarding golf as a metaphor for life, as I have been doing with my fellow travelers on Fairway to Heaven and elsewhere, is that I can look into the mirror of golf to see more clearly how I am right now; sometimes if I am lucky I may also catch a glimpse of the person I could be. I find that it takes courage, and a little help from my friends, to play and live in a way that challenges how I think I am supposed to behave.

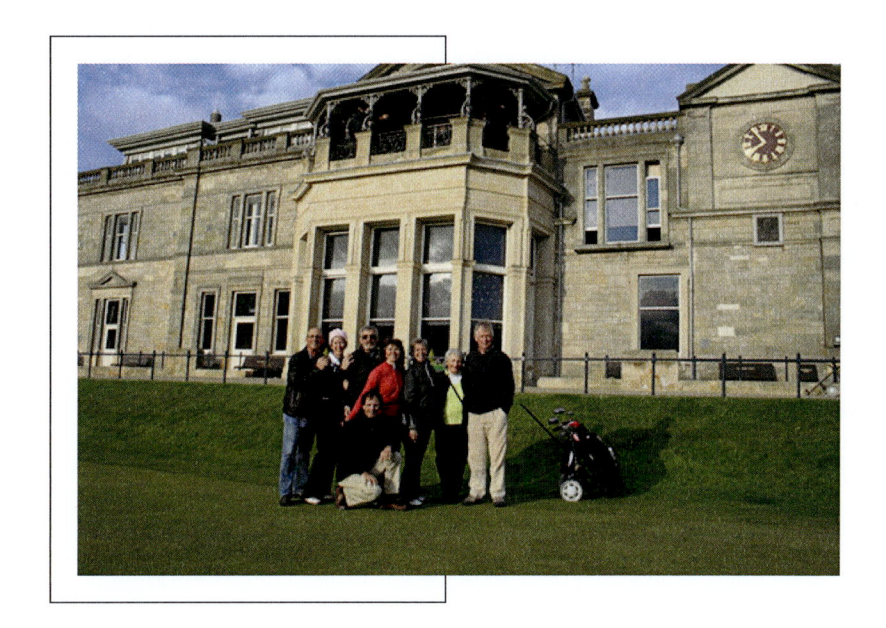

Figure 2: Fairway to Heaven in St Andrews the Home of Golf. Photo © Mitch Laurance 2012

PERFORMANCE AND LEARNING AND EXPERIENCE

In our modern society there is an implicit and rarely questioned assumption that if we humans get more of what we believe we want, we will inevitably experience satisfaction. And so our failure to clarify what we truly want permits the advertising industry to thrive. "After a time, you may find that having is not so pleasing a thing after all as wanting. It is not logical but, is often true." (Spock, 1967) Golfers are not immune to this dis-ease. Fred Shoemaker says:

> After twenty years of teaching golf, I have learned that if you lower your handicap, get the correct form, get out of bunkers in one shot rather than two, etc., it will have no effect on your overall happiness and fulfillment from the game (Shoemaker, 1997, p.26).

Yet most of us strive to improve our performance and feel with absolute certainty that if we succeed we will be happy. Timothy Gallwey developed his famous inner game method of coaching initially for tennis, then for golf and subsequently he applied the same principles in the corporate world (Gallwey, 1975,1986, undated). He suggests that taking the time to be really clear about our goals is necessary in whatever we undertake. Otherwise we may go out of our way to achieve external success without finding inner fulfillment:

> Essentially, any human activity offers three different kinds of benefits: the rewards that come from performance, or the external results of the action; those produced by the experience of performing the activity; and the learning or growth that takes place during the action (Gallwey, 1986, p.119).

This model of the "performance triangle" supports a balanced approach to the pursuit of happiness and excellence.

As Fred Shoemaker reminds us, the outer goal of playing golf remains very simple:

> The rules of golf say only that we should try to score as low as possible. They do not say what the purpose of the game is. That is for each person to determine (Shoemaker, 1997, p.4).

My reasons for playing golf are many, and they change from time to time. If I fail to keep this in mind and focus only on performance whilst neglecting my inner purpose, I risk missing out on the opportunities for enjoyment and learning; as an ironic consequence of this imbalance, performance invariably suffers. This may be more obvious on the golf course than in other areas of life. Sometimes I wonder does golf imitate life or does life imitate golf?

Pause and Reflect – Performance Triangle

Sit quietly and bring to mind something you do: your job or a project you are involved with or perhaps one of your hobbies.

Imagine you are observing yourself at work or at play.

Within the triangle of Performance-Learning-Experience, where would you say most of your energy is directed?

What would change if you gave more attention to the aspects of your activity that you tend to neglect?

What might happen if you engage in activity with awareness of the need to perform but also with an intention to keep learning and to enjoy the experience?

WHY DO I PLAY GOLF?

A perfect day, beautiful weather, I was with my friends playing one of my favourite holes at Moffat Golf Club. But I was not having fun! Score going badly, trying to figure out what I'm doing wrong, getting impatient, everything feels a bit tight, too serious. On a golf course there is a lot of time and space available for reflection; as long as I don't get lost in the dense undergrowth of my own rumination. From nowhere a question popped into my mind, "ok Vin…so why do you play golf?" My heart responded, "because I like to feel young and free". I felt myself smile at the recognition of this truth I had forgotten.

Acknowledging why I play, I remembered how to play. Eight years old, messing about, being outside with my pals, mood was different and physical movements felt free, less cautious. Fred Shoemaker articulates the impact that a shift of perspective can have as follows:

> *Extraordinary changes come from a new point of view – a new way of being.* In this as in all aspects of the game, "being" precedes "doing" (Shoemaker, 1997, p.80).

I wanted to know more about this inside-out approach. Is it really possible that being aware of my aspirations could transform my game? Could paying attention to my attitude change the flight of my golf ball and have an effect on the course of my life? An exciting prospect but it seems too good to be true.

> **Pause and Reflect – Why before How?**
>
> It is very easy to get caught up in the technical aspects of what we do.
>
> Of course, it is necessary to know How to do our job, practice mindfulness or play sport. Now may be a good time to reflect on Why you do what you do.
>
> Sit and rest for a while and ask yourself one or more of these questions:
>
> Why did I choose the work I do?
> Why do I practice mindfulness?
> Why do I spend time on my leisure activities?
>
> When you clarify your sense of purpose does it change how you will choose to work, rest and play?

WHAT ABOUT RESULTS?

When checking in to play a round of golf one day, I noticed a sign that said: "We are here to write down numbers – not to paint pictures". Basically, they were trying to encourage golfers to maintain a reasonable pace of play on the course. I wouldn't be too surprised if I was the only person who saw this and thought of Iain McGilchrist's description of the divided brain:

> The left hemisphere is not in touch with reality but with its representation of reality, which turns out to be a remarkably self-enclosed, self-referring system of tokens (McGilchrist, 2012, p.252).

This limited version of reality is reflected in the way golfers become obsessed with the numbers on the scorecard and forget how to fully appreciate the game we love.

As the famous motivational speaker Tony Robbins says, "Where focus goes, energy flows" (Robbins, undated). That's all very well, but focus usually gravitates towards the measurable results of performance. The problem is that we tend to ignore the enjoyment that can be derived from fully experiencing what we are doing, and we often neglect the learning that flows from participating fully in the activity. I suppose this is to be expected in the busyness of working life, but it is a pity when the same old habits play out in other areas of life where we are supposedly free to be off duty. Even though results do matter, let's not mistake them for the sole purpose of the game. Numbers never lie; they don't always tell the whole truth.

During a conversation about golf and life with Andrew Greig, I once said that I see golf as an opportunity to "invest in outcomes in a protected space" (Greig, 2006, p.237). Playing in this space, where results matter enough but not too much, serves to remind me that all is well when I get out of my own way and give up trying to control what happens: it does seem to be possible to let go of worrying about outcomes whilst still caring passionately about what I am doing. Why not value the numbers and the pictures? Of course, changing the habits of a lifetime is easier said than done and takes practice; on the meditation cushion, on the golf course, in daily life.

REMEMBERING TO REMEMBER

The word mindfulness is now part of our everyday language. Are we all talking about the same thing? According to Holmes (2013), the modern conception of mindfulness is perhaps closer to what Buddhists refer to as awareness which, without any particular ethical connotations, is simply being fully aware of what is happening. However, in Buddhism mindfulness involves knowing what we are doing and remembering or keeping in mind the commitment to a noble purpose (Holmes, 2013). It seems to me that the term mindfulness is being used to describe both of these two distinct yet interrelated qualities of attention:

- A non-judgemental awareness of the present moment.
- Noticing whether or not we are being true to our chosen purpose.

Mindfulness teachers often promote a non-judgemental attitude towards experience. Rob Nairn considers expectations to be a major obstacle (Nairn, 1998). Chasing after results tends to create assumptions about what is supposed to happen; what is actually happening is neglected or even suppressed. Perhaps an emphasis on acceptance is necessary to counteract the guilt and striving that are prevalent in our culture. However, according to Jon Kabat-Zinn, in order to consistently pay attention to what is happening in the present moment, we will need a compelling reason for our practice (Kabat-Zinn, 1994). How else can we hope to override the addictive fascination with past and future?

It appears that we need to cultivate our innate capacity to recognise distraction and return to open presence. A commitment to what is truly important guides us home when we get lost. The challenge is to give it our best shot without indulging in counterproductive self-judgement if it doesn't work out as we had hoped. This requires practice. When the golf course becomes a playground of learning and growth, each game offers an opportunity to challenge the patterns that hold me back and to establish the conditions that set me free. I have nothing to lose except a few golf balls: a small price to pay for an experience that might change my life for good.

Pause and Practice – Intention and Awareness

Sit comfortably and give yourself time to notice how it feels to simply be in your body and become aware of your breathing.

For the next couple of minutes, sit in silence with the intention to be aware of your breath coming and going.

When you notice that you are lost in thinking and are no longer aware of breath, regard this as a moment of mindfulness – you have remembered your intention. Now without making it a big deal, just return to being aware of your breath.

Getting carried away and finding your way back again and again. How do awareness of the present moment and mindfulness of intention support each other?

A TESTING GROUND FOR MINDFULNESS

As a long-term meditator, entrepreneur, mindfulness tutor and amateur golfer, I have found that the themes we have been exploring apply both on and off the golf course:

- Finding a balance between performance and learning and experience.
- Being clear about my intentions.
- Seeing that results are not an end in themselves.
- Keeping in mind my sense of direction.

Through regarding golf as a mindfulness practice as well as a metaphor for life, I recognise the possibilities for growth in this field of activity and I wanted to share with others the joy to be discovered in a game worth playing. This was what I had in mind when designing my golfing research project.

Sixteen amateur golfers had gathered in St Andrews to participate in a Fairway to Heaven golf week. We were there to explore the famous courses at the Home of Golf and the equally important but less well-known course to be found between our ears. What better people to ask to participate in my research? I distilled the issues I have been reflecting on into this one question:

"What happens if you keep in mind why you play golf when you play golf?"

Stage 1 – Knowing why you play golf

Fourteen golfers took part in a preliminary exercise, presented by myself and another programme facilitator. Through a guided reflection practice, they were asked to find a succinct expression of why they play golf. Participants were invited to complete the following statement "I play golf because I want to……" Rather than trying to look for the right answer, they allowed a statement with personal resonance to emerge and they wrote it down.

Everyone then chose a partner they felt drawn to work with. I reminded them to be curious and listen; mindful of any urge to judge or offer advice. The partners took turns to support each other in getting below the surface of their initial answers. They inquired into the completed sentence by asking "why do you want to…." This refined the original statement and the process was repeated until each participant felt that they had found a clear statement representing their own intention for playing golf. With consent from the participants I kept a written record of their stated intentions.

I introduced this exercise because I wanted to give people the time and space to look deeper and find out what really matters to them; to be clear why they play golf. I felt it was important to encourage participants to identify a purpose that had emerged from within. In my own experience and based on what I have understood from reading and conversations with friends, an off the shelf motivational slogan might seem attractive at first, but it is likely to be discarded sooner than a few simple words that resonate with our actual aspirations.

Stage 2 – Keeping in mind why you play golf

The process of helping people clarify why they play golf was interesting in itself but it was also a preparation for the next stage of my research. I suggested to all fourteen participants that they keep their reason for playing golf in mind when playing golf each day during the week of Fairway to Heaven and notice what happens.

Towards the end of the week, I invited four participants to be interviewed for the second stage of my research. They were told that the responses would be anonymous and that their experiences would be used to improve understanding of: "What happens if you keep in mind why you play golf when you play golf play?" Each of the four participants who were invited agreed to take part.

I held a one to one interview lasting between thirty and forty-five minutes with each of the four participants to find out what had happened. At the beginning of our meeting they shared their personal reasons for playing golf they had discovered during the initial inquiry. Then they were simply invited to reflect on how their experience had been when playing golf and keeping their personal sense of purpose in mind. I did my best to listen in a spirit of mindful inquiry; doing little more than asking for clarification when required.

I wanted to give people the opportunity to see what it would be like to take their own clearly articulated purpose for playing golf with them onto the course. I was curious to know what difference if any it might make to their overall experience of playing golf. Participants for this second stage of the research were selected because they had expressed an interest in mindfulness. They received some mindfulness practice training during Fairway to Heaven but they were by no means experienced practitioners.

Results of Stage 1

Seven pairs of participants helped each other to clarify individual reasons for playing golf. This resulted in fourteen statements of intention that fitted into one or more of the following four main categories:

- Letting Go
- Enjoyment and Fun
- Learning and Effectiveness
- Feeling Alive and Connected

Throughout the Stage 1 exercise there was a consensus that golf can be a vehicle for personal transformation. One golfer commented "golf helps me reconnect with life" and another expressed the intention to "become a better golfer and a better human being".

Results of Stage 2

The four golfers who took part in Stage 2 of my research are referred to as Players A, B, C & D. They shared with me their reflections and the key themes or insights that had emerged as they explored the question: "What happens if you keep in mind why you play golf when you play golf?"

- Player A - *"Reconnect with Life"*

Player A spoke of "golf as a mirror" for other issues in life: reflecting in particular how honest the player was being about personal challenges such as unresolved anger/intolerance, wishing for respect and after a period of illness wanting to reconnect with a sense of fun.

The experience of playing with awareness of purpose had brought perceived benefits such as: increased resilience, not bailing out or giving up, bringing back a sense of fun when too serious and not being too concerned about what others may think or say. Player A described the intention to remember the motivation for playing as "a magnet that draws me back".

- Player B - *"Relax, Perform, Interact"*

The wish to interact had the meaning for Player B of engaging with and learning about other people when playing golf. Player B noticed that the competitive nature of sport sometimes led to a "blurring of the intention to relax, perform and interact" and that when this happened, poor results followed. It had been difficult, but sometimes possible, to deliberately use staying with breathing as a means of returning to the original intention: the experience was described as "wonderful…when connected to breath, the golf swing takes care of itself". Player B found that the ability to use awareness of breathing to "get back into the zone" was supported by acceptance of "human frailty" rather than self-blame for having lost sight of the intended focus.

- Player C - *"No Expectations"*

The intention to play golf with "no expectations" was seen by Player C as an antidote to the feeling of having something to prove or wanting to please others which was perceived to lead to anger and frustration. An insight had arisen that "trying to prove is not about others" and reflecting on this further Player C stated that "golf shows you what you are...golf magnifies the best and worst".

Player C found that using the intention to let go of results helped to work with integrity and honesty on the issue of excessive striving and that this process incidentally brought about better results. There was an exploration of the dynamic between the inner and outer environment and an acknowledgement of the importance of self-acceptance: "it is internal supportive conditions that set me free".

- Player D – *"Swing Freely with Joy"*

For Player D the intention to "swing freely with joy" was a reminder to be aware of "the magic of being alive". The benefits of playing with this intention were described as "planting a seed". It was possible to "touch base with it" as a way to "recognise and observe doubts, anxiety and fears". There was a sense that by noticing the departures from the intention brought about increased awareness which seemed to facilitate "playful learning without judgment" and performance improvement.

Player D considered that there are many parallels between golf and life regarding golf as a vehicle for self-improvement; a way of using the external to work on the internal. An insight arising from playing with awareness of intention: "I play and work better when I laugh and smile".

BRINGING IT ALL BACK HOME

TIME TO REFLECT

I must confess that I did have some reservations about asking people to participate in my research. I was concerned that both the first exercise to clarify why they played golf and the subsequent inquiry into what happened when playing would be an invitation to over complicate the game. The last thing I wanted was to detract from the fun of play. As it turns out the invitation to keep their chosen purpose in mind helped the players to simplify their approach. I was pleasantly surprised when players A, B, C and D all found that difficulties were minimised, their enjoyment and learning was enhanced.

Players B and D in particular were able to use their intention as a support in the same way that breath or sound can be used in mindfulness practice. Player B noticed the "blurring of the intention to relax, perform and interact" and Player D was able to "recognise and observe doubts, anxiety and fears". By becoming aware of when they had lost sight of their intended focus they were able to return to their present moment awareness; what is more they both did so with acceptance and a joyful attitude.

The stated intentions of players B, C and D did not include specific performance related goals, yet in each case improvement happened coincidentally. This certainly reflects my own understanding and the ideas that were explored earlier. Focus on results to the exclusion of all other aspects of the game gets in the way. When paying attention to learning and the experience of playing, performance takes care of itself. I am becoming increasingly convinced that in mindfulness practice and in golf, expectations of results inhibit our natural capacity for excellence.

Playing golf whilst keeping in mind why they play golf enabled Players A, B, C, and D to notice when they had departed from their intention and to gain insights into their habitual tendencies which were diverting them away from their personally meaningful purpose. The golfers had the courage of heroes to take an honest look at their all too familiar patterns reflected in the mirror of golf. Perhaps even more impressive was how the players could then play golf as an expression of the freedom that had emerged.

So now what?

The participants in both stages of the study found the experience to be beneficial. However, all of them cited reasons for playing golf that included learning and enjoyment rather than performance alone; this is hardly surprising since Fairway to Heaven golf workshops attract players who are interested in personal transformation. You might then ask how mindfulness could benefit the majority of people who play sports, since they are certainly likely to be more concerned about performance and results than my fellow golfing pilgrims.

It would be naïve to apply a standardised form of mindfulness practice across different sporting disciplines without understanding the specific mental and physical strengths they each require. For example, in a round of golf very little time is actually spent playing shots. Golf's particular challenge is that it takes three or more hours to play. Mindfulness practiced in the playing of the game rather than as preparation for the game becomes particularly relevant. Dealing with our own reactions to the inevitable moments of success and failure is an intrinsic part of any sport played at any level. However, golf gives us more time than most sports to get lost in thought.

Although the players in my research received a relatively small amount of mindfulness training, they were able to notice when the familiar stories appeared. They reconnected with their intentions; they returned to the field of awareness where the game is played. I suggest this was made possible through the commitment to remain in alignment with their heartfelt reasons for playing. Without establishing a personally meaningful sense of direction how could they have stayed out of the hazards? Our heroes went further and noticed what was blowing them off course.

If you find out why you love to play golf, you will find a game that is really worth playing. When you have a reason for playing that resonates with the core of your being, you will want to hear this harmony more than you want to listen to the endless inner chatter that interferes with your latent talents. There can be no right or wrong reason for playing golf, and so I feel the approach I used in my research could have value for any golfer who is ready and willing to discover the game they have always wanted to play. I hope to have more opportunities to share what I have learnt; not least since I believe this has implications that extend far beyond the golf course.

Pause and Reflect – Back to the Future

Before you move on, please do take a moment to look back over the time we have shared together exploring the inner game of golf, mindfulness and life.

What have you discovered?

What will you take home with you to apply in your world?

Mindfulness practice may already help you to survive the inevitable challenges you face in your life: could mindfulness also enable you to thrive and express your potential?

Is it possible to see whatever you do as an opportunity for mindfulness practice: a way to become more familiar with your own mind?

THE 19TH HOLE

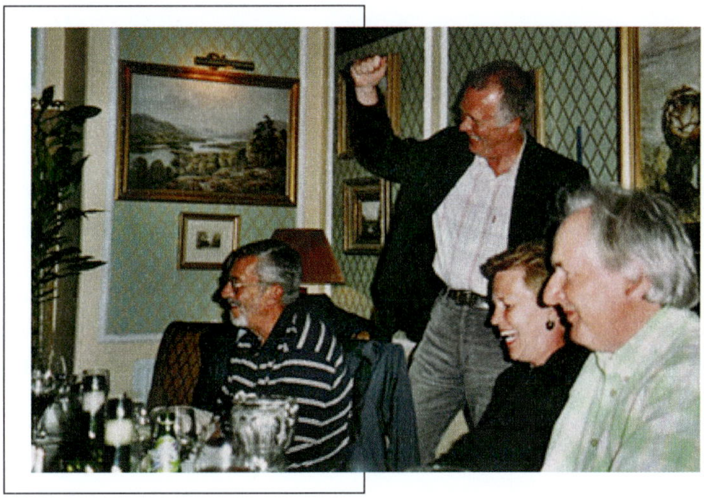

Figure 3: A place where golfing heroes tell their tales. Photo © Fairway to Heaven

Golf has its traditions and rituals. On the 1st tee, before the game begins it is common to wish each other "play well…. enjoy the game". As the last put is holed on the 18th green, players remove their caps, shake hands, congratulate or commiserate and thank their fellow competitors. And then there is the clubhouse, often known as the 19th hole; a place where conversation flows free. So afore ye go, let me get you a wee dram, make yourself comfortable and I'll tell you what I really think.

At first I felt a bit embarrassed to be writing about mindfulness and golf, knowing that my fellow mindful heroes were telling moving stories of how they had used mindfulness to help themselves and others when facing life's most difficult moments. To be honest I felt like my topic was insignificant, somewhat frivolous. As it turns out, it seems that wholehearted engagement with any activity, even golf, can show the way to wisdom.

I don't know how many times I've heard mindfulness teachers say to participants on their courses "you are ok as you are…. you don't need to fix anything….there is nothing wrong with you". Ultimately this may well be true. Provided we don't teach people to recite the jargon whilst forgetting the meaning, it is certainly good to remember that there is no point in making the situation worse than it has to be. However, particularly if we want to apply mindfulness in contexts such as sport, business, creativity and education, I think we must not forget that we humans like to improve ourselves. Like many people, I take great pleasure in the process of getting better at what I do. To take account of this common ambition, we may need to take a different approach to mindfulness teaching and practice when the emphasis shifts from facing our immediate problems towards seeking fulfillment and long term sustainable happiness.

And another thing…....if we are on a mission to become the best we can be then this may well be a very long journey and it will be easy to lose our way unless we allow ourselves to be guided by our own inner compass: by keeping the most distant horizon clear in the mind's eye we can appreciate each small step we take. Mindfulness resolves the paradox that it is possible to be content where we are now and at the same time prepared to settle for nothing less than our full potential.

FURTHER RESOURCES

For Information about Fairway to Heaven and upcoming workshops visit: https://www.spiritualgolf.com/index.html

Andrew Greig's book, Preferred Lies: A Journey to the Heart of Scottish Golf (2006), tells of Andrew's inner and outer golfing odyssey, featuring his experiences on Fairway to Heaven.

To hear my conversation with leading Performance coach Karl Morris about golf, life and more go to the Podcast. http://brainbooster.libsyn.com/ "Vin Harris, the Monk who drove a Ferrari – ep39"

REFERENCES

CHARIOTS OF FIRE. Film. Directed by Hugh Hudson. UK: Columbia, 1981.
GALLWEY, W. T., (1986). The Inner Game of Golf. London: Pan Books. (First published 1981 by Jonathan Cape Ltd).
GALLWEY, W.T., (1975). The Inner Game of Tennis. London: Jonathon Cape.
GALLWEY, W.T., (undated). The Inner Game. Available: http://theinnergame.com/
GREIG, A., (2006). Preferred Lies. A Journey to the Heart of Scottish Golf. Great Britain: Weidenfeld & Nicolson.
HERRIGEL, E., (2004). Zen in the Art of Archery. Training the Mind and Body to Become One. London: Penguin. (Translator not identified. Translation first published by Routledge& Kegan Paul 1953)
HOLMES, K., (2013). An Introduction to Buddhist Mindfulness. Available: http://www.calm-and-clear.eu/mindfulness.pdf
JACKSON, S. A. and CSIKSZENTMIHALYI, M., (1999). Flow in Sports. The keys to optimal experiences and performances. USA: Human Kinetics.
KABAT-ZINN, J., (1994). Wherever You Go There You Are. Mindfulness Meditation for Everyday Life. Great Britain: Piatkus Books.
McGILCHRIST, M., (2012) The Divided Brain and the Search for Meaning. Kindle Edition. USA: Yale University Press.
MURPHY, M. and WHITE, R. A., (1995). In the Zone. Transcendent Experience in Sports. England: Penguin.
MURPHY, M., (1997) Golf in the Kingdom. USA: Penguin.
NAIRN, N., (1998). Diamond Mind. Psychology of meditation. 2nd ed. South Africa: Kairon Press.
O'CONNOR, T., (1995). The Feeling of Gretness, the Moe Norman Story. Oklahoma: The Graves Golf Academy.
PRESSFIELD, S., (1996). The Legend of Bagger Vance. New York: Avon.
ROBBINS, T., (undated). Tony Robbins Blog. https://www.tonyrobbins.com/career-business/where-focus-goes-energy-flows/
SHAKESPEARE, W., (1605). Cited from (1980). The Complete Works of Shakespeare, The Alexander Text. London and Glasgow: Collins
SHOEMAKER, F., (1997). Extraordinary Golf. The Art of the Possible. New York: Perigee.
SPOCK, (1967). Star Trek, Amok Time. TV Series, Episode 34.
WODEHOUSE, P. G., (1999). The Golf Omnibus. London: Random House.

CHAPTER 18

THE MINDFUL CURLING OLYMPIC TEAM

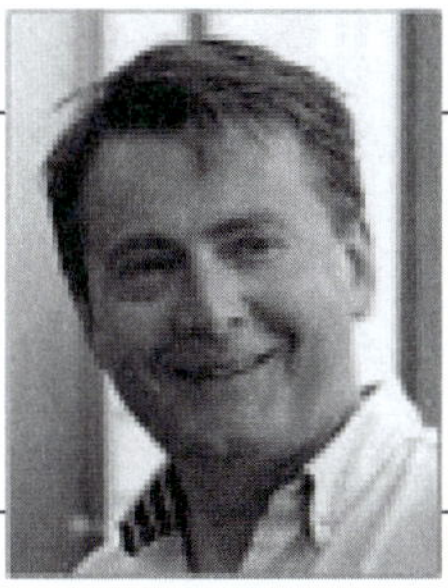

Misha Botting

mishabotting@gmail.com

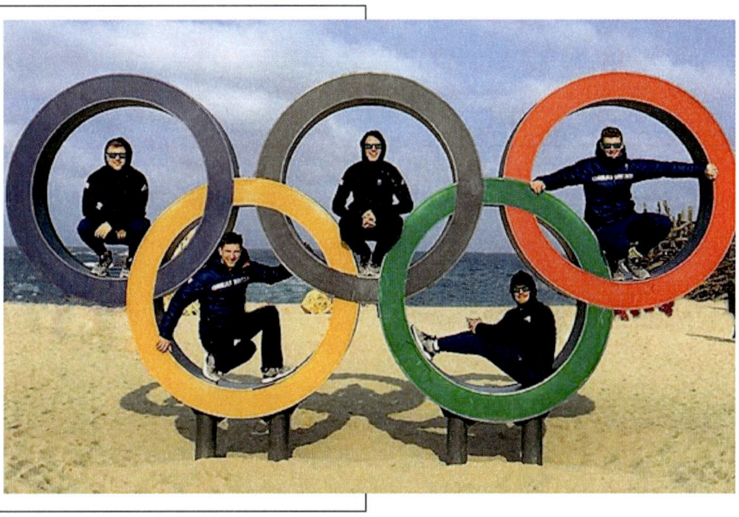

Figure 1: blue ring: Kyle Waddlle (2nd), black ring: Kyle Smith (skip), red ring: Thomas Muirhead (3rd), yellow ring: Glen Muirhead (ultinent), green ring: Cammy Smith (lead). Photo © the team at the Winter Olympic Games in PyeongChang 2018.

TRIALS AND TRIBULATIONS AT THE OLYMPICS

After the end of the last match at the Winter Olympic Games in PyeongChang 2018 we did not go through our usual routine of a debrief, we sat silently in the changing room drained of all energy trying to process what had just happened. We lost a tight match against the Swiss team which we had beaten earlier in the competition and consequently finished fifth overall. This was 'not bad', but was short of the team's expectations of their own performance. Something else happened too: not one player felt shame, no one walked away from his team-mates, not one of them was bitter about each other's efforts or pointed a finger for the loss at anyone else. There were no complaints about anyone's ability to support each other until the last stone was played. After a silent, heart breaking bus journey back to the Village, all of the players walked to the food hall for a bite to eat. You have to eat, even after the loss of an Olympic dream.

It is hard to describe the feeling when the most intense eight months journey ends with a loss. Your body experiences this dull and overpowering pain as if somebody has thumped you in the stomach. It does not kill you, but you cannot move, and your lungs don't draw enough breath for words. I was not even a player on this team, I was the team's sport psychologist, helping 'the boys' to get the best out of themselves. The terms 'the boys' is frequently used between players and is going to be used in this chapter with the utmost respect for the players.

Many months have passed since the last match and I still reflect on what else I could have done, what else I could have said that would have made a difference in the precision of the line trajectory of the last stone, or help the skip to make a better decision. Writing this chapter is an attempt to reflect on my choice to use mindfulness and team-compassion principles as cornerstones in the sport psychology intervention for the men's curling team on their journey to the Winter Olympics 2018.

MY CONTRIBUTION TO THE TEAM

In the ten months prior to being selected for Great Britain Team (Team GB) this young team of players managed to achieve unprecedented success and had a very impressive rise in the curling world rankings. The boys were winning against the most renowned and experienced teams from all over the world, but towards the end of the season they were unable to match the results they had demonstrated at the beginning of the season. This factor had an impact on the players unity, enjoyment of playing together, their communication and consequently the quality of their performance.

My job was to take a thorough look at the team, make an assessment of the causes of their performance slow down, and to determine the philosophy that would work for the team to embark on during the Olympic cycle and at the Olympic Games. The following stage was the delivery of psychological support to players and the team. At the core of this training was one very clear purpose: to assist the development of a team capable of winning a medal at the Winter Olympic Games in 2018. To contribute to this outcome, my sport psychology support focused on the team of players and their coach with a major emphasis on strengthening the boys' interpersonal skills, offering them deeper awareness of themselves and each-other and ultimately, to make them robust in the face of any adversity. To be successful again, the boys had to rediscover their love for curling, their love for the sport that they started playing at the age of eight, the sport that was passed to them through three or four generations of their family to a young and exceptionally gifted group of players.

I knew that if I use emotive rhetoric in my conversations with the team, it could potentially lead to emotional burn out before their first competitive match. Therefore, the philosophy of the work with the players had to be uplifting and charged with a solution focused attitude. The boys had to feel empowered – capable of sorting their own problems, enjoy each other's company and to cherish their friendship in the face of setbacks and successes.

> **Pause and Reflect**
>
> Imagine that a small group of very determined individuals (in any walk of life) asks you to help them to get the best out of themselves. What would you do first?
>
> How would you go about structuring and delivering your support?

THE OLYMPIC DREAM

The Olympic Games remains one of the ultimate challenges of human physicality, tenacity and courage. Many millions of people around the globe witness both the most devastating defeats which crush some athletes and the most incredible elevation of others. Victors become stars and are frequently called Olympic legends and heroes. The popularity of the modern Olympic Games has constantly grown and at the press of a button billions of people around the globe can watch dramatic battles between athletes from every corner of the planet.

Olympians frequently talk about the old generation of sporting heroes who inspired them. Hence the baton of inspiration keeps being passed forward to new generations. And so, the awe of the Olympics lives in young hearts who dare to dream big dreams and endeavour to walk in the footsteps of their heroes. Perhaps, these dreams become possible because of the blissful ignorance of the young. Or perhaps a young generation of athletes fully embrace the transcendental power of awe that was ignited in them by their role models. What they do not think about is the hardship and complexities of the Olympic journey. In order to qualify for their national team at the Olympics, they have to become faster, jump higher and be stronger than any other Olympian in the history of the games. Hence athletes have to step up in every aspect of their sport and use every possible (legal) advantage that would give them an opportunity to succeed and bring home a medal. Little wonder that the Olympics are considered by athletes and audiences as the ultimate sporting summit, requiring extraordinary physical and mental attributes to perform and succeed at the right time.

Pause and Reflect

When you think about your favourite Olympian, what three names arise in your memory first?

Reflect on what kind of qualities they have and what are you most impressed about their journey to sporting fame?

Do you think that the qualities you admire in these individuals are the qualities you would like to develop in yourself?

THE SPORT OF CURLING: CONSTANT CHANGE - CONSTANT READJUSTMENT

As a sport psychologist working with curling for many years, I have witnessed a tremendous change in the sport. Since curling secured its place in the Winter Olympic calendar, the business of winning medals has become a lot more than just having a laugh with friends 'throwing rocks' at the weekend whilst having a 'wee dram'. The opportunity of winning an Olympic medal has brought the prospect of being in the history books, attracting sponsorship deals and becoming a sporting legend. To achieve this sporting pinnacle, players commit to significant transformations. They move away from their homes; they embark on a long competition season; they constantly travel between comfortable and uncomfortable hotels, and for months they eat food that has been cooked by somebody else.

The life of a full-time curler consists of regular structured training with the aim of improving their technique and developing their tactical awareness. Players follow custom built strength and conditioning programmes, they have to do their individual injury prevention exercises, be mindful of what they eat and watch what they think.

Even though the landscape of the sport has drastically changed, the nature of the sport remains the same. It is still a target sport played on ice by a team of four players. Players throw a 20 kilogram polished granite stone (mined from a Scottish island called Ailsa Craig) towards the target called 'the house'. Each of the four players throw two stones intermittently with the opposition. Once a stone arrives at the house, it can be nudged or taken out by the opposition. This element creates a complex tactical choreography where any stones could be used as either obstacle or an aid. The number of points scored is calculated based on which stones are closest to the centre of the house and frequently are measured in millimetres.

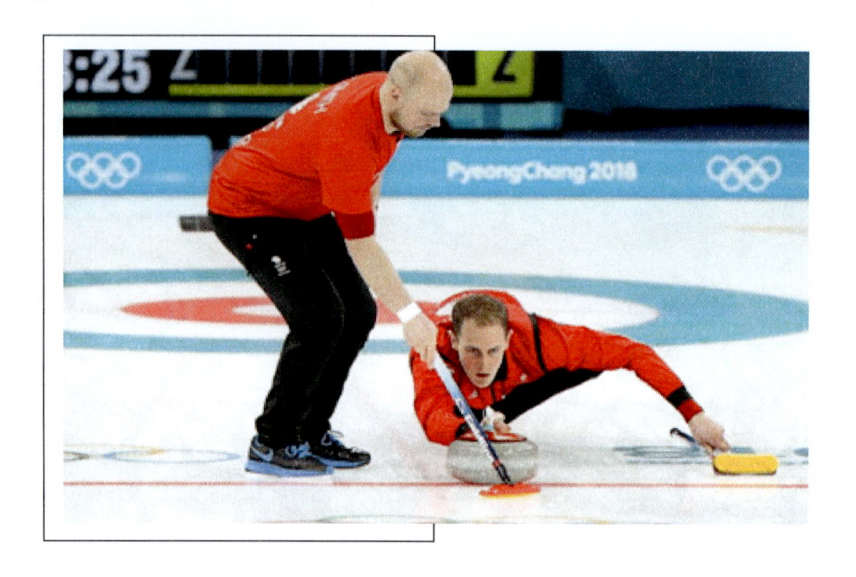

*Figure 2: Kyle Smith delivering the stone. Cameron Smith is the sweeper.
Photo © Richard Gray 2018*

PSYCHOLOGY OF CURLING: THE PROBLEM-SOLVING GAME

Curling is an exceptionally complex game and is frequently called 'chess on ice'. Every player must be fully alert to the changes in the conditions of the ice as these changes unfold stone after stone. If these changes are not noticed or somehow misinterpreted, a stone stops short of the target or goes right through the house. The most successful teams in curling are those who have a significant amount of experience picking up on the 'relevant cues', have knowledge of selecting the 'right' stones for the appropriate shots, those who are able to make relevant re-adjustments to the speed of the delivery. That is where curling matches are won and lost.

BATTLES WITH THINKING

Curlers constantly try to predict the future, driven by a strong desire of not wanting to lose and cling to the thought of winning. These powerful forces create battles inside players heads as they desperately try to retain their focus and avoid distractions. Ironically, these battles take up significant attention from the match and frequently this kind of struggle ends up in tears of defeat (Birrer and Morgan, 2012).

The technique of substituting the content of thoughts (cognitive re-structuring) is frequently used in sport and it comes from the Cognitive Behavioural Therapy (CBT) branch of psychology and now is deeply imbedded in sport psychology training (Teasdale, et al., 2000, p.616). One of the reasons why cognitive restructuring is so popular in sport, is because intuitively we know that having good thoughts is better than having bad ones and the positive rhetoric sounds very seductive ('we are winners', 'we are better than them'). Even though this shift may sound logical and intuitively right, the reality of this technique has a hidden irony: this restructuring process breaks down when curlers are under pressure, when they experience attention fatigue. In these conditions players get caught in escalating and self-perpetuating cycles of ruminative unwanted thinking. This type of thinking could quickly bring the diametrically opposite result from the desired positive outcome (Birrer, Röthlin, Morgan, 2012; Harris 2010). When I encountered the challenge of ironic thinking and cognitive restructuring, I was very keen to find alternative ways forward that may provide solutions to my clients in a competitive and stressful environment.

> **Pause and Reflect**
>
> When you find yourself in an anxious situation, what kind of thoughts do you have?
>
> Do you try to change them, avoid them or do you just drift along the stream of thinking with hope that everything will work out in the end?

MY HERO'S JOURNEY

FROM MINDFULNESS IN DANCE TO MINDFULNESS IN SPORT

My professional career started at the age of nine when I embarked on a long journey to become a professional classical ballet dancer. This journey took me through The Moscow Bolshoi Ballet Academy, where every day the students practiced awareness of the body for many hours. This training was slow, tedious and very competitive. For years I learnt how to point my toes and how to stretch my knees - properly(!). I learnt how to withstand physical pain and how to compete with others and with myself in a ballet class and on stage. It took me years of practice to develop a good proprioceptive awareness and develop the ability to internalise attention within the body in order to correct any deviations from 'perfect classical canons'. Nine years of training at the Ballet Academy prepared me well for a professional ballet career in Moscow and then in Scottish Ballet. Over the years I learned how to train my body, avoid injuries and get the best performance my body could produce in the most difficult circumstances.

DEPARTURE TO NEW TERRITORY

Only after the completion of my professional ballet career I realised that I had missed a trick. Everything that I was doing in my dance career was using lessons I acquired in the Bolshoi Ballet Academy: controlling the body and getting the best out of my physicality. At no stage during my ballet career did I come across the simple idea that the mind controls the body. I genuinely was not aware that there are some mental skills that could have helped me to produce my best performances. This realisation came to me years after I was 'killed' for the last time playing the role of the bereaved Paris in Romeo and Juliet.

DECENT: SEARCH FOR DEEPER MEANING

The quest to discover performance enhancing mental skills, took me on a journey through two universities and years of supervised training. Seven years after the final curtain on the ballet stage, I became a registered High Performance Sport Psychologist working with many professional and semi-professional athletes. I was a proud disciple of Cognitive Behavioural Therapeutic Philosophy. I felt that I had found the holy grail of secrets of optimum performance, which were universal and transferable between all performance expressions, whether in a theatre, on a pitch, on a court, in water or on ice. In my work I used the Psychological Skill Training approach (PST) which helped me to promote the development of self-regulation, including changing negative thoughts and emotions to positive ones (Thelwell & Greenlees, 2003; Birder, et al., 2012). The sport psychology path was clear: I was happily teaching my clients 'good' mental skills that were specifically designed to control thoughts, feelings and their bodies. For many years that was the direction, that was the content of my work and that was the method of the delivery of support to my clients.

Over the years I never stopped wondering and searching for connections within the science of sport psychology. I was reading about the subject and came across an interesting modality: Rational Emotive Behaviour Therapy (REBT). The founder of this branch of psychology, Albert Ellis was very open about the philosophical base for this modality which at the core had ideas of Stoicism and Buddhism:

> In essence these ancient philosophies, which stated that people are disturbed not by things but by their view of things, became the foundation of REBT... (Ellis and Dryden, 1997, p.2).

I decided to read on and go to the primary sources of these 'ancient philosophies'. There I discovered a cosmos of original ideas that have been so eloquently formulated thousands of years before psychology branched out from philosophy and became a separate entity. In my reading I was particularly taken by the Stoic philosopher Epictetus, who examined the causes of people's disturbed thinking:

> Some things are under our control, and others are not (though we may be able to influence them). If we are sufficiently healthy mentally, our decisions and behaviours are under our control. Outside of our control is everything else. We should concern ourselves with what is under our control and handle everything else with equanimity (Epictetus, sighted in Pigliucci, 2017, p.248).

To this day I find this quote most inspirational in my work and life. In this one short paragraph Epictetus sheds light on the fact that we need to shift our attention to what is within our control and not scatter it outwardly towards what we cannot control. When reading this discourse, I was encouraged to step outside of my perpetual need to control everything, including my thoughts and my body and have a more global perspective on the relationship between myself and the environment around me. My curiosity quickly extended towards Buddhism, where I found a lot of equivalent ideas to Stoicism, for example: "our natural tendency as human beings is always to find reasons outside ourselves, in our environment, to excuse what are really our own shortcomings" (Causton, 1995, p.15).

When reading about Buddhist and Stoic philosophies, I realised that one of the main concepts which unites them is the theme of striving towards equanimity in the face of adversity. These concepts captured my imagination and provided me with a platform to reflect on my former career in classical ballet and learn something new for my present profession – sport psychology. I decided to stick with my research and learn more.

I discovered that in Buddhism a prime example of equanimity was Prince Siddhartha Gautama (later known as the Buddha) who rejected a lifestyle of riches and fully engaged with the life of a travelling monk with no possessions. After reflecting on this story, I became more enthusiastic about the non-theistic base of Buddhism and I was very inspired by the Buddha's journey – the journey of awareness, courage, perseverance and finally achievement of his purpose. I then decided to learn more about this philosophy and signed up to workshops that had the word Buddhism in their titles. During these workshops I enthusiastically examined small details of a leaf and I was also asked to balance an egg on its sharp end. I was overwhelmed with joy when I managed to balance the egg on a table before everyone else! I also did a lot of breathing exercises, which I found interesting, but without a clear element of achievement, not necessarily as inspiring.

Despite my fascination with the subject, I still could not establish systematic practice and in-depth learning. Perhaps one of the reasons was that I was curious about this subject almost exclusively from the academic and professional point of view, this philosophy was certainly not a part of my daily practice. Over time my practical expeditions into Buddhism kept stalling, until one turning point of my life.

INITIATION: CHALLENGES AND SOLUTIONS

In a matter of two months I experienced a series of life changing blows that totally overwhelmed me. Everything I loved and treasured had been destroyed and everything I feared and desperately tried to avoid had become my daily nightmare. Very soon I lost any sense of perspective and motivation to carry on – at all. I was strongly advised to take anti-depressants and engage in a talking therapy. During this time, I decided to buy a book that could potentially help. In a big book store, I found a 'self-help' section; grabbed the thickest book that I could find and totally ignored the strange title and author's name. My murky, confused mind kept telling me: 'the thicker the book, the better… lots of words, very likely that the author knows what he is talking about... it'll do me.' At the time I simply lost any capacity of rational thinking and this kind of reasoning was the best that I could muster. I battled through the introduction until I was struck by the phrase:

> ...even if your mind is telling you constantly that it (meditation) is stupid or a waste of time, practise anyway, and as wholeheartedly as possible, as if your life depended on it. Because it does - in more ways than you think.

This sentence stunned me! In an instant I realised that I was standing on the brink. My life genuinely depended on what I did next. I decided to keep reading and followed the training, but with a different attitude and commitment. This 'thick book' was 'Full Catastrophe Living' by Jon Kabat-Zinn (above quote: 2013, p.xxxi). Gradually the 'thick book' was doing it's 'self-help' job and very slowly I started to pull myself out of the mire.

Reflecting on that time, I consider myself being pretty lucky that I encountered this incredible coincidence by randomly grabbing the 'thick book'. I had no idea that the author - Jon Kabat-Zinn managed to base his eight-week training programme on the Buddhist philosophy – the philosophy I was fascinated by, but previously unable to engage with. The 'thick book' offered me an easy to follow programme that inspired me to learn more about Buddhism and its modern incarnation - mindfulness. From then and to this day, a range of formal and informal meditative practices have become an integral part of my life. Now I meditate when I feel ok about myself and when I don't, when I was at the Olympics and also when at home before breakfast.

RETURN: LEARNING AND HELPING OTHERS

After I got better, I made a decision to take my progress with mindfulness to a different level. Supported by my employer (Sportscotland Institute of Sport), I embarked on an MSc course at the University of Aberdeen. Since then the degree has become an anchor in my life and work. It has enabled me to deepen my knowledge in this fast-growing domain of mindfulness and bring new knowledge and self-regulatory skills to a high performance sport of curling.

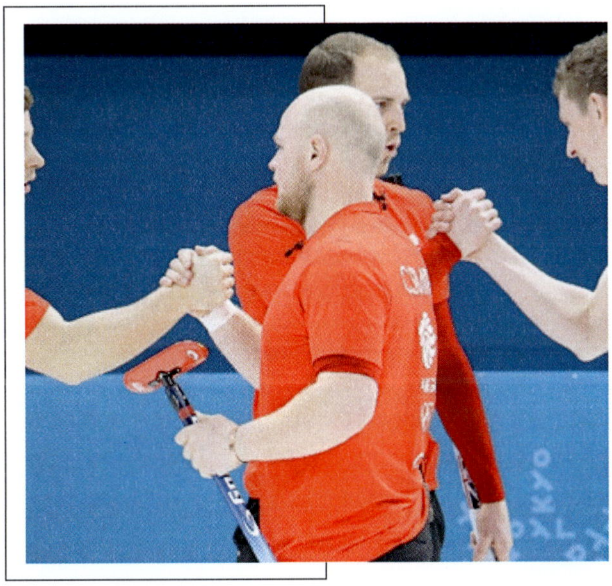

Figure 3: from left to right: Kyle Waddell, Cameron Smith, Kyle Smith, Thomas Muirhead. Photo © Richard Gray 2018

MINDFULNESS FOR THE OLYMPIANS

The second year on the MSc course coincided with my work with the men's curling Olympic team. I started working with the team eight months before their first match at the Winter Olympics. A big part of my job was to conceptualise the philosophy, structure the intervention and deliver the best sport psychology support I was capable of.

After careful consideration, I was reluctant to use a CBT approach in this intervention due to the main limiting factor associated with ironic thinking of players during competitive matches. When players become aware of their negative thoughts, they try to regain control and radically turn around their thinking from negative thoughts to positive ones. I observed that this process frequently leads players into a loop of battling against themselves. Consequently, players end up with the opposite state of mind from the one they desired to have (Birder, Röthlin, and Morgan, 2012). This state of mind is frequently charged with discontent, frustration and even hatred towards themselves.

Based on these considerations and a decade of work experience in sport psychology, I decided to depart the very familiar shores of CBT approach and embark on a mindfulness-based modality that offers a useful bypass to ironic thinking. Instead of being trapped in 'terror of thinking' (Kabat Zinn, 2013) mindfulness-based principle helps players to re-focus their attention on the relationship with the thoughts and emotions without changing them. Sharon Salzberg (2017, p.58) elegantly captured the potential consequence of trying to control thoughts in the following quote: "Often when we believe we are practicing self-control or self-discipline, we're actually confining ourselves inside an overly analytical, self-conscious mental chamber".

The 'mental chamber' is exactly what I tried to help the boys to get out off in order to play their best game, without being paralysed by over-analysis, self-criticism and suffocating perfectionism. It was very encouraging to learn that there were a lot of precedents of using the mindfulness approach in work with Olympians. In the mid-80's Jon Kabat-Zinn and his colleagues successfully delivered a mindfulness-based intervention for the USA Olympic rowers (Kabat-Zinn, et al., 1985). From then on there was a gradual increase of mindfulness-based interventions in sport and Kabat-Zinn's definition and his intervention framework is still widely quoted and used in mindfulness-based literature in the context of sport (Baltzell, and Summers, 2016).

"Paying attention in a particular way: on purpose, in the present moment, and non-judgmentally". (Kabat-Zinn, 1994, p.4) Even though this definition is very generic and needs to have a lot of clarity and shared understanding of every component amongst every member of the team, I felt very comfortable that this definition places 'attention' at the heart of the approach. Later, I came across another elegant definition of mindfulness: "…knowing what is happening while it is happening, no matter what it is." (Nairn, 2001, p.24) This succinct definition helped me to conceptualise the whole philosophy of my support to the team. When I think about the effectiveness of such a short definition, I use an analogy with a self-inflatable safety raft. When deflated, it is compact and shapeless, but when it hits the water, it unfolds into a vessel and reveals its substance and all the important safety features. The definition works in the same way - at first glance it may appear trivial, but when put into action, it reveals practical substance and demonstrates a conceptual shift from controlling thinking to just being aware, paying attention and knowing what is happening.

> **Pause and Reflect**
>
> In what way can mindfulness philosophy can fit in your work environment?

NOTICING AND KNOWING

'Being aware, noticing and knowing' – these concepts may sound a little passive and may feel intuitively 'not enough' for players who constantly strive to try to gain 'Stoic control' over their technique, tactics and their bodies. And yet, just paying attention to 'what is happening when it is happening' without changing it, offers a player an opportunity to genuinely understand what is going on in the environment and self. When the players become aware, they don't have to hurry to start changing anything or whipping themselves into the 'right' shape. Awareness is opposite to being 'spaced out' or being in an 'autopilot' state of mind. Noticing and knowing opens choices. It gives an opportunity for players to settle down their roller coaster of emotions and hold the ground of equanimity without panicky, rushed actions.

NO MATTER WHAT IT IS

In order to effectively use a mindfulness-based concept, it is appropriate to contextualise the non-judgemental element of the intervention in an appropriate way. The fundamental principle in any sport is a contest and its outcome, in other words, it matters that you win. It matters at any level and it certainly matters at the Olympics! From a very young age players progress in their sport based on the ratio between winning and losing. Those for whom winning is not that important, drop out from the sport. Most competitive players progress to the very top and only a few have an opportunity to be selected to participate at the Olympics. Therefore, the Olympic Games gathers quite an obsessive bunch of athletes for whom "victory means more than anything" (Pete Reed, triple Olympic champion. Presentation to British Curling, August 2018). However, if athletes get caught in a closed loop of thinking about their desire to win and avoid failure, this rumination has the darker side: "This leads to chronic stress, performance anxiety and burnout" (Harris, 2010, p.98).

It is not so unusual for a player to go on a long devastating rant about their poor performance. Frequently these rants are charged with abuse and negativity. After an unsuccessful shot I heard players tormenting themselves with sarcastic, self-attacking questions: "you are an absolute idiot, why did you do that?". It is not so unusual that elite level players expect a nearly perfect performance and if they fall below their 'nearly impossible standards', then self punishment is swift and devastating. These kinds of rants lead to more stress, more uncertainty and with this state of mind it is impossible to have a rational analysis of the causes of the error.

According to Birrer, Röthlin, Morgan (2012) a legendary Russian swimmer, Alexander Popov, said: "who thinks of winning loses." This poses an interesting dynamic: even though players are driven by desire to win they frequently get stuck on a negative ruminative loop which triggers performance anxiety and the fear of failure. Therefore, during a curling match, the non-judgemental attitude has a significant advantage that helps a player to maintain momentum to re-focus on the next task, without being stuck with 'self-defeating' comments (Baltzell and Summers, 2017, p.6).

In this context a mindful attitude does not prevent players from having negative thoughts, and neither does it give stern instructions to shift to positivity. With awareness and a non-judgemental state of mind, players have the choice to move forward regardless of their response in relation to what just happened. It offers them a choice of actions - not to get stressed about 'what if' scenarios, but re-focus on every shot independently from previous shots. 'No matter what it is'… if it is the first shot in a tournament or the last, if the team is are ahead or behind on points, if the match takes place in a local club or the final at the Olympics. The non-judgemental principle stays the same irrespective of the level of the competition. It helps to stay equanimous in the face of external challenges of all kinds, no matter what these challenges are. This principle is the bedrock of mindfulness approach and it is the key for successful performance in any competitive environment.

MINDFULNESS IN APPLIED SPORT PSYCHOLOGY SUPPORT

I encouraged players to hold on to their desire to win, but not at the expense of undermining their self-confidence that could lead to a deterioration of performance. We prioritised consistency of performance in the face of all challenges and called it 'bounce back'. This term stipulated enhancement of their frustration when things don't go according to the plan in a match, but with awareness and non-judgemental attitude to their negative responses. In order to present the boys an objective reflection of their responses, I asked them to wear radio microphones during matches and recorded their communication and self-talk. When re-playing the audio recording, boys were genuinely surprised to hear what kind of language (negative and at times dismissive) they used towards each-other and also themselves. That was an important lesson that helped players to practice 'letting go' of their negativity and re-directing their attention to the immediacy of the match and their next task.

In our conversations we specified steps:

> 1. Awareness was always the starting and the most important point. Without awareness, the autopilot of negative self-punishment was most likely but an undesirable outcome.
>
> 2. Acceptance was never an antithesis of giving up on the desire to win a match and perform at the optimum level. It helped the boys to move forward without being stuck in the past. Accepting thoughts and responses for what they are, meant accepting unsuccessful shots, accepting occasional miscommunication and feelings of anger and frustration. Communication based on acceptance helped the boys to maintain confidence in themselves, trust in their technique and shot-making ability.
>
> 3. Re-focus on the next task Once players accepted the situation and reflected of what they had to change (if anything), their job was to re-focus their attention on the next task (sweeping, decision making, etc).
>
> 4. With kindness This re-focusing transition had to be done with kindness and support from each player to himself and his team-mates. The reason for this style of transition was the reinforcement of acceptance and emotional equilibrium. We rejected the option of 'getting rid of negative thoughts'. Even though frustration responses like slamming brushes and kicking stones were detrimental behaviours for the team, we accepted them, reviewed during the audio/video session, learnt about causes of these responces and moved on.

When written down, this approach may look a bit formulaic, but all players really bought into it. They took individual responsibility to follow this path and helped their team-mates as much as they could. They stuck to their guns and embodied these principles in all matches at every level, including the very last match at the Olympic Games.

COMPASSION – THE MISSING LINK

One of the main influential figures in the emergence and subsequent growth of mindfulness-based modalities was Jon Kabat-Zin. In the late 70's he introduced the Mindfulness Based Stress Reduction (MBSR) programme, that was originally designed for patients who were recovering from significant operations and suffering from chronic pain. MBSR provided a rich environment for growth of a range of modalities including Mindfulness-Based Cognitive Therapy (MBCT). This modality also has a clinical and health base and it focuses on clients with clinical psychology conditions (Crane, 2012).

It is important to acknowledge that the origins of these modalities have roots in clinical environments where the focus of support is placed on individual patients. Consequently, these modalities do not have the team element in their content. It is a perfectly logical gap due to the fact that in a clinical set-up there is not an interdependent team, only individual patients. This is possibly why the team element of sport is not addressed in sport specific mindfulness-based interventions.

However, in Buddhist philosophy there is an element that extends beyond of self-regulatory practices of an individual towards the welfare of others. That is compassion. This philosophical concept has a tremendous depth and richness and could be applied for the benefit of growth and the effective performance of sports teams.

COMPASSION – THE CONCEPT AND APPLICATION

His Holiness Dalai Lama and Archbishop Desmond Tutu in the book 'The Best of Joy' offer a simple explanation of the term: Compassion is a sense of concern that arises when we are confronted with another's suffering and feel motivated to see that suffering is relieved". (2016, p.252). A well-known Buddhist and mindfulness teacher - Yongey Mingur Rinpoche describes compassion as: "a complete identification and active readiness to help others in any way" . (2007, p.174) In a more secular context offered by Boyatzis and colleagues this term is segmented into three distinct components: (a) noticing another's need, (b) feeling empathic concern for the other person, and (c) actively responding to enhance his or her well-being" (Boyatzis, 2012).

These definitions provide a perfect base for building team values and awareness that shifts players attention from 'I' towards empathetic and accepting 'we'. Based on the post-Olympics feedback from players, this element of mindfulness-based intervention was deemed the most beneficial for building the positive dynamic in the team.

COMPASSION IN APPLIED WORK

TEAM BACKGROUND

The team of the five players included two pairs of brothers who were also business partners in their respective farms. The farming background created an important positive element of common interest between brothers. The flip side was the fact that the siblings took each other for granted and did not work very hard at strengthening that bond between one another.

At the start of my work with players I observed a complex interplay of high competitiveness, high expectations coupled with taking each other for granted. The boys felt frustrated with each other and the level of enjoyment from the sport went down. Their good friendships and trust was slowly trickling away. Something had to be done to turn the team dynamics around. That is where the fundamental principles of compassion played a key role in taking the team to a new level of interaction for the benefit of each other.

STEP ONE

At the heart of our communication the boys were introduced to the concept of kindness to each other. In order to demonstrate this principle in action, I used the approach that was described by a Russian philosopher, Grigory Pomerants:

> The devil is born from an angel spitting in rage… the tone of the debate is more important than the object of the debate. Objects come and go, while manners form the building blocks of civilizations (Pomerants, undated).

This principle became the key building block of all communication in the team. All players started to be mindful of how they shared their feedback with each other irrespective of who was right or 'blindingly obviously' wrong. The key task of a communicator was to stick to the kind, non-judgemental tone that would ensure dampening down the 'passion' of the exchange. This style of tone helped the boys to have productive conversations even during emotionally charged match situations and thus ensure the preservation of the quality of their relationships.

STEP TWO

To extend awareness and empathy of each other, we used structured psychological profiles, which were conducted by a reputable company. Based on these profiles we ran a series of team sessions that focused on the players' contribution to the team and preferred communication styles. Since the boys were already equipped with the knowledge about the 'right' tone of conversation, the door was open to have an in-depth, non-judgemental conversations. That was something they had not done before, but something that gave them an opportunity to reflect on and share their preferred style of communication – not what a lot of boys typically do at their age.

STEP THREE

In the team sessions, I introduced a conversational self-disclosure exercise which was design to helping players to build relatedness, emotional intelligence, improve their active listening and compassion for each-other. During the exercise each player had to answer a series of open questions and tell a short story that related to their lives, their beliefs, and attitudes. The original exercise was designed by Arthur Aron and his team (1997) in a non-sport environment and therefore the nature of the questions had to be amended for the purpose of curling. The boys were encouraged to be open and honest with each other, make a lot of eye contact, share their stories and an occasional joke.

The boys took to this exercise like fish to water. Very soon it became the team's favourite activity where they learned a lot about each other and had a chance to share with their team-mates some experiences and reflections they never talked about with anyone else, including their respective brothers.

During these conversations I was taking a step back - just listening to the exchanges and rarely making comments. As conversations progressed, I started noticing an important transformation in every player. The boys became more secure talking about their feelings and they started to relate to the experiences that they shared with each other. It was very noticeable how In each of these sessions the boys were practicing kindness, empathy and compassion. They learnt to listen intently to their team-mates stories, they became less judgemental, and more appreciative and genuinely close with each other. I also started observing significant changes (verified by the team coach) in the boy's behaviour during matches. For example, they went an extra mile to support each other and had more important conversations whilst standing shoulder-to-shoulder. They carried an upbeat attitude to their pre-match warm-up's irrespective of their opposition. In post-match debriefs they created an atmosphere of support and kindness for each other. They knew how to maintain the appropriate tone in their conversations. This skill helped them to get to the causes of their defeats and errors, without irritation and feelings of guilt.

When entering the Olympic village, the boys knew how and when they needed to reach out for each other and how to make their team-mates and brothers feel more secure, irrespective of the outcomes of certain shots and certain matches. In the eight months before and during the Olympics, the boys managed to transform their team-dynamics and saturate their relationships with kindness and compassion.

POSTSCRIPT

Massimo Piglucci in his book 'How to be a stoic' (2017) describes a metaphor made by one of the stoic philosophers Cicero in relation to an archer and the controllable elements of a shot execution:

> If he has been a conscientious archer, he has done his best up to the moment when the arrow leaves his bow. Now the question is: will the arrow hit the target? That, very clearly, is not up to him (p. 35).

This thought is as important today as it was 2,000 years ago. Even though this passage was made about an archer and relates to every curler, the same can be said about a sport psychologist. I did what I could for the team, helped them to acquire new mindfulness-based skills and helped them to re-build a tight and joyful team guided by the principles of compassionate attitude for each other. They took mindfulness and compassion to their battles on ice and constantly reflected on and actioned all necessary improvements. I could not ask more from them. Now it is time for me to let go of this project and reflect on the boys' achievements.

Yes, we did not win a medal at the Olympics. That was a major disappointment that we all will carry with us for the rest of our lives. With this footnote, it is inevitable to reflect on the meaning of success and failure. The team threw their hats in the ice rink and gave their all. Each one of them loathed losing, but they were not afraid of it. Each one of the five players were brave enough to step outside of their comfort zone, take on board a new way of thinking, implement it in their lives and take it to their sport. It takes guts to do that, it is a true sign of bravery and courage.

In my eyes these five are the true heroes – heroes who dared to have big dreams, who embarked on one of the most difficult tasks that has culminated in one of the most challenging contests, who managed to deliver on every commitment they made to themselves and each other and stand up to the biggest disappointment in their lives. They stood together, they took responsibility for their actions and thanked those who walked with them from the first to the last stone. They learned the lessons about camaraderie and care for each other during their engagement at the Olympics. In my eyes this is a journey of heroes, by a bunch of guys with a farming background who did themselves proud during the most challenging contest in their sporting lives to date.

FURTHER RESOURCES

1. Headspace for sport training. https://www.headspace.com/sport/training
2. George Mumford. Mindfulness in Sports and Performance https://www.youtube.com/watch?v=A27EQ1YsJ_E
3. Arthur Aron. Self-disclosure exercise - building strong connection between people. https://www.youtube.com/watch?v=gVff7TjzF3A
4. Misha Botting, sport psychology support to men's curling Olympic team. TedxTalk: https://www.youtube.com/watch?v=fJ9GAel6bxY

REFERENCES

ARON, A., MELINAT, E., ARON, E., DARRIN, R., BAROR, R. (1997). The Experimental Generation of Interpersonal Closeness: A Procedure and Some Preliminary Findings. Personality and Social Psychology Bulletin. 23 (4), pp. 363-377.

BALTZELL, A.L. and SUMMERS, J., (2017). The Power of Mindfulness. Mindfulness Meditation Training in Sport (MMTS). Springer.

BALTZELL, A.L. and SUMMERS, J., (2016). The future of mindfulness and performance across disciplines. In: A.L. BALTZELL, ed., Mindfulness and Performance. Cambridge: University Press. pp. 515-541.

Baltzell, A.L. (2016) Self-Compassion, Distress Tolerance, and Mindfulness in Performance. In: A.L. BALTZELL, ed., Mindfulness and Performance. Cambridge: University Press. pp. 53-77.

BIRRER. D., RÖTHLIN. P., MORGAN, G., (2012). Mindfulness to Enhance Athletic Performance: Theoretical Considerations and Possible Impact Mechanisms. Springer Science+Business Media. LLC 2012.

BOYATZIS, R.E., SMITH, M.L., BEVERIDGE. A.J. (2012). Coaching with Compassion: Inspiring Health, Well-Being, and Development in Organizations. The Journal of Applied Behavioral Science, 49(2), pp.153-178.

CAUSTON, R., (1995). The Buddha in Daily Live. An Introduction to the Buddhism of Nichiren Daishonin. London, Auckland, Johannesburg: Rider.

CRANE. R.S., KUYKEN. W., WILLIAMS. M.J., HASTINGS. R.P. COOPER. L., MELANIE J. V., and FENNELL. M.J., (2012). Mindfulness. Mindfulness in practice. 3, pp. 76-84.

DALAI LAMA, TUTU, D., AND ABRAMS, D. (2016). The book of JOY. Hutchinson. London.

ELLIS, A., DRYDEN, W, (2007). The Practice of Rational Emotive Behavior Therapy. Second Edition. Springer Publishing Company, LLC.

GOULD, D., MAYNARD, I., (2009). The use of sports science in preparation for Olympic Games. Journal of Sports Sciences. 27(13). pp. 1393-1408.

HARRIS, R., (2010). The confidence gap. From fear to freedom. Robinson.

KABAT-ZINN, J., BEALL, B., AND RIPPE, J., (1985). A systematic mental training program based on mindfulness meditation to optimize performance in collegiate and Olympic rowers. Poster presented at the World Congress in Sport Psychology, Copenhagen, Denmark.

KABAT-ZINN, J., (2013). Full catastrophe living: Using the wisdom of your body and mind to face stress, pain and illness. New York: Delacorte.

KABAT-ZINN., J., (1994). Wherever you go, there you are: Mindfulness meditation in everyday life. New York, NY: Hyperion.

KABAT-ZINN, J., (2004). Wherever You Go, There You Are. London: Piatkus Books Ltd.

NAIRN, R., (2001). Diamond Mind, A Psychology of Meditation. Boston & London: Massachusetts Shambhala.

PIGLUCCI, M., (2017). How to be a stoic. Basic Book. New York.

POMERANTS, G., Undated. The dogma of polimic. http://www.pomeranz.ru/p/pub_dogmats.htm [Date Accessed: 22nd November, 2018].

TEASDALE, J.D., SEGAL, Z.V., WILLIAMS, M., JUDITH M. SOULSBY, J.M., LAU, M.A., (2000). Prevention of Relapse/Recurrence in Major Depression by Mindfulness-Based Cognitive Therapy. Journal of Consulting and Clinical Psychology. 68/4, pp. 615-623

THELWELL, R. C., AND GREENLEES, I.A., (2003). Developing Competitive Endurance Performance Using Mental Skills Training. The Sport Psychologist. 17, pp. 318-317.

CHAPTER 19

INTRODUCTION TO STORIES OF MINDFUL HEROES IN CREATIVE ARTS SETTINGS

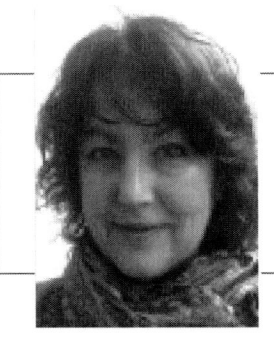

Sarah Moore (Fitzgerald)

sarah.moore@ul.ie

It's a pleasure to have been asked to provide an introductory response to the creative arts section of this book. I'm an academic and creative practitioner with a lifelong interest in teaching, learning and creative writing. More generally, I believe strongly that formal education needs to engage consistently and supportively with learners' natural propensity to think and act creatively and to produce new work.

As a teacher in higher education, I've been involved in many projects focused on enhancing learning, and to me, creativity is at the very heart of learning. As a novelist, with a longing to write, it was only when I removed barriers to my own creativity that I was able to bring my creative work and practice out into the light. Since then I have published four novels with a fifth due for publication shortly. My creative work has sustained me, has supported and informed my academic work as a researcher and teacher and has provided insights and lessons that have shed light on the conditions in which people learn most effectively and with the greatest sense of self-direction and agency.

And so, it is hugely encouraging to read the accounts both of Susanne Olbrich and David Waring whose insights on their own creative work and lives very much chime with my experience and research in the areas of learning and creative practice. From both these accounts we see the importance in creative work of being entirely present in order to engage. From presence comes a real sense of focus and the experience of 'flow' that is much-talked about in creative theory and much sought after in creative practice (Csikszentmahalyi 1992). A real sense of presence is increasingly elusive in a world that is so distracting, and in an age where people's attention has become commodified. More and more, the decision to be present is a defiant act, requiring agency and proactive decision making in order to confront a world that competes for attention in a mystifying range of ways. The act of unplugging, of disconnecting, of closing oneself off from the world in order to access one's own creative spark or energy is more important now than it has ever been and arguably more difficult. Both Susanne and David's fascinating accounts speak to this imperative.

Other themes that transcend both chapters include the following: the importance of authenticity as an essential dimension of the creative act; how essential it is to be receptive, to have one's creative radar attuned to possibilities and to creative potential. Another key theme in this section focuses on what needs to be done to overcome self-doubt, limiting beliefs and fear of failure. While we must hold ourselves to account as creative practitioners and aim for standards that can be difficult to reach, all too often we risk sabotaging our earliest efforts, being intimidated by 'the canon', being silenced by voices of 'the masters' that make us somehow feel inadequate or unworthy. The real secret is of course that everyone is creative, and that by worrying about talent or entitlement we close ourselves off to the creative territory that belongs to every human being. I love how Susanna and David both assert that creative practice takes a leap of faith and often requires that we actively silence the voices of doubt that might stop us from realising our creative dreams. 'Dare to create!' invites Susanna, with her wise implication that creativity does take courage and commitment but that we should engage with it all the same. And, 'take time to (re) focus' is one of the key elements of

David's creative insights which also demonstrates that focus can be knocked off balance, often by such obstructing forces as self-doubt and fear. Armed with these insights, as a teacher, one of my primary responsibilities is to create environments in which students feel supported enough to take the leap into their own creative practice. My lifelong commitment to creating time and space for creative work (for example, the UL Creative Writing Winter School. https://smoorefitzgerald.wixsite.com/ulcwwinterschool) reflects this responsibility.

But for me, the most resonant of the insights I have read in these chapters are the accounts from both writers about how creativity requires us to be comfortable with ambiguity and uncertainty – or as Susanna puts it: of 'not knowing'. She argues convincingly that 'rather than being uncomfortable with not knowing, as creators we could regard uncertainty as 'the seedbed in which ideas germinate' (Claxton,1997). This is a powerful idea, also reflected in David's assertion that creative practitioners need to find ways of trusting their own abilities to embody creative work. These creative principles apply across different disciplines. Creative writers for example, often report that there comes a point in a creative project when everything feels hopelessly lost, when the piece they are working on feels broken and incoherent and unsalvageable. It is a feeling that often comes before a major breakthrough in the work. Persistence and grit are the orientations required, and without a tolerance for ambiguity and uncertainty it would be impossible to hold one's nerve. In current highly codified educational environments, a tolerance for not knowing is not always prioritised. Systems, teachers and students are increasingly becoming accustomed to curricula which articulate and demand certainty when it comes to specifying such things as learning outcomes, assessment criteria and learning content. With highly specified and fine-grained curricula the risk is that learners and teachers may not be afforded the joy of the uncharted path and may become unaccustomed to the experience of ambiguity.

Being 'lost in a forest' can feel dangerous, but it is often an experience that mobilises our creative energies in all sorts of interesting ways, helping us to discover things about ourselves that we might never have known. Authentic creative practice helps us to put ourselves to the test, to think in new ways, to venture beyond the well-worn path. It's been a privilege to have Susanna and David's accounts – which have both reminded me of such important ideas.

REFERENCE

CLAXTON, G., (1997). Hare Brain, Tortoise Mind. How Intelligence increases when you think less. New York: HarperCollins.
CSIKSZENTMIHALY, M., (1992). Flow: The Psychology of Happiness. London: Rider

CHAPTER 20

DARE TO CREATE! MEDITATION, INSIGHT AND CREATIVE PROCESSES IN MUSIC

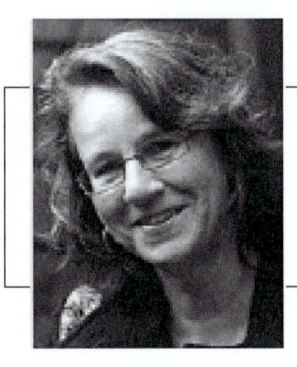

Susanne Olbrich

creativepiano@tutamail.com

INTRODUCTION

Some decades ago my mother was clearing out old paperwork. A music notebook emerged from the bottom of a drawer with two pieces of music inside, lovingly written by a child's hand. The tunes were titled 'Minuet' and 'Wedding Dance' and were skillfully set for the piano with a right and left-hand part. I had composed these delightful little pieces around age eight, we reckoned, in the style of the classical music I was learning to play in my piano lessons. However, the remainder of the book was empty.

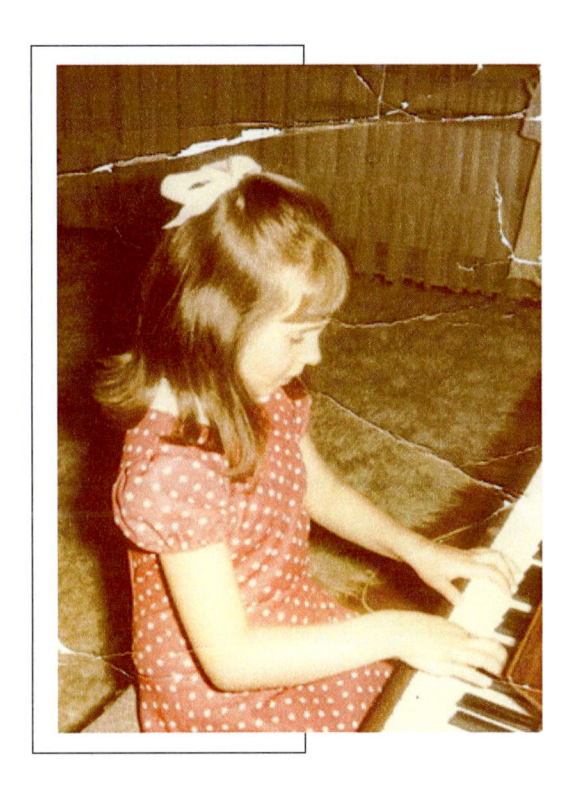

Figure 1: Myself age eight, preparing for my first public performance
© Susanne Olbrich 2018

We can only speculate why this young girl's creative flow dried up so quickly. Creative exploration in the form of composing or improvising certainly was not part of the piano tuition of my childhood and youth. I still remember the austere atmosphere of my early lessons. Male composers of the past were revered as genius creators, in keeping with the cultural paradigm of the time, and quite possibly this young girl's creative outpouring was not valued or encouraged.

Fast forward some forty years. I now work as an independent music educator, performing musician and mindfulness teacher, and musical creativity has come to the fore in both my educational and artistic work. In my piano tuition and music workshops, one of my main interests and concerns is how to engage students of all ages creatively in music-making. Creating music through improvising and composing is commonly part of lessons from the very early stages of learning music. As a pianist one of my greatest joys has been to produce a CD of my own compositions, played with my band Marama Trio. And as part of my mindfulness teaching, I particularly enjoy offering 'Sounds and Silence' retreats where participants engage in mindfulness and intuitive music making as mutually supportive experiences. Clearly, a transformation has happened: from the girl whose self-penned tunes were not valued, who grew into a young woman believing that she is not creative, to living the varied life of a music practitioner. I believe that one of the key ingredients of this journey of transformation has been my mindfulness practice of over twenty years.

> **Pause and Reflect**
>
> What was your favourite way of being playfully creative in your childhood? Allow some memories to come up, engaging your senses. What did it look, feel, sound, smell like to be in engaged in your creative explorations?

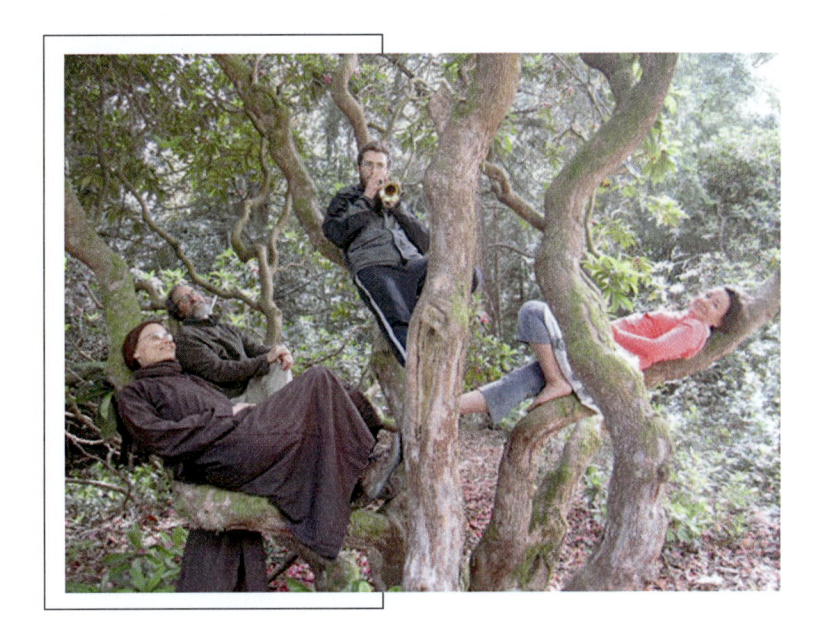

Figure 2: Mindfulness and Creativity retreat, photo © Aleksandra Kumorek 2018

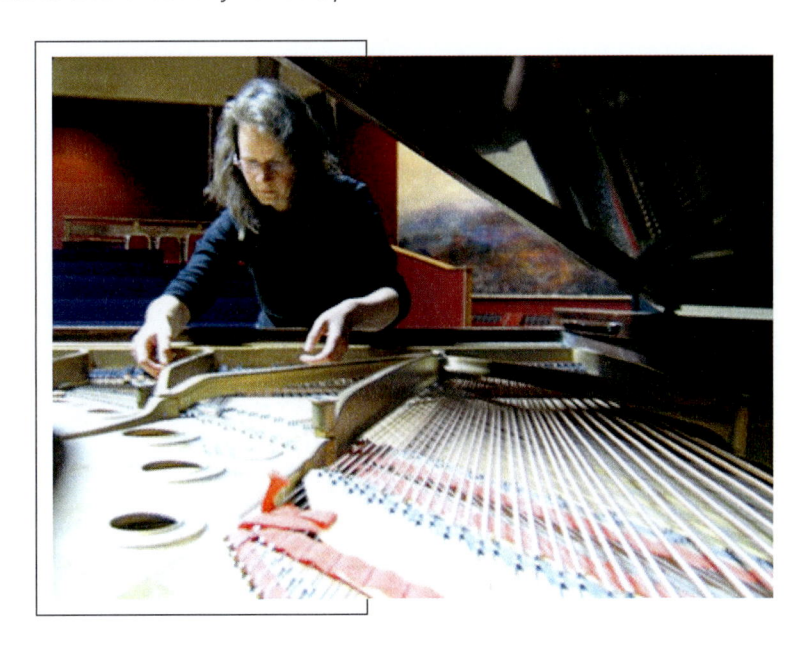

Figure 3: Myself using extended playing techniques © Susannne Olbrich 2018

PERSONAL AND CULTURAL OBSTACLES TO CREATIVE EXPRESSION, AND HOW MINDFULNESS HELPED ME TACKLE THEM

When reflecting on my past obstructions to creative expression, I find that they manifested as tension on the physical level and as limiting beliefs on the mental level. My many years of old-school music lessons resulted in somatic frozenness while playing the piano and performing. And I was convinced that creative expression through composition or improvisation involves genius talent; it was for others but not for me. As I know now, this devaluation of one's own creative potential is very common in our culture and I regularly witness it in my students and workshop participants. It is rooted in the romantic myth of the composer as a genius creator who possesses (and is possessed by) otherworldly musical powers, someone who is removed from conventional ways of living, and most likely male. Over time, mindfulness practice has provided me with an antidote to those blockages. My perception has widened to include the senses and bodily awareness. Simple awareness of breathing, as I discovered, is conducive to presence, aliveness and musical expression in the moment. When tensions arise during rehearsing, performing or teaching, they now can be worked with productively. I have learned to recognise tightness as it forms, accepting rather than fighting it, and allowing it to soften through conscious breathing.

Sustained mindfulness practice over the years also helped me to get to know the underlying mental processes that give rise to those bodily tensions. Discouraging memories and fantasies, the inner critic sneering "not good enough", voices from the past of teachers and parents, all of those can be observed in the mind as they arise and pass away. Through learning to see them as mental events rather than the truth, they loosen their grip. In addition, as part of mindfulness training we cultivate attitudes of curiosity, openness, acceptance, non-striving and kindness, and may I add humour? They all add up to a mindset that has proven conducive to creative work, resulting in inner space for ideas to germinate without premature judgment getting in the way.

Mindfulness does not just mean looking inward, but also at the world around us. Looking deeply at social and cultural conditions, we can see that they have an impact on people's creativity and expression, too. To give an example, when I took up the piano as a six-year- old, music education was narrowly defined by the European classical paradigm. It involved studying a restricted canon of historical music, was exclusively reproductive, and perfectionism was the all-pervasive attitude. Clearly, this was a cultural climate where creative exploration was stifled rather than encouraged. Seeing and understanding those conditions helped me gain perspective on my inner verdict of not being creative, and to transform it over time. These examples illustrate how long-term mindfulness practice has played an important part in liberating my creative energy as a musician. Additionally, mindfulness has found its way into my work in many ways big and small. When I do my accounts or book concerts, when I perform, prepare a workshop or speak with piano pupils' parents, when I work on a new piece of music or rehearse with other musicians, my intention and practice is to do so with presence and heart: to care, to notice, and to be fully alive in the process.

As we have seen in Chapter 3 by Graeme Nixon, the practice of mindfulness does not only offer new possibilities for working fruitfully with pathologies and for ameliorating difficulties, it also opens up new avenues towards actualising human potential. Expanding on this aspect, this chapter explores the connections between mindfulness and creative processes in music. I specifically look at insight practice as taught in the MSc Studies in MIndfulness, where in module three called Insight the basic mindfulness and compassion practices are taken to another level. In what ways can skills and attitudes trained through insight meditation become supportive of creative processes? Taking four of my own compositions as case studies, I explore the procedures by which they evolved, and I investigate the role of insight.

While this chapter focuses on music, I invite you to see whether any of my descriptions resonate with your own creative path, whatever your chosen medium might be. My wish is that through sharing my own experiences and relevant literature you may be inspired to explore your own creative impulses, and that meditation practice may become a resource on the creative path.

> **Pause and Reflect**
>
> In what way would you like to be creative? What makes you feel fully alive?
> In what way might you be able to express this more in your life?

MEDITATION, INSIGHT PRACTICE AND THE CREATIVE PROCESS

INSIGHT PRACTICE

Mindfulness practice does not stop at the development of stable present-moment awareness, as Graeme Nixon explained in Chapter 3. In fact, a settled mind may be seen as only the start and the foundation for a lifelong deepening. Through sustained practice over time we cultivate an inner environment where our mindfulness and compassion serve as conditions for insight to arise (Rosenberg, 1999). What kind of insight is this? In the MSc Studies in Mindfulness, insight is taught as direct and experiential seeing of our own mental conditions, which include subtle thoughts and feelings below the threshold of the conscious everyday mind - manifestations of the unconscious attitudes, assumptions and expectations that shape our experience.

In the simplest, most direct understanding of the word, insights are 'aha' moments. Additionally, in meditation practice insight describes a clear seeing into the nature of reality, including the nature of our own mind (Nairn, 2001). Through reduced distraction and the slowing down of mental activity we get intimately acquainted with the arising and passing of our mental patterns. The more we sit quietly and watch them play out, the more obvious it becomes that mental patterns are not solid but fleeting, not permanent but everchanging, not objective reality but mental events, and to some extent not even a given but a matter of choice (Rosenberg, 1999). We can watch the mind as it is constructing reality without being tricked into identifying with it.

One of those mental habits is our belief in a separate self. Based on perceived separateness from the world, a narrow sense of 'me' becomes the main reference point, driving self-centred behaviours and destructive emotions (Tsoknyi Rinpoche, 2012). This "Story of Separation" (Eisenstein, 2013, p.6) is deeply entrenched in our Western world view as a cultural narrative and is at the root of much personal and global suffering. Through the practice of mindfulness and compassion, however, insight can illuminate the new (and ancient) story of 'interbeing', the intimate interconnectedness of everyone and everything (Hanh, 1998).

Insight is not linear and does not come about through reasoning, analysis, logic or 'doing' of any kind; all we can do is create conditions for insight to arise on its own terms (Claxton, 1997). In meditation, the embodied resting in a panoramic awareness of experience creates conditions for direct seeing, the discovery and exploration of subtle layers of mental activity that normally go unnoticed. Almost casually we are aware of moment-to-moment experience as it presents itself. With an attitude of gentle curiosity, we tune into our inner landscape, allowing what we find to be there right now and meeting it with unconditional friendliness. "The attitude to sit with is one of total receptivity and openness. You lay the calculating mind to rest and allow life to come to you..." (Rosenberg, 1999, p.155).

> **Pause and Reflect**
>
> **Resting in the Midst of it All**
>
> Settle into your posture, upright, alert and at ease. In a relaxed way, find the movement of your breathing within your body.
>
> Become aware of the weight of your body on the ground and gradually broaden your focus to include other bodily sensations.
>
> Now open up to the space around your body, noticing sounds, and then rest loosely in the midst of what you are experiencing now – noticing thoughts, feelings and sensations.
>
> Cultivate a sense of gentle curiosity, being receptive and open to your experience in this moment – not moving towards what is happening with thinking and analysis, but simply holding whatever arises as an open question – resting in the midst of it all.
>
> Tune into your emotional world, sensing where feelings may be reflected in your body sensations, and meeting it with warmth and allowing – resting in the midst of it all.
>
> If you notice reactivity in the mind, either resistance and pushing away or grasping and contracting, make space for it, allowing this to be present, too – resting in the midst of it all.
>
> If you find your mind drifting away into thinking, then come back to your body as a light support – mind resting in the body and body resting on the ground.
>
> Nothing to fix, nowhere to go, and nothing to achieve…

CONTEMPLATIVE APPROACHES TO CREATIVE PRACTICE

When I discovered collective music improvisation in my thirties, I found to my surprise that my state of mind while improvising music showed similarities to my experiences in mindfulness meditation. Acute listening and spontaneous responding in the present moment, a heightened receptivity, curiosity and alertness, a surrendering to not knowing, a sense of wonder and connection to something larger than 'me', these were all familiar to me from my meditation practice. My experience is echoed by professional violinist Sarah Neufeld. When she moved into improvising music, she discovered that it evoked the same open, expansive quality of awareness she knew from her meditation practice, which led her to state in her online talk: "Oh my God, this is the same thing!" (2013).

The link between musical creativity and meditation has not received much attention from researchers yet. I am currently engaged in a Masters thesis as part of which I am developing a "Mindfulness for Musicians" course, to be delivered to music students at the University of Aberdeen. After completion of the course I intend to examine the connection between mindfulness and musical creativity through interviews with the students.

Tentative findings from the few existing studies suggest a promising field for further research. Newton (2015) interviewed three composers after they had received some introductory mindfulness training. They all stated that their increased awareness had a positive effect on their ability to focus and express, both while composing and during live performance. Especially the attitude of non-striving cultivated during their meditation practice was experienced as helpful. This attitude was linked to a lessening of negative self-judgment, allowing the composers to express themselves more openly and intuitively.

Two further studies highlight the benefits of attitudes developed in meditation practice especially for creativity in performance situations. Oyan (2006) in her theoretical study argues that an important part of mindfulness practice, the non-avoidance of difficult feelings, can be utilised with performance nerves. She emphasises the importance of an accepting approach: "The flow state, or creative act, comes about when one is willing to risk failure by struggling through the anxiety" (p.29). Engaging in present-moment experience as it is, including the audience, difficulties, and feelings of anxiety, is a key skill here, a skill honed through mindfulness training. Czajkowski and Greasley in their study with singers report that musicians experienced a slowing of time perception during performance in response to mindful breathing, with the effect of "allowing them to be more creative in the areas of dynamics, expression, vocal tone and feeling in control of the performance" (2015, p.17).

These examples show that even after a short period of introductory mindfulness training musicians perceived a positive impact on their creativity. This is supported by accounts from artist-meditators themselves (see for example Nachmanovitch, 1990; Hind, 2011; Sarath, 2013; Alexander, 2014). Pianist Mark Tanner calls piano playing a "practical meditation" (2016, p.18). In his book "The Mindful Pianist" he quotes jazz pianist Nikki Iles:

> Mindfulness is clearly a fundamental part of jazz, and is at the core of the process of improvisation. To be truly free and 'in the moment' it is important to take risks - without fear of judgment - in search of a heightened creative state (2016, p.108).

Singer, composer, dancer and filmmaker Meredith Monk, who has been a long-term meditator, wrote about the convergence of her meditation practice and creative work:

> Creativity means staying present throughout the process; when desperation and anxiety enter, one remembers to go back to the breath, the space, stillness. One moves through delusions of success and failure, fame and humiliation, to an intent to create a work that is of benefit (2010, paragraph 11).

For the late Zen teacher and photographer John Daido Loori, creative and meditative practices have common attributes: "The creative process, like a spiritual journey, is intuitive, non-linear, and experiential" (2005, p.1). He highlights that in the Zen arts, which include poetry, painting, tea ceremony, flower arranging and calligraphy, among others, meditation historically has been an integral part of the creative process. He explains this way of making art as follows:

> Its only purpose was to point to the nature of reality. It suggested a new way of seeing, and a new way of being that cut to the core of what it meant to be human and fully alive. Zen art… expressed the ineffable, and helped to transform the way we see ourselves in the world (Loori, 2005, p.4).

In the world of music, composer John Cage notably has brought a meditative mindset to the creative process. For him, the function of music was "to change the mind so that it does become open to experience" (cited in Buzzarte and Bickley, 2012, p.101), which could just as well be a description of mindfulness practice. His notorious piece 4'33" from 1952 simply consists of the instruction to the musician to sit quietly at the piano for four minutes and thirty-three seconds, which for the audience potentially becomes a meditation on ambient sounds (Larson, 2013).

NOT KNOWING AND BEGINNER'S MIND

Every aesthetic product starts with a 'blank canvas'. Rather than being uncomfortable with not knowing, as creators we could regard uncertainty as "the seedbed in which ideas germinate" (Claxton, 1997, p.6). Meredith Monk explains:

> At the beginning of every new work - and every day of work - is the unknown. Being an artist is being unsure, asking questions, stumbling around with only an inkling of what will manifest and tolerating the fear of hanging out in the unknown. When curiosity and interest become more present than discomfort, the mystery becomes enjoyable and its exploration vivid and vibrant (Monk, 2010, paragraph 1).

On a similar note, the violinist Stephen Nachmanovitch states:

> As an improvising musician, ... I am in the surrender business... Surrender means cultivating a comfortable attitude toward not knowing, being nurtured by the mystery of moments that are dependably surprising, ever fresh (1990, pp.21-22).

What he describes here is an attitude of 'beginner's mind', which also is one of the core attributes of mindfulness practice (Kabat-Zinn, 1990). Every time we choose to tap into the freshness of beginner's mind, we can experience the essential uniqueness of that moment. The letting go of preconceived notions allows the mind to open up to new possibilities - in life, in art and in meditation.

Learning to become comfortable with not knowing is also part of the Insight module of the MSc Studies in Mindfulness, because insight cannot be willed or forced, as we have seen earlier. In a culture that highly values a mindset of active problem solving and being in control, this might feel counterintuitive. However, in insight practice we learn to let go of goal orientation and cultivate an attitude of non-striving. This is not the same as passivity. It takes a relaxed, yet concentrated and receptive mind.

RECEPTIVITY, INTUITIVE WAYS OF KNOWING AND THE FELT SENSE

To be comfortable with not knowing, it helps to trust emergence and learning to be receptive to inner prompts. Again, these skills are trained in insight practice, and they prove useful for the creative process, too. Meredith Monk writes about "working with an 'anything-is-possible' mind, allowing whatever arises to be, knowing that discovery comes when least expected" (2010, paragraph 6). This frame of mind transcends our human habits of grasping and seeking, for which Claxton gives an example from poetry: "By allowing the poem to suck us in, we are drawn into a mode of perception that is situated upstream of our usual habits of conceptualization and self-reference" (1997, p.177). Composer and performer Pauline Oliveros gave a description of her state of mind during improvised performance, which is characterised by a similar sense of immersion and emergence: "The music comes through as if I have nothing to do with it but allow it to emerge through my instrument and voice" (2005, p. xix).

While in improvising music this process is immediate, composing involves engaging with the raw material of sound and music over a period of time, perhaps trying out different versions, and making choices by engaging a "visceral and aesthetic response" (Claxton, 1997, p.177). How does the artist know which choices to make from an infinite range of possibilities? And how does she know when a piece is complete? In my own composing, I have encountered an intuitive knowing that sometimes manifests as just a hint, and at other times is clear without doubt. As Claxton explains:

> There is a kind of knowing which is essentially indirect, sideways, allusive and symbolic; which hints and evokes, touches and moves, in ways that resist explication (Claxton, 1997, p.173).

Intuitive knowing and the aesthetic response both seem to involve a felt sense: "The body feels something that the mind may not understand" (Claxton, 1997, p.177). As Newton describes in his study, while composing he experiences "visceral reactions when playing music and discovering a new musical idea" (2015, p.174). They help him discern whether or not a musical idea is worth pursuing. Through mindfulness practice he developed a heightened awareness of those bodily cues.

Pause and Reflect

Whether you are a musician or not, do you recognise some of the attributes described above from your own creative processes? Have you at times encountered beginner's mind, a felt sense of intuitive knowing, a sense of transcending the self?

The felt sense is located in a border zone between conscious and unconscious that often goes unnoticed (Rome, 2014). Here, another parallel between insight practice and the creative process becomes apparent: both draw on layers of the mind beyond everyday consciousness, on subliminal insights that arise on their own accord. All the practitioner can do is create supportive conditions, watering the seeds.

DEEP LISTENING®

Composer Pauline Oliveros developed a pioneering framework that aims at creating such supportive conditions for creative processes, by linking meditation and sound practices with body awareness and dream work. Deep Listening evolved since the 1980s as a body of sound pieces and practices to facilitate creativity in art and life:

> Deep Listening is a form of meditation. Attention is directed to the inter-play of sounds and silences... Sound is not limited to musical or speaking sounds but is inclusive of all perceptible vibrations... Compassion and understanding comes from listening impartially to the whole space/time continuum of sound, not just what one is presently concerned about. In this way, discovery and exploration can take place (Oliveros, 2005, p.xxiv).

The attentive listening described here parallels the panoramic awareness we cultivate in insight meditation. Here it is the all-inclusive awareness of sounds that is supportive of transcending narrow self-concern, opening the imagination to new possibilities.

While Deep Listening uses its own terminology without reference to 'mindfulness' or 'insight', there clearly is an overlap of perspectives and approaches between those pathways. Similar to mindfulness training, Deep Listening includes body and breathing practices that are aimed at becoming grounded in somatic awareness. Heightened awareness is achieved through sounding and listening to sounds and silence. Working creatively and intuitively with dreams is a way of tapping into the unconscious mind that might serve the creative process.
In 2005 I had the good fortune to experience a week-long Deep Listening retreat with Pauline Oliveros and her co-teachers Heloise Gold and Ione, which had a significant impact on both my teaching and creating of music. In Deep Listening practices, meditation becomes music and music becomes meditation. One of my compositions examined later in this chapter, "Beyond Gone", grew directly out of my applying the Deep Listening approach.

FOUR EXAMPLES OF CREATIVE PROCESSES IN MUSIC

While my masters degree in music provided me with a foundation in music theory and a basic understanding of compositional techniques, I received no formal training in composition. In my composing I meet emerging sounds and structures with beginner's mind and playful experimentation, guided by listening, intuition, and sometimes serendipity. My approach is reflected in this statement by Meredith Monk: "Each piece presents its own world. Part of making a piece is exploring its principles, listening to what it wants" (2010, paragraph 3). We now will look at four of my compositions and the creative processes by which they emerged.

BEYOND GONE (OLBRICH, 2009)

This piano piece evolved in response to bereavement, the traumatic event of the suicide of a close friend. In the aftermath I experienced a period of intense dreams where I was communicating with my deceased friend. An urge to play the piano tied in with my need to express things that had been left unsaid. It felt natural to use Deep Listening, which can be summarised as an acute, meditative listening to sounds, to the body and to creative impulses. Sitting at the grand piano, I switched on a recorder, took time to connect with my breathing and listening, then started improvising. At that time there was no conscious intention to create an aesthetic product beyond the momentary playing, so after I had finished I forgot about the recording and didn't listen to it until months later. But when I did, what I heard felt of both personal and musical value. So, I decided to give the material a reproducible form through transcribing and editing.

"Beyond Gone" evolves over an oscillating left-hand drone, with the right hand taking on the rhythm of speech, the phrases resembling penetrating questions. The tonality is ambiguous, and the spectrum of expressions ranges from despair and rage to inquisitiveness and tenderness. The piece has a raw quality and is a reflection of my grappling with the pain of loss and coming to terms with it.

The work was completed in only two sessions a few months apart. During the first session, musical material was generated through Deep Listening and improvisation in a deeply personal and intuitive process. In the later stage of editing and transcribing I brought in my aesthetic judgment, drawing on both intuition and musical knowledge. Some years later, another dimension was added to the piece when it became part of the repertoire of my band Marama Trio. In keeping with its quality of immediacy and edginess, the saxophone and double bass parts are completely improvised every time, so each performance is new and different.

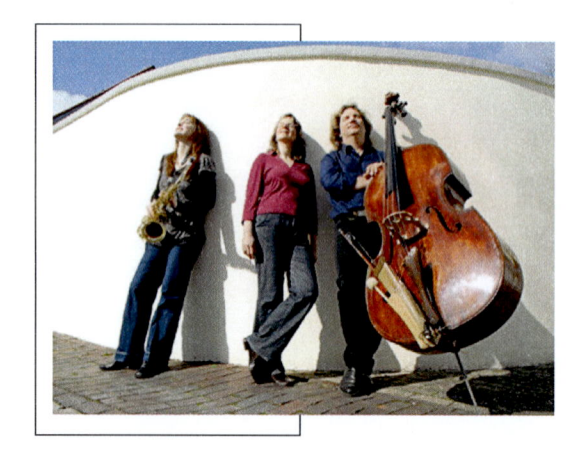

Figure 4: Marama Trio, © Julia Jasionowski 2018

This is an example for what creativity research calls a "Beyond-Domain" process (Katz and Gardner, 2012, p.108). Inspiration comes from associations outside of the realm of music, with the subject matter being intensely personal to the composer. The fact that initially no creative product was intended reflects an attitude of non-striving, which allowed me to experience complete freedom of expression in that moment. My Deep Listening practice resulted in heightened receptivity and a sense of music emerging from my hands without the intellect being involved at that stage. The conscious shaping into a final piece happened as a second step.

Pause and Listen

https://store.cdbaby.com/cd/maramatriosusanneolbrich

MAGIE DE LA PLUIE (OLBRICH, 2009)

Another compositional strategy is "Within-Domain" (Katz and Gardner, 2012, p.108), where the inspiration for a piece comes predominantly from musical material. For "Magie De La Pluie", the impulse came from listening to a song with an entrancing repetitive bass line, which inspired me to create something with a similar feel. I also had wanted to make a piece with the sound of rain, a sound which I find deeply evocative. Those two ideas combined for this piece.

My intention was to write something simple and spacious for the piano, in contrast to our strong cultural bias toward virtuosity. I came up with a single repeated line in the odd time signature of 7/8, played on the keys while muffling the strings with the other hand. This results in a spacious, reverberating sound that doesn't resemble a piano at all. Playing on the strings and other parts inside of the grand piano is termed "extended playing techniques". Originating from contemporary classical music, these are unorthodox methods of playing musical instruments that result in unusual sounds and timbres, opening up a new range of possibilities to players and composers.

To the regular, repeated piano pattern a slow saxophone melody and a double bass part were added. The music follows a simple standard structure in jazz: a musical theme is followed by an improvised section and a (slightly embellished) repeat of the theme. The continuous backdrop of my field recording of rain is adding to the overall entrancing quality. During the improvised part the saxophone and double bass players also experiment with extended playing techniques. The bass is played with a variety of hard and soft drum sticks for percussive sounds. These are echoed by the saxophone player, who creates rhythms on the saxophone keys. "Magie De La Pluie" is characterised by a combination of simplicity and unexpected sounds, using musical language from jazz and contemporary classical.

Like "Beyond Gone", this piece came together in only a short time, which is atypical for my work where pieces usually go through a process of gestation lasting weeks or months. Here, the process flowed harmoniously back and forth between structural considerations and intuitive playing with ideas, leading to a satisfying result right away.

Pause and Listen

https://susanneolbrich.net/live-performance/

ON THE HILL OF MY LIFE... (OLBRICH, 2009)

This piece took me eight years to complete. The music was prompted by a poetic passage from a letter written to me by a friend, and the musical theme manifested in a burst of inspiration on the piano right after receiving the letter. To my surprise I realised that the emerging melody line formed a twelve-tone row - not a structure I was very familiar with or would choose deliberately. I welcomed the quirky sound of it and went on to harmonise it with quite complex jazz chords in a steady rhythm. Though I have done some study of jazz harmonies in the past, I am no expert in the field. I was simply enjoying experimenting with sounds and finding chord structures I liked. The resulting '12-tone jazz' turned out to follow neither common jazz chord changes nor the tight procedures of 12-tone composing, but formed its own intriguing sonic cosmos.

Now there was a distinct theme, but I had no idea how to continue. For eight years, neither approaching the piece intuitively nor structurally brought any satisfactory results. It would have ended unfinished in a drawer, had it not been for a colleague and friend who was so fond of the beginning that year after year he demanded to hear the completed work. At one point I had the chance to take my fragment to a one-to-one session with composer Fred Frith. He was very positive and suggested that this may be the complete piece, albeit very short, which should be complemented by other miniatures. I appreciated his encouraging comments, but intuitively knew without a doubt that the piece wasn't finished yet. It took me another year to finally find the solution. It evolved around repeated left-hand bass notes, a technique used in a cycle of contemporary piano pieces which I was playing at the time. I combined the repetitive bass notes with variations of the 12-tone tune, which appeared inverted and then in reverse in the right hand. The piece later was awarded first prize in a composers competition, which I took as a validation of my sincere longterm persevering efforts.

Initially written as a piano piece, I later arranged "On the Hill of My Life…" for my trio and included an improvised solo part each for the saxophone and double bass. The unconventional harmonies happened to pose quite some challenge to the musicians. None of what they had learned about improvising on standard jazz chord changes was applicable here; the unique sound world needed their complete listening and responding in the moment.

In the categories of Katz and Gardner (2012), this example is a "Hybrid", where the process of composing reflects both Within-Domain and Beyond-Domain approaches. While the initial inspiration came from a letter (Beyond-Domain), subsequently my composing evolved largely around musical-structural considerations (Within-Domain). In addition, this example shows how social aspects can influence creative work. While in the past creativity was seen as an individual ability and process, more recently creativity research has acknowledged the numerous sociocultural factors that play a part (Sawyer, 2012). Rarely does creative work happen in complete isolation; the artist is part of a larger network of people and circumstances that will influence the process in subtle or direct ways. In the case of "On the Hill of My Life…", there was input from a friend, from other composers by way of direct feedback and through inspiration from their music, and later from my band members and from adjudicators.

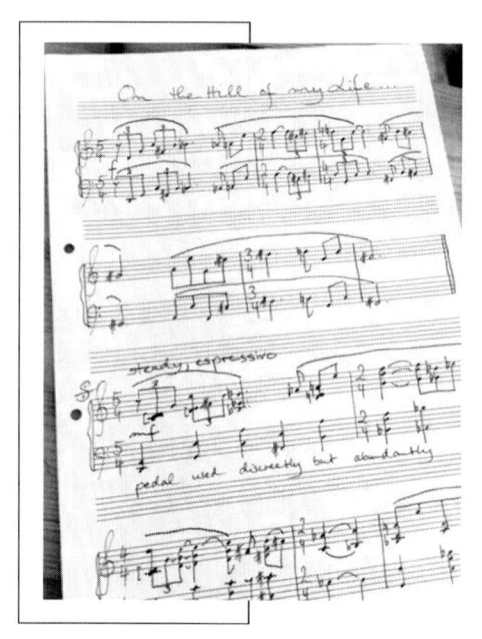

Figure 8: Score of "On the Hill of My Life…" © Susanne Olbrich 2018

Pause and Listen

https://store.cdbaby.com/cd/maramatriosusanneolbrich

ON HIS JOURNEY TO THE STARS (OLBRICH, 2012)

This piece again was prompted by the sad news of a suicide by someone I had known a while ago. As with "Beyond Gone", initially I had no intention to compose a piece of music.

A need to process my feelings and thoughts led me to the piano every day, and while improvising I found that my hands kept coming back to the same pattern of music. Although it was comforting, I didn't like it very much in aesthetic terms. I tried to abandon the pattern and consciously play other things, but the music kept coming back and even started to 'in- habit' my inner listening while away from the piano. There was a curious sense of music almost imposing itself on me - something I had not experienced before. Eventually I surrendered to the momentum and decided to give the pattern the chance to develop into a piece.

In the course of further piano improvising and playing with the musical pattern, I indeed warmed up to it. At the same time, I felt that the music was working on me, soothing me and helping me come to terms with the situation and my own feelings. At the heart of the piece is a basso ostinato, a repeated bass line, above which the right hand is playing variations developing from simple long single notes to fast complex passagework. Being in the key of C major, the piece has a gentle, warm, friendly and even bright quality that is very different from the emotional rawness of "Beyond Gone", my other piece about loss. I now have grown very fond of "On His Journey to the Stars", which for me is an expression of friendship, of embracing sadness, and of learning to let go. The title was taken from an online comment made by a friend.

This work initially evolved against my aesthetic response and judgment; at a certain point, it involved moving beyond my likes and dislikes. Meredith Monk writes about "simply engaging in a process and getting out of the way of the work… The sense is that the piece already exists – it's just a matter of uncovering it" (2010, paragraphs 2 & 3). This captures a quality of selflessness, something we also aspire to in insight practice. There we work with the reactivity of the mind, making space for wanting and grasping as well as not wanting and resistance without identifying with those mental states, but resting in the midst of it all.

Pause and Listen

https://store.cdbaby.com/cd/susanneolbrich

CONCLUSION

Insight means different things in different contexts. In everyday day life, insights manifest as 'aha' moments. During the creative process, creative insights mark the progression of a project towards its final shape. At the most profound level, insight also stands for clear seeing of the nature of reality, an understanding of the relationship between self and world beyond our conditioned views.

This chapter has explored the analogies and links between insight practice and creative practice. Both processes unfold between the polarities of 'letting be' and non-doing on the one side, and of conscious active choice on the other. The creative work involves being receptive to intuitive insights, which then get shaped into an aesthetic product by way of skill and craft. Insight meditation calls for resting in the midst of experience; yet time and again we actively choose not to jump onto a train of thought. This allows conditioned concepts of self and the world to become less rigid over time and be replaced by clear seeing of the impermanent and interconnected nature of everything.

Meditation practice and creative work both engage subliminal layers of mind, they both draw on intuitive ways of knowing. Neither can be forced or willed, but insights occur in their own time. All the practitioner can do is create supportive conditions. This includes cultivating attitudes of receptivity, inner listening, non-striving, patience, and perseverance.

As we have seen in the four case studies, creative processes can vary greatly. In my experience they often are messy and multilayered, to a much greater extent than is suggested by linear scientific models of the creative process. Each work could be seen as a 'hero's journey' unto itself, to use the mythological metaphor introduced by Vin Harris in Chapter 2. The 'departure' of inspiration can come in many guises, be it from music or art or life. It is followed by the 'initiation' through meeting the challenges and going through the ups and down of the creative process. Here, as practitioners we utilise a variety of skills and ways of knowing: receptivity, intuition, intellect, training and craft. The 'return' finally brings a completed piece of work that can be shared with others, work that hopefully touches and enriches others.

Insight training leads toward transcending self-concern, personal likes and dislikes, in the direction of a felt sense of interconnection with a larger whole. The creative path has this potential, too. As the poet and philosopher Mark Nepo describes it poetically:

> truth, each of us is a tiny conduit connecting everything. Each living being, a hair-like filament in the fabric of existence... Carl Jung thought of poets and artists as filaments who, against their will, find themselves used as lightning rods for the collective unconscious... It's all a writer or artist can hope for – to be a medic of consciousness (2012, p.205-207).

FURTHER RESOURCES

My homepage gives an overview of my work in music, music education and mindfulness.
https://susanneolbrich.net/
Sharon Stewart's article "Listening to Deep Listening – Reflection on the 1988 Recording and the Lifework of Pauline Oliveros" is a good introduction to Deep Listening with many links to sound recordings and video footage.
https://www.researchcatalogue.net/view/261881/261882

REFERENCES

ALEXANDER, R., (2014). Mindfulness, Musicians and the Creative Flow. Huffington Post. Available: https://www.huffingtonpost.com/ronald-alexander-phd/mindfulness-musicians-and_b_5160931.html [Date Accessed: 2nd January 2018].

BURNARD, P., (2012). Musical creativities in practice. Oxford University Press. BUZZARTE, M. and BICKLEY, T., eds. (2012). Anthology of Essays on Deep Listening. Kingston: Deep Listening Publications.

CLAXTON, G., (1997). Hare Brain, Tortoise Mind. How Intelligence increases when you think less. New York: HarperCollins.

CZAJKOWSKI, A.-M. and GREASLEY, A., (2015). Mindfulness for singers: The effects of a targeted mindfulness course on learning vocal technique. British Journal of Music Education, 32 (2), pp. 211-233.

EISENSTEIN, C., (2013). The More Beautiful World Our Heart Knows Is Possible. Berkeley: North Atlantic Books.

HANH, T. N., (1998). The Heart of the Buddha's Teachings: Transforming Suffering into Peace, Joy and Liberation. New York: Rider.

HIND, R., (2011). Head first: mindfulness and music. The Guardian, Thursday 16th June. Available: https://www.theguardian.com/music/2011/jun/16/mindfulness-meditation-music [Date Accessed: 30th May 2018].

KABAT-ZINN, J., (1990). Full Catastrophe Living: How to Cope with Stress, Pain and Illness using Mindfulness Meditation. Edition 2004. London: Piatkus.

KATZ, S.L. and GARDNER, H., (2012). Musical materials or metaphorical models? A psychological investigation of what inspires composers. In: HARGREAVES, D. J., MIELL, D. E., and MACDONALD, R. A., (2012). Musical Imaginations. Multidisciplinary perspectives on creativity, performance, and perception. New York: Oxford University Press. pp.107-123.

LARSON, K., (2013). Where the Heart Beats: John Cage, Zen Buddhism, and the Inner Life of Artists. New York: Penguin.

LOORI, J. D., (2005). The Zen of Creativity: Cultivating Your Artistic Life. New York: Ballantine Books.

MONK, M., (2010). The Art of Being Present. Lion's Roar. Buddhist Wisdom for our Time, 11th September. Available: http://www.lionsroar.com/the-art-of-being-present/ [Date accessed: 3rd May 2018].

NACHMANOVITCH, S., (1990). Free Play: Improvisation in Life and Art. New York: Penguin.

NAIRN, R., (2001). Diamond Mind: A Psychology of Meditation. Boston and London: Shambala.

NEPO, M., (2012). Seven Thousand Ways to Listen: Staying Close to What is Sacred. New York: Simon & Schuster.

NEUFELD, S., (2013). The Intersection of Meditation and the Musician's Path. Available: https://wanderlust.com/journal/watch-arcade-fire-violinist-sarah-neufeld-uses-yoga-inspire- art/ [Date Accessed: 29th May 2018].

NEWTON, J.Z., (2015). Musical Creativity and Mindfulness Meditation: Can the Practice of Mindfulness Meditation Enhance Perceived Musical Creativity? International Journal of Transpersonal Studies, 34(1), pp.172-186.

OLBRICH, S. with MARAMA TRIO (2009). CD Continuations. Marama Music. OLIVEROS, P., (2005). Deep Listening: A Composer's Sound Practice. Lincoln: iUniverse.

OYAN, S. (2006). Mindfulness meditation: Creative musical performance through awareness. (Doctoral dissertation). Louisiana State University, USA. Available: https://pdf- s.semanticscholar.org/fcba/1d9eab70fe3791d1b28398420d80adde5659.pdf [Date Accessed: 26th October 2017].

ROME, D. I., (2014). Your Body Knows the Answer: Using Your Felt Sense to Solve Problems, Effect Change, and Liberate Creativity. Boston: Shambala.

ROSENBERG, L., (1999). Breath by Breath.The Liberating Practice of Insight Meditation. London: Thorsons.

SARATH, E. W., (2013). Improvisation, Creativity, and Consciousness. Jazz as Integral Template for Music, Education, and Society. Albany: State University of New York Press.

SAWYER, R. K., (2012). Explaining Creativity: The Science of Human Innovation. Second edition. New York: Oxford University Press.

TANNER, M., (2106). The Mindful Pianist. Focus, practise, perform, engage. London: Faber Music.

TSOKNYI RINPOCHE, and SWANSON, E., (2012). Open Heart, Open Mind. A Guide to Inner Transformation. London: Rider.

CHAPTER 21

HEROES OF THE STAGE: CONNECTING WITH THE JOY OF PERFORMING

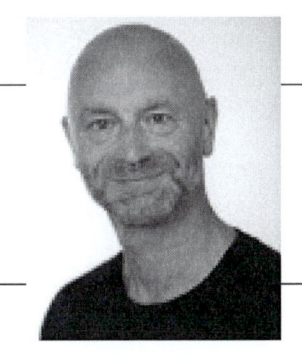

David Waring

dpwaring@btopenworld.com

WAY IN

I'll begin by making a declaration - All artists are heroes! I consider all performers to be especially heroic as they are present, literally, in front of people expressing their art and creativity.

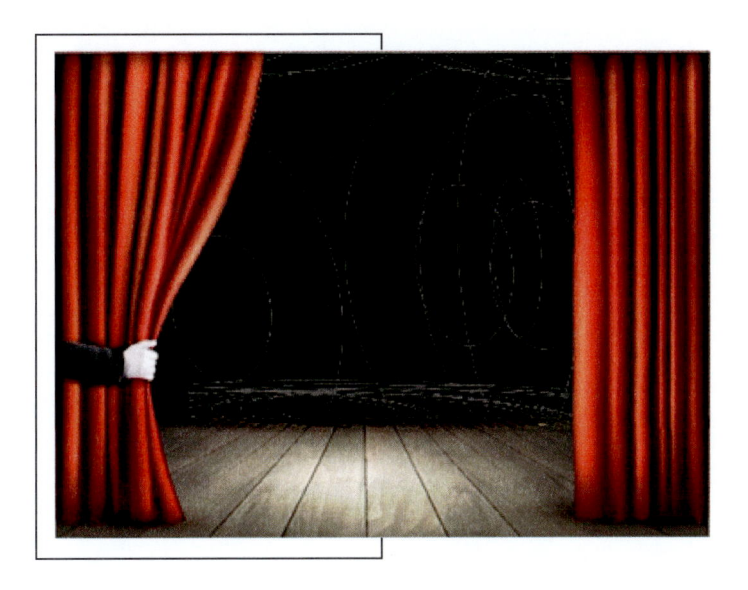

Figure 1: Revealing the process
Photo by Vladimir Galantsev, Colourbox

We prepare the ingredients in order to make a tasty meal. We prepare machinery in order that it functions well by oiling it. Mindfulness prepares me for living and being in my life, daily, helping me to focus on being present. It stands to reason, therefore, that performing on stage, as a way of expressing ourselves creatively and artistically, and communicating with an audience, needs considered preparation.

One New Year's Eve a number of years ago, I found myself in a Buddhist meeting. The meditation practice offered was focused on compassion as a way to take us, and those we brought to mind, from the old year into the new with love and care. What I discovered was a welcoming and non-judgmental environment. A seed was sown in me to search for more of the same – kind and compassionate people who were concerned with their growth and engagement with and experience of, and in, the world.

My experience on that fateful evening encouraged me to join a Mindfulness Association diploma programme, which further led to my enrolment on University of Aberdeen's MSc Studies in Mindfulness. I was excited to see that the way of relating to oneself and the world in which one lives from the inside – out, the embodied place from which mindfulness operates, is extremely similar in principle to the somatic methods I use in my professional teaching and personal performing practices. The term 'somatic', meaning 'of the body', asks that the performer connects to their expressivity, impulses and knowledge from inside themselves, as opposed to say from a more conventionally aesthetic, or outside perspective. By which I mean that movement decisions might then arise from a deeper place as opposed to moving or performing to satisfy another's criteria or needs. In this way I feel that the work the practitioner produces is more personal, more authentic.

As a dance artist, performer and teacher I wanted to find a regular meeting where people were exploring principles and developing a practice that spoke to my heart and nature as a person and professional. I've learned that mindfulness practice is very much about being in the world and, in my experience, is taught in an open and very human way. It celebrates authenticity and is framed by creativity and humour. As I said earlier, both dance performance and mindfulness practices are embodied processes of 'being' and 'doing', so, I would define dance performance and mindfulness practice as attentiveness to being present. Dance is intrinsically of the present for at its most pure it deals with the immediate expression of sensations experienced by the body/mind, says Steinman (1995, p.10).

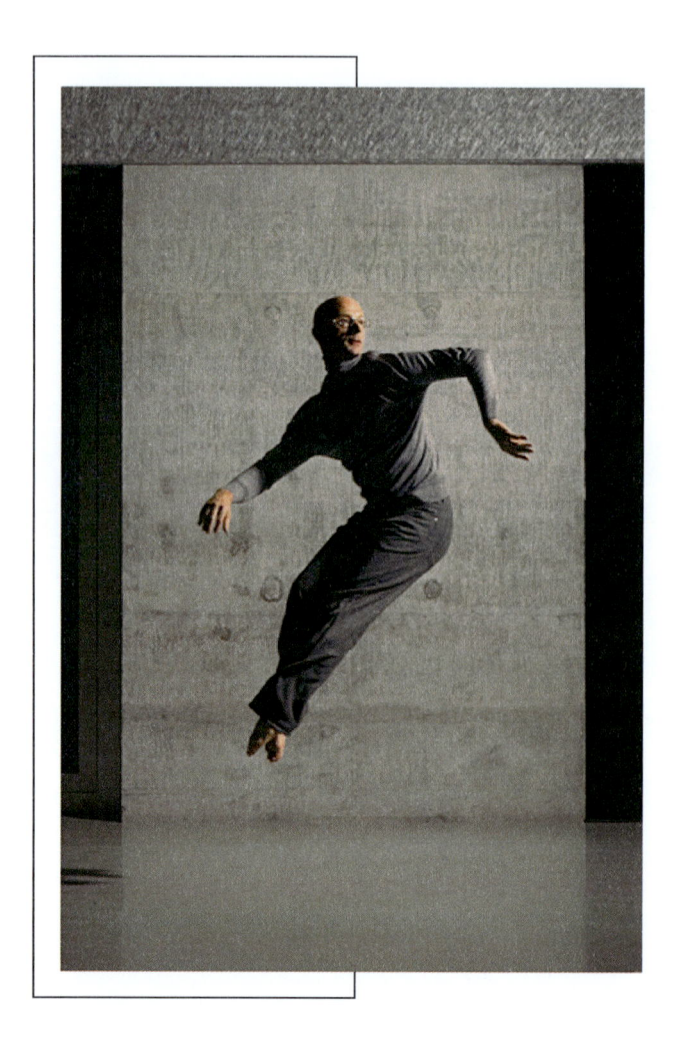

Figure 2: Me, dancing
Photo © Chris Nash 2018

PRESENCE

Presence is arguably a most elusive topic, an alchemic process, according to Goodall (2008) and immeasurable. In my role as Artistic Director of Transitions Dance Company (TDC), I've found that a performer has presence and is watchable when he/she appears to be there, doing it, in that moment. It's authentic, coming from the heart and with a fullness of being let's say. I wondered: If mindfulness meditation practice encourages awareness of one's presence and inhabiting the present moment, could performers benefit from integrating mindfulness principles into their practice? The pre-show preparation or 'warm-up' seemed the best starting point. As a newly professional performer, and certainly before coaching younger performers and studying mindfulness, my own understanding of warming-up and preparing was very self-directed and came from observing others, doing what I needed in relation to how I felt and any particular needs of the choreography. Performers recognize and acknowledge the need to 'warm-up' prior to going onstage, and I believe that a mindful approach to pre-performance preparation (PPP) could be effective in allowing the dance performer to remember to be present when performing - initiating 'presence' through a stronger somatic awareness and embodiment. This could enable performers to attend to themselves in order to give the best they can in that moment onstage.

Any performance event is stressful, according to Pargman (2006), and, given the live nature of performance, 'success' could depend on a balanced, open perspective and impetus, which is also reflexive and focused. Alongside the latter, this live element is a most clear connection to my experience of studying and practicing mindfulness and, as Nairn et al. (2009, p.4) state, "knowing what's happening, whilst it's happening, without preference". The inherent use of self-acceptance in mindfulness practice could support a reduction in any sense of self-criticism, stress, or distraction prior to performance. A mindfulness preparation method could support clarity and groundedness of practice for dance performers in such events. Edinborough (2011) advocates mindfully embodied performance practice and training, and Cotterill (2015) states the efficacy of including meditation within performance preparation to create attentional focus.

Performance events are demanding, publicly scrutinized by audience, critics, other practitioners and possible future employers, and could create feelings of vulnerability and insecurity. The body - the dancer's tool - in meditation can be used as, "an anchor in the present that is a source of stability in the midst of the whirlwind of life", according to Tart (1994, p.33). As a performer and TDC's Artistic Director, I'm very aware of the pressures of performing - feeling the need to do a good job, to want to represent both the choreographer's ideas and one's own artistry during a performance, to satisfy the needs of all those involved in the production as well as the audience, on some level. There is possibly a need to present oneself as the very best one can and demonstrate many different skills and the highest standard of work. This is no mean feat! Sometimes I liken it to a first date - have breath fresh, be 'presentable', be the funniest I can be, the best listener I can be, show my personality, try to overcome a level of shyness and the possibility of rejection. To be able to settle yourself enough to feel that you can be brave and face your audience, to know that you've connected with yourself, checked in, so that you're clear enough that you're actually there, seems really crucial to giving yourself a good chance to 'pull it off'. The audience, the choreographer, your fellow performers and you yourself deserve the very best you can give in that one-off show. Of course, this is also true of any type of event that could be considered a 'performance', whether in the creative arts or indeed one's social life, so I hope that the ideas and approaches I present here could be supportive to everyone in such a situation.

> **Pause and Reflect**
>
> How did you stay focused when you last had to prepare yourself for an important event, in order to do it as best you could?

You'll notice that I've used weigh and way as headings for my chapter. The way part concerns direction and path, and the weigh part concerns the substantive nature of mindfulness in my experience – how it supports a resonance, authenticity and quality to my life, and also could be given gravitas as a tool in all areas of life for everyone. They signify the journey through my ideas but also reflect the importance I've found in practising mindfulness and connecting it with my professional life. I also want to return to the idea of the "one-off show" and connect it with the notion that mindfulness teaches us that, indeed there is only the present and we could, therefore, agree that everything only happens once. Now.

WEIGHING IN

What do researchers and practitioners say about my topic? Surprisingly, research into dance performance preparation is almost non-existent. This infers the idea that one instinctively knows what to do to be ready to perform, which seems dismissive of the importance of finding methods to support such a highly demanding event. So, in order to explore how my interests of dance performance preparation and mindfulness might fit together, I explored ideas from dance, as well as psychological well-being and mindfulness. These ideas included: preparation, attention, intention and motivation, authentic presence and embodiment. In sport psychology, event preparation is called Pre-Performance Routine (PPR) (Clowes & Knowles, 2013). I decided on Pre-Performance Preparation (PPP), as the word routine suggests something more repetitious than that for an artistic practice, when the performer might not always do exactly the same thing in the same way to be stage-ready. There is an apparent paradox in preparing to be present, but I'm sure that we can all recognize that we drift off, daydream or become distracted, and when one's role is to be present then using a method helping or reminding us to be there seems useful. In my initial research of PPP, I felt that there was a connection to what is known in sport psychology theory as 'Flow' (Csikszentmihalyi, 1992). However, in my understanding it is actually not the same as being engaged in dance performance. The broader aspect of dance performance is to be immersed in what one is doing, yes, but not so focused that one is unaware of everything else in the environment. The audience is the crucial partner to the performer in the act of performance, so in my opinion, there is actually a duality of engagement with what one is doing when performing, which doesn't quite seem to fit with 'Flow'.

MINDFULNESS

Mindfulness is written about as connecting to a sense of self and authenticity that it is embodied and creates presence. Mindfulness meditation engages one in being present in the here and now, both within and outside of oneself, with attention and awareness. It is a practice concerned with being and experience. Alongside focusing on present experience, one cultivates kindness and self-acceptance, a care of and for self, so that a knowing observation of one's mental processes and behaviour signifies being in the moment, here, present, say Nairn et al. (2009).

The Mindfulness Based Living Course (MBLC) programme developed by the Mindfulness Association directs an embodied approach from the outset. Body awareness through posture is addressed in the opening session, and from the second session onwards the body is designated a site for self understanding and experience, acting as an anchor and place of mindful enquiry. The breath is proposed as the connection between body and mind. In parallel, dance is exceptionally concerned with the body as the focus and medium of expression. Somatic dance practices rely on more internal processes, and especially emphasise the use of breath, to create and support physical expression. With particular focus on the body, the 'body scan', mindful movement and mindful walking are part of the Mindfulness Based Living Course (MBLC) programme taught so as to find holistic, experiential and embodied connections to one's self. One dancer researcher, Caldwell (2014), advocates elevating the importance of the body within meditation practices. Her contention is that dancing contributes to fulfilling one's potential, is self-realising and creates enhanced attentional focus, that the body is who we are and how we experience. "Bodyfulness" is the term she uses.

> **Pause and Practice**
>
> Walk either clockwise in a circle or in a long channel forward and back for 3 minutes. Take your time to walk with awareness. Be aware of your contact with the ground beneath you, the shift of weight from one foot to the other, each foot leaving the ground and then touching the ground as you step. Give your attention to what you're doing as you move. Be aware of any bodily sensations that arise as you move without judging them. Accept what you notice as kindly as you can.

Whatley and Lefebvre Sell's (2014) research in creating mindful dance work found that student dancers professed to an authentic and deeply embodied creation and performance period, leading to clarity of presence, detailed attention and heightened awareness due to mindfulness practices. Researching into mindfulness and performance with student athletes, Gardner and Moore (2004) found that mindfulness supported an open attention useful for live events. The Mindfulness-Acceptance-Commitment (MAC) model they advocate would engender improved attentional awareness and focus and emphasise process over goals.

Vago's (2014) theoretical model, with motivation and intention as key components, based on evidence from neurocognition studies created to understand self-awareness in mindfulness practice, proposes therapeutic benefits. He states that mindfulness creates a more positive view of self, is psychologically transformative, and affords attentional capacity, allowing clarity and positive cognitive strength. Kabat-Zinn (2004) and Brach (2015) discuss intention in relation to a heart connection, which, they say, creates presence. Considering that dance performers may need to feel a positive, attentive, aware and clear sense of self support ahead of a performance, with all its potential stresses, it seems reasonable to apply a method which could bring this to the fore. To be present from the heart suggests authentic performance for me.

MOTIVATION, INTENTION AND SELF-CARE

In mindfulness practice, motivation is embodied – an energy – meaningful and personal, which should be used beyond the individual and in support of others say Nairn et al. (2009). It is concerned with sharing, doing and communicating from a heartfelt place, but without attachment to any goal. Nairn et al. (2009) also believe that clear cognitive intention creates focus and direction for mindfulness practice. Simply acknowledging an intention, even without a felt or bodily sense, in mindfulness compassion practices is said to create positive outcomes, according to the Mindfulness Association (2012). Jack Kornfield (2008) sees a common lack of conscious application to intention and notes how repeated intention to create positive outcomes results in new neural pathways in the brain.

Mindfulness meditation allows practitioners to focus on their present moment experience with acceptance and non-judgment. This opportunity to focus on oneself and be aware of one's internal and external experience, could arguably be seen as 'self-care' and formed the basis of Kabat-Zinn's (2004) influential and pioneering work using mindfulness at its core to support well-being and health. In summary, Mindfulness, dance and sports literatures discuss mindfulness as an embodied practice supporting a sense of authentic presence and 'being'. Using awareness and attention, founded upon intention and motivation, has been found to be greatly beneficial to promoting self-care and well-being mostly due to the inclusion of self-compassion and acceptance. Considering the needs of dance performance, as I see it, dance performers would do well to take care of themselves prior to performing in order to perform at their best.

DANCE

As a physical act of expression, the body dancing could be said to represent the 'whole' dancer, the totality of that person as they move in the moment – an embodied dancer. This "totality" and wholeness clearly relates to the concerns of mindfulness, I would say. Preston-Dunlop and Sanchez-

Colberg (2002) note the performer's 'lived' experience as informing and presenting his embodied work. Furthermore, Critien and Ollis (2006) propose the 'live' and 'lived' moment and strong sense of self in reference to peak and authentic performance. Again, this is true of mindfulness – the living, present moment experience proposes authentic presence. I suggest that an unembodied performer is more of a shadow on stage, a sketch of himself, and I would say likely distracted. Mindfulness teaches us to be aware of when we are distracted as this means not being present.

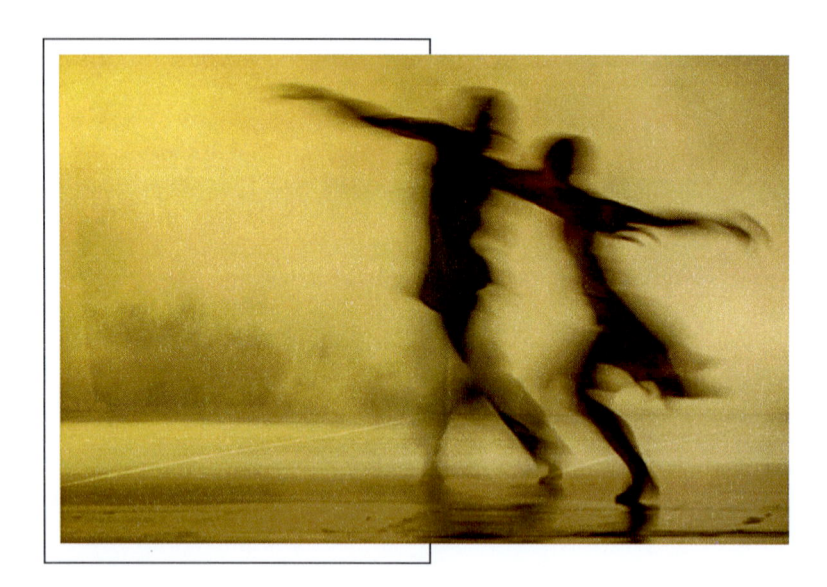

Figure 3: Shadowy dancers
Photo by Emiral Kokai, Colourbox

Authentic dance work resulted from teaching students to be more in process, embodied, somatically aware and experiential (Smith, 2002) and Batson and Wilson (2014) note the experiential body as communicative due to the performing, embodied dancer's body relating both to self and audience. They insist that somatic awareness creates powerful presence. Dance improviser Dilley asserts, "embodied practices are incredible personal laboratories for working with attention and developing a stronger sense of presence [...] So attention is an essential training" (de Spain, 2014, p.171). In agreement, Batson and Wilson (2014) writing on dance, somatic practice and neuroscience discuss attention as an imperative in the act of performing, noting how developing and heightening attentiveness supports technique and expression. They also discuss emergence as a key element of the 'beingness' of dance-embodied communication, which suggests a clear synergy with the qualities of mindfulness to me – person-centred moment-to-moment experience, awareness and attention – and fits with my proposed mindfulness method for dance PPP. The emphasis on an experiential process governed by attentiveness to lead one into a performance, which will itself be processual, also supports my method.

MOTIVATION, INTENTION AND ATTENTION

Cotterill (2015) and Lazaroff (2001) note the importance of motivation to consistently engage the performer in performance situations and Chua (2014) found that motivation was critical to outstanding outcomes for expert dancers. Alongside this, intention creates embodied, communicative and 'lived moment' performance according to Preston-Dunlop and Sanchez Colberg (2002), and Critien and Ollis' (2006) study proposed that one important element of a professional dancer's performance practice was having an intention or goal, which could be "lived" onstage. I suggest that the latter's point demonstrates the significance of intention for embodied performance presence. Finally, attention is defined by Krasnow and Wilmerding (2015) as "concentrated mental activity" – a necessary onstage skill that allows a performer to deal with all variables.

In summary, developing mental skills and PPP by engendering a sense of 'being' and presence through embodied practice in order to perform authentically is clearly important. Motivation, goal-setting and intention could support a holistic approach in this.

> **Pause and Reflect**
>
> What is your intention for reading this book?

WHICH WAY?

My motivation and intention were to offer a method and tools to effect positive and useful change. The self-compassion aspects of the mindfulness programme as well as the opportunity to understand and develop 'everyday' presence and self awareness have been so beneficial for me, that I knew there was an opportunity to give succor to those under stress and managing significant events in their lives and studies. In my experience, performing, regardless of how much or how little rehearsal one has, is incredibly revealing – one can feel vulnerable and open to very public failure – so a performer may need 'anchors' of sorts. These anchors would offer a possibility to feel assured and clear in order to precipitate a truthful and authentic rendering and 'in the moment' experience. Performing of any kind is a creative journey and opportunity. I would argue that everyone is creative in one way or another and could apply the ideas I'm suggesting in order to be present in moments of 'performance'. So that means you as a teacher, as a best man or woman giving your wedding speech, as a surgeon, dentist, dog walker.

I chose a constructivist Grounded Theory methodological framework as the way to focus my research. Simply put, this methodology necessitates exploring the topic from within the field itself – an investigative dialogue between the participants and me. A supportive attribute of this methodology is in its engagement with emergent data using the gerund, the 'ing', so it is a present, ongoing methodology of process – just like mindfulness! For instance, coding data would be done like this: "practising mindfulness" or "needing time alone for warming up". To begin my data gathering I created an online pilot study for final year undergraduate students at Trinity Laban Conservatoire for Music and Dance, where I teach. I asked questions about experience and understanding of performance presence, perfectionism, somatic training, and component aspects of PPP and how this was developed. I also asked their views on the possible efficacy of mindfulness in supporting onstage work. From this cohort, a small, self-selected group were interested in being involved in my research, learning mindfulness with a view to an intervention as part of their final degree shows. I taught them mindfulness based on the eight-week MBLC programme developed by the Mindfulness Association and used as part of the Aberdeen University Mindfulness programme. The programme is founded on the core practice of 'settling, grounding, resting and support' (SGRS). The stages of SGRS are as follows:

- Settling – focusing attention on posture; set personal intention and motivation; focusing attention on breath and breathing to help settle the mind
- Grounding – focusing attention on the body and its connection to the ground; awareness of the body and physical sensations
- Resting – letting go of any focused attention
- Support – allowing a mindful attention to one's present experience using the breath or sound to support this

Knowing the demands and rigours of a dance performer's daily training and to emphasise a necessary self-caring and generosity, I made an addition. Alongside the usual MBLC mindfulness practices of 'loving kindness' and the 'self compassion break' I added the 'compassionate body-scan' practice that Neff (2011) recommends. I also emphasised employment of the 'setting of intention and motivation' - an opening stage of mindfulness practice that I had seized on as essential on beginning my own mindfulness training. It struck me that without this there is neither heart nor grounding to mindfulness.

The intervention consisted of using sitting, walking or movement mindfulness practices, or a blend of any, as part of these performers' PPP for their two degree show performances - a courageous undertaking on their behalf given the special importance of these events. Based on emergent data, the performers were very clear that they wanted to enjoy their performance, and they felt that the audiences would appreciate it too. So, we agreed that the sentiment of intention and motivation should be as follows: "My intention is to connect with my joy in performing" and "My motivation is to share my experience with the audience", or something very similar of their own wording.

Pause and Reflect

How might you use a similar phrase in your life, as a way to recognise and embody your joy in doing whatever it is in that moment?

Having coded all data gathered from pre and post-intervention questionnaires and a focus group discussion, where other new sub-themes such as investment and immersion, and attention and awareness in onstage work had emerged, I formed three categories. I found an overlap between all categories with embodiment, personal focus, and pleasure in performing for and commitment to the audience all interconnected. Fig.4 (below) illustrates these connections and demonstrates how integrating mindfulness into PPP supported my heroes in feeling and working more positively onstage.

Taking time to (Re)Focus
- this can be a physical thing and a deliberate mental thing too
- intention is remembered and physicalised
- this helps confidence
- not being too internal
- connecting with self
- creating awareness
- using Mindfulness

Needing to be Embodied
- this needs time and application, therefore preparation
- creates authenticity
- this gives presence

The Joy in Connecting
- Mindfulness aspects (like non judgment etc) are implied here
- this needs confidence, therefore preparation
- feeling supported and authentic
- intention is demonstrated

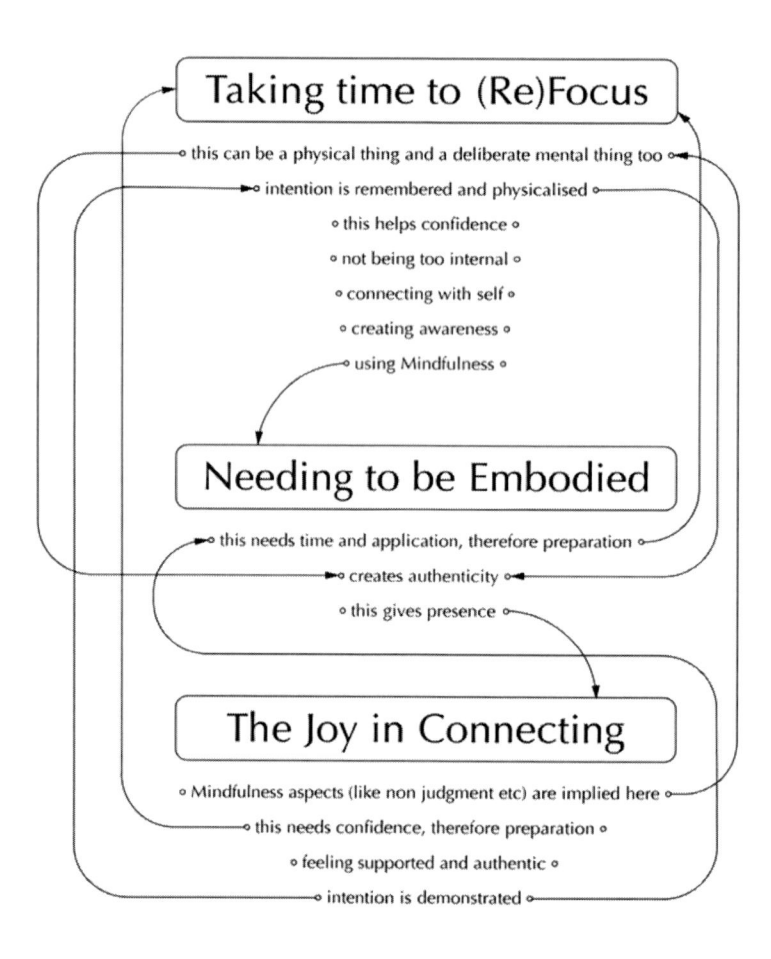

Figure 4: Three emergent categories and the interconnections between them

WAY THROUGH

The question central to my study was, 'Is mindfulness a suitable support mechanism for dancers' pre-performance preparation (PPP), and might this support a sense of embodied presence onstage?' My study participants had clear ideas about what they felt the requirements of being and being onstage with presence are, as one states here:

> It is when you realise you are here right now doing this. But sometimes it is also being so present with the movement of your body that you don't see yourself from the outside, but experience the situation from within your body.

Figure 4 presents the three categories I created: Taking Time to (Re)Focus, Needing to be Embodied and The Joy in Connecting. They represent recognition of a performer's need to be embodied for performing effectively and foreground the importance of prioritising time to prepare to access this state of being; a state supportive to feeling confident and ready to dance before an audience. I believe they could represent the essential cornerstones of a contemporary dancer's PPP and suggest a complex mind-body process and an activity more substantial than, say, a physical tuning.

What emerged from the data, simply speaking was this:

> **Preparing to perform** – by taking time to (re)focus – from inside to out – using mindful intention and motivation – and attention and awareness – to be authentic

TAKING TIME TO (RE)FOCUS

Prior to the intervention and early on in learning and practising mindfulness, I asked my heroes what their preparation had been so far, what they needed it to be, and how they imagined mindfulness could possibly be useful during preparation time. They said:

> Pre-performance routine is very important as it allows me to become fully invested in the work so that the movement is embodied and the mind is focused and directed towards the choreographic process (Participant 8)
> Being both mentally and physically prepared before any performance allows me to tap into the correct state needed for the piece (Participant 8)
> Think about yourself, ground (Participant 2)
> [...] concur with the word investment, invest before you even go onstage (Participant 3)
> [...] nerves…settle…relax…will feel grounded onstage (Participant 9)

Figure 5: Pre-intervention participant comments

Considering PPP as highly individual and personal processes, I distilled all data concerning this down to i) self prioritisation and care ii) facilitation of awareness and engagement and iii) mindfulness as a way to self, as key elements to consider.

Following the PPP intervention participants stated:

> I feel that this was very useful because as soon as I stepped on to the stage I felt very clear on what I was aiming to achieve when performing the piece and what impression and ideas I wanted to share with the audience (Participant 8)
> I felt like I was moving wholly and fully without getting lost within my self (Participant 7)
> I enjoyed having that moment to myself just focusing on me, something that I don't think I do enough (Participant 5)
> Support confidence to perform. It allowed me to stay calm and find time for myself, to channel my thought process, deviating any negative thoughts that may have impacted my confidence onstage (Participant 6)

Figure 6: Post-intervention participant comments

My interpretation of this is that unstable and pressured circumstances or the inability to prioritise personal needs could lead to performers being too distracted to prepare effectively, creating a need to (re)focus. Setting aside time pre-show for this, to determine needs, seemed to offer a deep sense of self-prioritisation and care, with the participants reporting confident, embodied, self connected positive experiences prior to the performance and onstage. Being able to create supportive space and time for themselves in which to focus their attention on becoming embodied and present prior to performing clearly helped. It seemed that taking time to (re)focus could lead young dance performers to deeper commitment, embodiment, and perhaps most importantly, help them to fulfill their potential.

USING MINDFUL INTENTION AND MOTIVATION

Central to Vago's (2014) theory is creating intention and motivation as a way to gain effective personal strength and well-being. A cornerstone of mindfulness practice, setting intention and motivation proved beneficial to the study participants, and significant in creating a fuller sense of embodiment; focus; connection to the audience; presence and aliveness due to the awareness that the PPP provided. One participant reported,

> The sentences of my intention and motivation appeared in my mind during both performances and reminded me to keep focusing on the joy of performing and of sharing my experience with the audience within the performance.

My heroic participants believed that 'intention' helped to create, support and maintain an embodied presence. One said, "I wasn't ever thinking 'be present now !!!' - it was a more lighter [sic] reminder of physical awarenesses [sic] that would stimulate my feeling of presence" and, for another setting the intention and motivation, "[...] provided a focus, something to be striving toward. Fuelling my performance with a more personal intention".

ATTENTION AND AWARENESS

Rob Nairn (1999), a mindfulness teacher, says that the focus of awareness and attention in mindfulness practice gives time to be present, to become embodied - the participants' aim for the stage! Performers need to train in developing and improving effective attentional capacity according to Cotterill (2015) and Ehrenberg (2015) and using mindfulness as a tool for this has shown positive outcomes in studies. The attention and awareness created by the mindfulness PPP led to focusing on self experientially, engendering a meaningful engagement with performance activity. A participant relayed this experience:

> The first night I felt very ready after doing the practice and it gave me time to really focus on myself and be in the moment which I felt I could bring onto the stage.

Another participant stated, "[the PPP intervention allowed] me to assess, and thus ultimately care for, the conditions of my body and mind-state prior to performance".

TO BE AUTHENTIC

Mind-body, focus, motivation and goal-setting are important for positive performance outcomes, according to Taylor and Estanol (2015). All of these aspects are encompassed within the umbrella of mindfulness training, to a greater or lesser extent, and are consistent with my findings. One participant's experiential perspective of working with the intervention and its benefit is defined significantly here:

> [W]as noticing how present I was, present in a way I had not experienced before. I honestly felt that I was in the moment and at the time of performance I noticed that the time felt slower and that I felt in control of what I was doing.

I think that this statement reflects an authentically present performance. A sense of personal authenticity is arguably a consequence of practising mindfulness, and, together with confidence, authenticity was a reported outcome of Sander's (2013) study, which proffered the importance of mindfulness training in developing non-judgmental and engaged performance practice.

My exploration of preparation for the stage led me to another category, Needing to be Embodied, which I'm summarizing in this way:

Embodied Preparation – from inner to outer – supports authenticity and presence

---

In relation to their understanding of the importance of embodiment, being embodied, and how they perceived embodiment in their PPP pre-intervention, the participants said:

Being both mentally and physically prepared before any performance allows me to tap into the correct state needed for the piece. (Participant 8)

Pre-performance routine is very important as it allows me to become fully invested in the work so that the movement is embodied and the mind is focused and directed towards the choreographic process. (Participant 8)

I believe [it] is being true to the moment you are presenting. To my experience I would say I feel present when I'm fully engaged mentally and physically with what I'm doing. (Participant 1)

Being calm and work on the breath before a performance helps me doing that. If I don't focus on my PPR I feel less able to sustain mentally and physically the flow of the performance and things that can go differently than what expected. (Participant 1)

[doing] yoga poses …the whole body is involved and my mind rests on that…something that takes me entirely and engages my body entirely. (Participant 1)

I feel most present when there is a sense of flow and the movement and my intention (mind) is fully embodying and focused on what is being asked. (Participant 4)

About 5 years ago I entered the stage not prepared or warm and I got badly injured, this has made me really aware of how important it is to make sure the body is warm as well as the mind being in the right place. (Participant 2)

Figure 7: Participants pre-intervention perception of embodiment

Post-intervention, my heroes stated:

> My more relaxed state through my PPR and gave me room for my mind to encompass more than if I had not engaged in the practice, where just my hyped/nervous body and energy would pre-occupy me. (Participant 3)
> My practice did alleviate nervous energy as I had the awareness of my mind-state and I could then address my body/mind state, it supported my confidence, enjoyment and non-judgement onstage - through the body scan, I was able to inhabit the performance without distraction as to any other thought than the work, and employing my body's potential. (Participant 3)
> I felt like I was moving wholly and fully without getting lost within myself. (Participant 7)
> Okay was very aware of what I was doing I was indulging each movement I was doing it felt good to me. I felt aware of everything even when I was off stage I had a clear understanding of my body throughout the whole performance. […] I was paying attention to the largest and smallest of detail during the piece and the attention to my body during the performance. I was aware of what I wanted my body to do and because I was paying attention to my body when I was doing it, it felt great. (Participant 5)
> I feel that my performance presence raised I was aware of everything that was happening and I felt engaged, ready and present. (Participant 5)
> I can recall specific moments and experiences within the performance when I can remember was [sic] I felt or saw and also recall drifting. (Participant 4)
> I definitely felt an enhanced embodied experience where my attention to execution was heightened. (Participant 4)
> Once performing on stage the breath control centred me in the faster and more intricate movement especially as we had to wear heels in the piece. Also my focus was very clear and I felt very in the moment and fully engaged with the audience. (Participant 8)

Figure 8: Post-intervention participant awareness of embodiment in performance

One performer beautifully summarised this whole idea of embodied preparation and the effect it had on them onstage here:

> I felt very connected and true to what I was doing, I was really embodying the movements and tasks in the work, I also felt very connected to the rest of the group and enjoyed performing. My awareness was alive I would say and as mentioned earlier I think it happened naturally as I had been practicing this before entering the stage, it became a part of the performance without forcing it to be.

FROM INNER TO OUTER

Hanna (1979, p.24) states, "[a]ll dance has purpose or intent", which could suggest that one might not need to examine or create an intention for onstage work in order to perform in an embodied way. However, the particular mindfulness intention used by each performer originated in their personal intention, rather than that of the choreography or its origins and is thus potentially more heartfelt, embodied. Interestingly, this mindfulness PPP did also facilitate a positive and clarifying re-examination of the choreographic origins, creating confidence in some participants. Batson and Wilson (2014) believe that embodied dancers are expressive, communicative and profoundly present. A participant experienced the following:

> I felt I was very much in the moment of what I was doing, and the embodiment came very naturally […] I think when being aware of myself before going on stage it naturally became a part of my performance. Also, I felt a lot more relaxed with myself when entering the stage and I was able to be more honest in the way I approached the work.

AUTHENTIC PRESENCE

The honesty reflected in the performer's comment above suggests authenticity to me. Interestingly, directly before going onstage some participants reported using a practice called the '3 Minute Breathing Space' (3MBS). The purpose of '3MBS' is to notice one's present experience from a wider focus/external, then narrow into an internal focus (the breath), then open out into an external focus once more. I see this as a 'top up', a reminder of their mindfulness PPP to re-embody, to reconnect with themselves, to be present, and it reminds me of my personal experience of the 3MBS - it brings me "back to me", an authentic, embodied and present moment sense of myself. Prioritising time for self-care, then, was central to facilitating an embodied sense and presence in PPP.

> **Pause and Practice**
>
> **3 Minute Breathing Space**
>
> - Find a quiet space, sit comfortably and close your eyes
> - Without judging, analysing or dwelling, simply notice what is arising or what you're aware of in i) your thinking ii) your body iii) your emotions. Let go of your awareness of these as soon as you notice what is there
> - Begin to equalise and lengthen your in-breath and out-breath (counting to three or four for each) and continue this for around 2 minutes. Then let your breathing be the rhythm and length it wants to be
> - Gently open your eyes and allow yourself to become aware of your surroundings
>
> Continue with what you were doing.

Overall, post-intervention, performance presence was expressed as an augmented sense of being present, engaged and ready, as well as security in awareness and connection to the work, others and self. I would say that this relates to the idea of 'being 'inside' and/then 'out' whilst moving' as expressed here:

> [...] renewed energy, but at the same time I felt very grounded [...] I felt like I had some sort of overview over the evening, our performance and myself in my body. Throughout the performance I thought many times that I felt extraordinarily calm and grounded and I noticed that my eyes were open and that I was actually seeing my fellow performers and the audience.

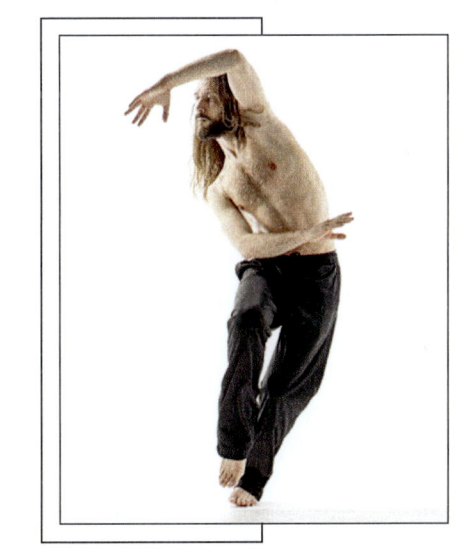

Figure 9: Embodied and present dancing
Photo by Alexander Yakovlev, Colourbox

WAY FORWARD

Over many years, I have spoken with young performers who discuss stage fright, perfectionism, lack of self-esteem and other challenges to their practice. I've seen fear in their eyes as they panic towards the start of a show or become blank and robot-like onstage as a coping mechanism for the pressure they feel. Knowing that these people are, or have the potential to be, great performers but hearing and seeing their (di)stress has focused my desire to share the personal support that I have found in practising mindfulness. To be more relaxed or at ease, to be breathing more comfortably, to feel grounded and more 'me' through mindfulness practice was an offer worth extending. If performers could check in with themselves prior to a show to understand their state of body-mind, and not in a 'routine' way, I believed, would give them a better chance to gather themselves and prepare in a most personal, attentive and caring way using what they needed at that particular time.

Training dance students with a PPP that could give them confidence, clarity and purpose to enhance their skills for being and living in their performance onstage is vital. I feel that my mindfulness PPP intervention was wholly supportive to the young contemporary dance performers involved, creating enhanced performance capability and equipping the artists with an adaptable and individually tailored practise. With a heartfelt emphasis on intention and motivation it facilitated a positive PPP experience and could be an ongoing tool for those performers to further explore and adapt as they develop their careers. The significant benefits of it derive from the reported strong sense of support, confidence and authenticity. I contend that it offered a framework or method with which to understand, develop and practise being, or becoming, present.

A real sense of energy and clarity in the participants' setting intention and motivation was apparent to me, echoing my own daily practice. It seemed to act as a positive support and as a signpost to find focus and purpose. To be able to relax into the PPP process by creating a framework for it arguably added potency its development and allowed a particularly useful self awareness. This seems to relate strongly to Kabat-Zinn's definition of motivation as, "what is most important to you, what you believe is most fundamental to your ability to be your best self, […] be whole" (2004, p.46). My intention now is to promote the idea that prioritising the contemporary dance student's personal pre-show time to focus on their needs at that moment, and to become embodied mindfully, can create an appropriately keen and strong sense of focus.

I thoroughly enjoyed the opportunity to share and research new ideas and ways to work for the stage with my newfound stage heroes. In the same sense that Vin Harris in Chapter 2 discusses in "passing the baton", so to speak, it was extremely satisfying to explore my knowledge, practice and experience more deeply and find an application for it that nurtured and enabled those young performers. I am now intent on making mindfulness part of dance education. I said to my boss, "Mindfulness needs to be part of creative studies because it allows time for making choices rather than following one's usual habits or being reactive." I believe that this is true of any creative endeavor.

FURTHER RESOURCES

Tara Brach
https://www.tarabrach.com
Transitions Dance Company
www.trinitylaban.ac.uk/transitionsdc

REFERENCES

BATSON, G. and WILSON, M., (2014). Body and Mind in Motion Dance and Neuroscience in Conversation. Bristol UK: Intellect

BRACH, T., (2015). Listening to the Calling of our Hearts. tarabrach.com. 01/21/2015. Available: www.tarabrach.com [Date Accessed: 10/01/16]

CALDWELL, C., (2014). Mindfulness & Bodyfulness: A New Paradigm, The Journal of Contemplative Inquiry, 1, pp.77-96.

CHUA, J., (2014) Dance talent development across the lifespan: a review of current research. Research in Dance Education, 15 (1), pp.23-53. DOI: 10.1080/14647893.2013.825749 (Date Accessed 22/10/15)

CLOWES, H. and KNOWLES, Z., (2013). Exploring the effectiveness of pre-performance routines in elite artistic gymnasts: A mixed method investigation, Science of Gymnastics Journal, 5 (2), pp.27-40.

COLOURBOX Photos. Stage and curtains (Revealing the process) by Vladimir Galantsev - https://www.colourbox.com/vector/theater-stage-with-wooden-floor-and-open-red-curtains-vector-vector-15096559

Single man dancing -barechested (Embodied and present dancing) by Alexander Yakovlev - https://www.colourbox.com/image/young-beautiful-dancer-posing-in-the-studio-image-33733941

The two dancers (shadowy dancers) by Emiral Kokai   https://www.colourbox.com/image/group-of-contemporary-dancers-performing-on-stage-image-11128222   All Photos purchased 10.10.2018 by author.

COTTERILL, S., (2015). Preparing for Performance: Strategies Adopted Across Performance Domains. The Sport Psychologist, 29, pp.158-170. http://dx.doi.org/10.1123/tsp.2014-0035 © 2015 Human Kinetics, Inc. (Date Accessed 9/9/15)

CRITIEN, N. & OLLIS, S., (2006). Multiple engagement of self in the development of talent in professional dancers, Research in Dance Education, 7 (2), pp.179-200. DOI: 10.1080/14647890601029584

CSIKSZENTMIHALY, M., (1992). Flow: The Psychology of Happiness. London: Rider

DE SPAIN, K., (2014). Landscape of the now. A topography of Movement Improvisation. UK: Oxford Press

EDINBOROUGH, C., (2011). Developing decision-making skills for performance through the practice of mindfulness in somatic training, Theatre, Dance and Performance Training, 2 (1), pp.18-33. DOI: 10.1080/19443927.2010.543917

EHRENBERG, S., (2015). A Kinesthetic Mode of Attention in Contemporary Dance Practice. Dance Research Journal, 47 (2), pp.43-61. DOI:10.1017/S0149767715000212 (Date Accessed 6/10/15)

GARDNER, F.L. and MOORE, Z. E., (2004). A Mindfulness-Acceptance- Commitment-Based Approach to Athletic Performance Enhancement: Theoretical Considerations, Behaviour Therapy, 35, pp.707-723. DOI 005- 7894/04/0707-0723

GOODALL, J., (2008). Stage Presence. UK: Routledge

HANNA, J. L., (1979). To Dance is Human. USA: University of Texas Press

KABAT-ZINN, J., (2004). Full Catastrophe Living. 15th Edition. USA: Dell Publishing

KORNFIELD, J., (2008). THE WISE HEART. London: Rider

KRASNOW, D. H., and WILMERDING, M. D., (2015). Motor Learning and Control for Dance. USA, Champaign, IL: Human Kinetics

LAZAROFF, E. M., (2001). Performance and Motivation in Dance Education. Arts Education Policy Review, 103 (2), pp.23-29. DOI: 10.1080/10632910109600284

MINDFULNESS ASSOCIATION © COMPASSIONATE MIND ASSOCIATION © 2012 Manual

NAIRN, R., (1999). Diamond Mind A Psychology of Meditation. USA: Shambala Publications Inc.

NAIRN, R., CHODEN, REGAN-ADDIS, H., NEVEJAN, A., MCMURTRY, D., and CRAIG, L. (2009). Mindfulness Handbook Module 1. Aberdeen University and Mindfulness Association.

NEFF, K., (2011). Self Compassion. London: Hodder & Stoughton

PARGMAN, D., (2006). Managing Performance Stress. Oxon, UK: Routledge

PRESTON-DUNLOP, V. and SANCHEZ-COLBERG, A., (2002). Dance and the performative a choreological perspective Laban and beyond. London: Verve Publishing

SANDERS, L. A., (2013). Integrating Contemplative Education and Contemporary Performance NEW DIRECTIONS FOR TEACHING AND LEARNING, 134, DOI: 10.1002/tl.20054

SMITH, M. L., (2002). Moving Self: The thread which bridges dance and theatre. Research in Dance Education, 3 (2), pp.123-141. DOI:10.1080/1464789022000034695

STEINMAN, L., (1995). The Artist as Storyteller in Contemporary Performance. Berkley USA: North Atlantic Books

TART, C. T., (1994). Living the mindful life. A handbook for living in the present moment. Boston, USA: Shambhala

TAYLOR, J. and ESTANOL, E., (2015). Dance Psychology for Artistic and Performance Excellence. USA, Champaign. IL: Human Kinetics

VAGO, D. R., (2014). Mapping modalities of self-awareness in mindfulness practice: a potential mechanism for clarifying habits of mind, Annals of the New York Academy of Sciences, 1307, pp.28-42. doi: 10.1111/nyas.12270

WHATLEY, S. and LEFEBVRE SELL, N., (2014). Dancing and Flourishing: Mindful Meditation in Dance Making and Performing. In: A. WILLIAMSON, G. BATSON, S. WHATLEY and R. WEBER, Editors, Dance, Somatics and Spiritualities Contemporary Sacred Narratives. Bristol: Intellect. pp.437-458.

CHAPTER 22

INTRODUCTION TO STORIES OF MINDFUL HEROES IN COMMUNITY

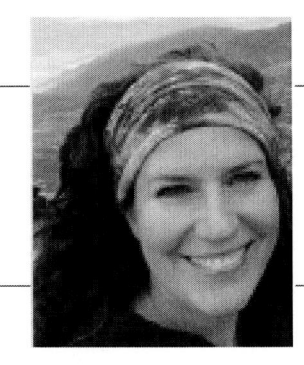

Jane Negrych

janenegrych@sanctuary.ie

Community has always been important to me. Not only through my journey with mindfulness but also in relation to my mental wellbeing. Whether it was a book club, a women's group, a Plum Village sangha or the communities that I have helped build and foster through my role as a 'mindfulness teacher', I have always found that it has been the presence of others that has helped sustain my balance and even picked me up off of the floor, in times of need.

Therefore, as I read about Jacky's work with family care caregivers, John's ability to help those who are ageing find a place to belong and to be valued, and the many bridges built and communities created as a result of the Everyone Project, I was struck with a sense of admiration and deep privilege to be able to witness all of the ways connection through communities of mindfulness practitioners has helped so many.

My own introduction to mindfulness was very much born out of a need for wellbeing and community. I can still remember the morning that I was struggling with anxiety and post-traumatic stress disorder (PTSD). When I dropped my children to school, I could see all the other parents laughing and visiting at the school gate. As I sat in my car, I felt so alone. In my mind, there was no way that any of them could relate to what I was experiencing. The same thought kept repeating in my mind- "I am alone. I am alone. I am alone". It wasn't until I trained in compassion- based mindfulness that I learned that this is what the mind does, and if anything, my sense of 'alone' was a shared experience.

Kristin Neff, author of the book "Self-Compassion", identifies this as an "irrational but pervasive sense of isolation" (www.self-compassion.org, 2019) that contributes to suffering. In fact, one of the steps in her practice the Self Compassion Break addresses this by inviting the practitioner to reflect that, in all actuality, the one thing that unites us as humans is the fact that we suffer (Neff, 2011). And this is what I discovered as I came to know mindfulness and the many communities of practitioners that followed suit. We all suffer and somehow, we can take comfort in this knowledge. Now, don't get me wrong, I don't want others to suffer. Instead, I simply needed and continue to need to feel a little less alone. My anxiety and PTSD became all encompassing; therefore, I decided to learn mindfulness as a means of helping me cope. What I didn't realize at the time was that it would ultimately address this sense of isolation that had been plaguing me.

Interestingly, while I was not a caregiver (indeed, I probably need to be cared for!), Jacky identifies this sense of isolation as something that caregivers may experience and can be a contributing factor to the grief and anguish that many caregivers go through (Seery, Chapter 24). Moreover, this theme is reflected, if not a bit more indirectly, in both John's description of the self -marginalization, or the "self-stereotyping" (Darwin, Chapter 23) of the ageing population. In the Everyone Project's focus on bringing mindfulness to "groups that are currently excluded" (Harris, Hughes and McColl, Chapter 25). So, just like me, mindfulness became a catalyst for community for the participants who took part in these projects as a means of managing difficulty.

My own mindfulness community started as a small group of people meeting to practice in the Plum Village (Thich Nhat Hanh's Zen Buddhist) tradition, which led me to the MSc: Studies in Mindfulness with the University of Aberdeen. I then went on to work for the Mindfulness Association as their communications and membership manager; and most recently, I have undertaken the role of Programme Manager at the Sanctuary in Dublin, Ireland. In each of these contexts, community has been integral and has contributed to not only my own wellbeing, but to those who were part of the group experience. For instance, in my deepest despair, practicing together in sangha brought me out of my house, connected me with other practitioners, all the while arming me with breath practices that create the conditions for my mind to become more still and for my mind to open, allowing alternative perspectives. Maybe I wasn't so alone after all?

John writes about the broadening of viewpoints when he states that in the Mindful Ageing course that he ran with Mike Pupius, they explored ways in which mindfulness practices might help participants "[re]align toward the positive – challenging stereotypes…open to new possibilities and beginnings" (Darwin, Chapter 23). This is incredibly important for whether you are suffering with PTSD, part of the ageing population, a caregiver confined to the house or an asylum seeker, our minds can become fixed on our stories. To highlight this, one of the participants in Jacky's study shares "I've been making up stories as I have been going along. I used to worry about what people think but now I am different. I realised I didn't need to make up a story" (Seery, Chapter 24). Just like this participant, I had been making up stories that felt very real.

Indeed, that morning in the car at the school drop, my story was that I was alone. There was nothing anyone could say to convince me otherwise. Thankfully, I now know this not to be true. However, it took my mindfulness practice to uncover this lie. Eventually, I became someone who helped create community through mindfulness when I became a mindfulness teacher. As soon as I started teaching, I decided to teach a mindfulness course in my local village. To my surprise, the people who attended were the very people at that school gate all those years earlier. I had not been alone. They too were trying to manage fear, anxiety, depression and loneliness. And just like me, they too found that mindfulness and the communities that we create around practice helped them feel less isolated.

As my career progressed, I started to create community for the Mindfulness Association (MA) in the form of its membership. We needed to find a way to unite all of the people in various locations throughout the UK who had and continue to take the courses ran by the MA. In short, we really felt a deep need to find a way of sustaining practice and wellbeing through community, something I could relate to. Due to the nature of the work of the MA being UK wide, we decided to create an online membership platform, alongside weekly online meditation sits and monthly online teachings. We also held various face-to face membership events in the form of practice weekends and conferences. In this way, we hoped to provide a structure to support our members beyond an 8- week course, beyond an 8- month course, beyond an event. We hoped to provide a structure to support the practice of mindfulness for life. In fact, it was at one of our membership weekends in which the Everyone Project was launched. Moreover, it has been the members of the MA who have helped deliver the mindfulness courses ran by the Everyone Project: community creating community.

Most recently, I decided to take on the role of Programme Manager at the Sanctuary in Dublin, Ireland. The Sanctuary is a meditation and mindfulness centre that was founded by Sr. Stan Kennedy. Her vision for the Sanctuary was to provide a reflective contemplative, beautiful place for people in the midst of our frantic busy, world. A place and space where they could be re-energised and nourished in body, mind and soul. In this way, her hope is to help people to live to their full potential, and community plays an important role. At the Sanctuary, we run mindfulness and compassion courses for all walks of life. However, the work at the Sanctuary also hopes to transform society through mindfulness courses for youth, caregivers and those working on the frontlines. In this way, we hope to create a more compassionate and resilient Irish society.

Similar to the MA, we also recognize the need for community and aim to help sustain and support the lifelong practice of mindfulness and compassion. However, the Sanctuary differs in that it provides a physical place to come to. At the Sanctuary, we foster community through our daily (morning/lunch/evening) practice sessions, our monthly days of practice and the many day and evening courses available for all: whether a teacher, a caregiver, one whose cared for, a lawyer, an advertising exec or a mother struggling to contain her anxiety, PTSD and sense of being alone.

Mindfulness is so much more than 8- week programme. It is not a quick fix, rather a practice for life; and it is through the communities that these programmes can create, that real change and ease of suffering can take place. So, if you find yourself feeling alone, reach out and find a community to practice in! As Helen Keller once said, "Alone we can do little, together we can do so much".

FURTHER RESOURCES

The Sanctuary, Dublin
www.sanctuary.ie
The Mindfulness Association
www.mindfulnessassociation.net

REFERENCES

NEFF, K., (2011). Self-Compassion: Stop Beating Yourself Up and Leave Insecurity Behind. London: Hodder & Stoughton.
NEFF, K., (2019). The Three Elements of Self-Compassion. Available: https://self-compassion.org/the-three-elements-of-self-compassion-2/ [Date Accessed: 15th April 2019].

CHAPTER 23

THE AUTOBIOGRAPHY OF A MINDFULNESS COMMUNITY IN EIGHT SHORT CHAPTERS

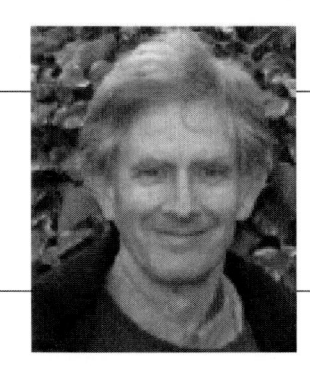

John Darwin

johnadarwin@aol.com

There are many heroes in this story, and I can best tell it, paraphrasing the title of Portia Nelson's popular poem, as the *Autobiography In Eight Short Chapters of our Mindfulness Community*.

> **Pause and Read**
>
> If you are not familiar with it, take a look at Portia Nelson's excellent poem
> http://www.doorway-to-self-esteem.com/autobiography-in-five-short-chapters.html

CHAPTER ONE: STUDYING MINDFULNESS

I had a stuttering start to my meditation practice. When I was 16 I became fascinated by Buddhism and read extensively. But at University I became politically active and the spiritual side dropped away. It was another 25 years before I realised that I had set the political and the spiritual as either-or. The political dimension had been very important to me, leading to a career first as a community worker, then a local government officer, and ultimately a Chief Officer in Sheffield City Council. But this realisation, so obvious in retrospect, that I had set up an unnecessary dualism in my mind, led me to revisit the spiritual. I made several visits to Throssel Hole Buddhist Abbey and developed a daily practice in SotoZen meditation.

Years later came the time I stopped working full time (by then I was an academic at Sheffield Business School). Jubilación, as the Spanish say, so much better than the pejorative English term 'retired'. I had read Kabat-Zinn (1990) and other authors on mindfulness, and now was a good opportunity to explore this further. So I did a Postgraduate Certificate in Mindfulness Based Approaches at Bangor University, which introduced me to new practices, including the bodyscan and different meditative approaches. By the end of this I had decided that if I ever did teach mindfulness I would:

- Not run it as a therapy course such as MBSR or MBCT – after all, I am not a therapist.
- Put a greater emphasis on mindful movement. I had also taken up yoga in my jubilación, and could already see the benefits, including greater flexibility and enhanced balance.
- Incorporate the Four Immeasurables (Loving Kindness, Compassion, Empathetic Joy and Equanimity). Although I had previously read about them, I had never explored them in depth. An excellent module at Bangor on 'The Buddhist

Foundations of Mindfulness' by Michael Chaskalson led me to revisit this and discover the beauty of the Brahma Viharas.
- Emphasise positive aspects as well as the negative, for example gratitude and savouring, drawing on the rapidly expanding study of positive psychology.
- Include mindful learning, drawing on the writings of Ellen Langer (1997, 2009) and others who have explored this.

CHAPTER TWO: MINDFULNESS BASED LIFE ENHANCEMENT IS BORN

Despite these reflections, I still had no intention of teaching mindfulness - I just wanted to learn about it. When people at my University (where I was still doing some postgraduate teaching) asked what I was up to, I would say I was studying mindfulness and in 2010 you could still get the response, 'What is that?' So I did a couple of seminars on the theme which attracted far more people than I had expected, and I was then asked to provide some guidance in mindfulness, initially for staff in the University library who were under stress. Others in the University heard about this and asked me to take it further. An email to people attending the two lectures, inviting expressions of interest in an eight-week course, brought more than 16 applicants (the number I have found best for a course).

And so Mindfulness Based Life Enhancement (MBLE) was born, using an eight week structure like MBSR, but incorporating the provisos above. I was fortunate in knowing an expert in positive psychology, Ann Macaskill, so I took advice from her on the central themes from this emerging discipline which could be incorporated into the course. I was also fortunate in getting strong support from fellow members of the University's Multifaith Centre, which meant that I could use a room there to run the courses – support that has been unwavering ever since.

I mentioned in the previous Chapter that I wanted to include the Four Immeasurables. Initially MBIs did not explicitly address these, although a loving-kindness meditation was included in the day of practice. Their role was seen as "implicit and embodied in all of the practices and teaching" (McCown et al, 2010, p.185). Subsequently, McCown et al note, MBSR teachers "have developed curriculum adaptations that include loving-kindness and other compassion-oriented practices, and/or include such practices in ongoing home practice". 'Cultivating kindness' is the main theme in week seven (ibid.138). More recently we have seen the development of MBIs emphasising compassion, including Compassion Focused Therapy (Gilbert 2010) and Mindful Self-Compassion.

My conviction that more than mindfulness is needed stemmed initially from my investigation of Zen's sometimes dark history, in particular reading Victoria's analysis of the complicity of Japanese Zen masters in war crimes, and the subsequent use of zazen by corporations to engender "discipline, obedience, conformity and physical and mental endurance" (2006, p.184). From this, and a review of events in various Western Buddhist traditions, I concluded that:

- The Zen tradition, Zen centres and other Buddhist communities are as susceptible to corruption and malpractice as other organisations
- Whether the malpractice involves violence, intimidation or sexual misconduct, the common factor is the pervasive role of power and influence, leading to conformity and obedience, and de-individuation
- The Buddhist teachings on compassion are open to distortion, primarily by being presented in a partial manner – compassion only for 'us', and not 'them'
- Therefore while loving-kindness and compassion should be explicitly addressed, so too should Joy and Equanimity. For example, compassion needs the support of equanimity, addressing the dangers of preference and prejudice. Empathetic joy – joy in the well-being of others - links well with my desire to stress positive enhancement. Nyaponika Thera argues this "has not received sufficient attention either in expositions of Buddhist ethics, or in the meditative development of the four sublime states" (2005). (A detailed discussion of these points can be found in Darwin 2014)

Further support is given in Wallace's contention that a sniper can be mindful; "When mindfulness is equated with bare attention, it can easily lead to the misconception that the cultivation of mindfulness has nothing to do with ethics or with the cultivation of wholesome states of mind and the attenuation of unwholesome states" (2008). Mindfulness needs to be underscored and supported by the qualities expressed in the Four Immeasurables. And I also realised that one of the beauties of these four qualities is the way they reinforce and support each other, as shown in Figure 1, which gives the Far Enemies, the opposites, of each quality, as well as the Near Enemies, the deceptive substitutes for which they can be mistaken. One of the most significant of these concerns Compassion, defined in the Oxford Living Dictionary as "Sympathetic pity and concern for the sufferings or misfortunes of others". Compassion and pity are very different, but this is often not recognised. Each of the Immeasurables has a role in countering the Near Enemies of the others.

Loving Kindness	Far Enemies: Hatred, ill will, anger Near Enemies: Attachment, greed, conditional love
Compassion	Compassion prevents loving-kindness from forgetting that, while both are enjoying or giving temporary and limited happiness, there still exists much suffering in the world.
Empathetic Joy	Empathetic Joy brings a sense of power, setting boundaries externally and internally.
Equanimity	Equanimity guards love from being dissipated and from going astray in uncontrolled emotion. It helps us recognise that our concerns and interests are with all living beings, challenging any tendency to self-centred attachment.

Compassion	Far Enemies: Cruelty Near Enemies: Pity, grief
Loving Kindness	Loving-kindness guards against partiality, prevents compassion from discrimination by selecting and excluding and thus protects it from falling into partiality or aversion against the excluded side.
Empathetic Joy	Empathetic Joy helps to recognise that it is not all suffering and grief, and that we can attend also to the joys and virtues of ourselves and others.; it holds compassion back from becoming overwhelmed by the sight of the world's suffering, from being absorbed by it to the exclusion of everything else.
Equanimity	Equanimity guards compassion from being dissipated and from going astray in uncontrolled emotion. It helps develop composure and internal calm allowing one to know what can or cannot be done.

Empathetic Joy	Far Enemies: Envy, jealousy, aversion Near Enemies: Joy tinged with insincerity or personal identification; frivolity and hedonism; schadenfreude
Loving Kindness	Loving-kindness brings us back to the desire that all beings will find genuine happiness and its causes, avoiding frivolity and hedonism.
Compassion	Compassion prevents empathetic joy from forgetting that, while both are enjoying or giving temporary and limited happiness, there still exists much suffering in the world. Empathetic joy needs understanding and compassion and equanimity if you are to avoid becoming a Pollyanna.
Equanimity	Equanimity addresses elation by bringing attention to the tendency to react to whatever arises in experience; acting with vigilant self-control for the sake of the final goal, does not allow empathetic joy to rest content with humble results, forgetting the real aims we have to strive for.

Equanimity	Far Enemies: Greed, resentment, partiality Near Enemies: Indifference, foolish unknowing
Loving Kindness	Loving-kindness addresses indifference and detachment, which is a form of shutting down. It imparts to equanimity its selflessness, its boundless nature and even its fervour. For fervour, too, transformed and controlled, is part of perfect equanimity, strengthening its power of keen penetration and wise restraint.
Compassion	Compassion attends to and reminds us of the suffering in the world; it guards equanimity from falling into a cold indifference, and keeps it from indolent or selfish isolation.
Empathetic Joy	Empathetic joy gives to equanimity the mild serenity that softens its stern appearance. It is the smile that persists in spite of our knowledge of the world's suffering, a smile that gives solace and hope, fearlessness and confidence.

Figure 1: Supporting Links between the Four Immeasurables

Pause and Watch

The Four Immeasurables
https://www.youtube.com/watch?v=gxgtPLMPQaQ&feature=youtu.be

All these considerations led to the basic eight-week structure of MBLE (Figure 2). There have been minor changes and improvements as we learnt from experience, but the basic structure has proved sound.

	Theme	The Four Immeasurables	Positive Psychology
1	Introducing Mindfulness		Overview Negativity bias; Broaden and Build
2	Acceptance	Introduce the Four Immeasurables	Savouring
3	The Power of Being Present – The Mindful Space	Loving Kindness	Optimism
4	Thoughts are not facts – Challenging Negative Thinking	Compassion	Hope
5	Mindful Change	Empathetic Joy	Gratitude
6	Cultivating patience and kindness – the Four Immeasurables	Equanimity	Forgiveness (Self)
	DAY OF PRACTICE		
7	Relationships, Communication and Insight Dialogue	The Four Immeasurables and Communication	Spirituality Strengths of Wisdom and Knowledge
8	Using what has been learned – Life Enhancement		Happiness activities/ A new toolkit for positivity

Figure 2: Mindfulness Based Life Enhancement

Since I approach MBIs as an educator, I drew on my experience as a University lecturer and adult education tutor. The overall process I chose was Reflective Experiential Action Learning. Alongside conventional lecturing, I have been extensively involved in action learning. On an integrated masters' programme which I led for ten years, action learning has always been a central component. This is explained to participants in the MBLE Home Activity Booklet (Figure 3).

> The course is REAL: Reflective Experiential Action Learning (forgive my weakness for acronyms!) Action Learning has four stages:
>
> - Identifying the problems
> - Identifying the causes of the problems
> - Identifying the solution
> - Putting into practice the solution
>
> In an action learning set:
>
> - We learn from experience and share that experience with others.
> - We are open to the views of colleagues and listen to alternative suggestions.
> - We have time where we are listened to in a non-judgemental atmosphere.
> - We generate more choices about the way forward.
> - We review the outcome of actions with the support of fellow set members and share the lessons learned.
>
> In most action learning sets the action takes place outside the meeting. In this course it takes place also during each session, through formal and informal practices - hence the term Experiential. Reflection is the ability to think and consider "experiences, perceptions, ideas (values and beliefs), etc, with a view to the discovery of new relations of the drawings of conclusions for the guidance of future action" (Quinn 1980). Thus the group will be working as an Action Learning set, reflecting on the experience you have during the sessions and in your home practice between the sessions, and through this drawing new insights into the practice.

Figure 3: Reflective Experiential Action Learning

Support for this way of using Action Learning is to be found in the writings of Revans, founder of action learning. When asked the origin of the ideas that inform it, he replied "they form the logical support to the teachings of the Buddha" (1982, p.534). Since the primary motivation of MBIs is the same as that espoused by the Buddha, this relationship is an important – and inspiring – one (Figure 4).

We may interpret the Four Noble Truths in the light of action learning theory as this has been presented in the modern literature. ...
The first: "This is suffering - this have I declared"; it is the first principle of action learning that men learn only of their own volition, and not at the will of others.
The second truth: "This is the arising of suffering - this have I declared." Our first task, having become aware of our suffering, is to identify its cause. Without diagnosis, without being able to recognise the arising of the problem, we cannot cure it.
The third noble truth set forth by the Buddha: "This is the cessation of suffering - this have I declared", has its counterpart in action learning: the proposed solution to the problem that is the arising of the suffering.
It is, perhaps, the fourth truth enunciated by the Buddha that awakens the greatest interest in the student of action learning: "This is the path leading to the cessation of suffering - this have I declared." It was he who, probably for the first time in the history of mankind, taught that salvation - or at least deliverance from adversity - must be achieved by each individual by his own actions.
Revans 1982,pp.535-538

Figure 4: Action Learning and Buddhism

The stress on the experiential was also very important to me. In his exploration of the Hero's Journey in Chapter Two Vin Harris recalls his initiation into the woodwork craft, his tutor saying that 'you can't get it from a book'. Years ago, I did an intensive 10-day course in Traditional Thai Massage with the Theravada monk Asokananda. The first morning he went through the two-hour process of a full massage, and I took copious notes. In the afternoon we began practicing, and I immediately realised that the notes were useless – the only way to learn and develop the skills was to embody each movement – his book (Asokananda 1990) then provided support. I had the same experience when learning Tai Chi – we had an excellent book (Wu Ying-hua and Ma Yueh-liang 1993), but it served only as an aide memoire – each of the 89 movements needed to be practised repeatedly until it was thoroughly embodied (involving three years of weekly classes). So MBLE was to be strongly experiential, a sharp contrast to my conventional teaching on masters' and doctoral programmes, where I had sometimes earned the title Dr Death-by-PowerPoint!

Much to my surprise, MBLE developed a life of its own. By the time I had run the first course I had a long waiting list, and so course followed course (it has now run more than 60 times). And while the first two courses involved participants from the University, this soon widened. Previous participants asked if their friends and relatives could attend; people at yoga classes I attended at my local gym asked if they could join. News was spreading by word of mouth.

I decided that if I was going to run the course several times, it would be important to monitor and evaluate MBLE, both for my own benefit, to improve the programme, and because I wanted to know whether it actually made a difference to participants. Having been involved in research projects (often action research) throughout my three careers (community activist, local government chief officer and University academic), I decided to approach this in the same spirit, by designing a wider action research project, incorporating evaluation and feedback methods into it. This involves repeated cycles of Action (running the course), Experience (my own and that of participants), Reflection (personal reflection and the views of participants, obtained through discussion and evaluation forms), and Integration and Theorisation (making revisions, and explaining why).

I learnt much from this process, which continues to the present day. A few examples of learning are given in Figure 5.

In Zen we move quickly from one activity - shikantaza - to the next - kinhin - and back. Without thinking, I did the same in the course, until several participants said they found this abruptness unsettling. I changed to slower, smoother transitions between activities.
One participant found the shift from the discussion of the Unpleasant Events diary to walking meditation abrupt. I adopted her suggestion of a short silent meditation following that discussion to allow matters to settle.
As the weeks progressed people were increasingly willing to participate in discussion, and modifications to the timings were made to allow this.
Because my practice has been rooted in Zazen, I have made minimal use of visualisation. Recognising the importance of different learning styles, I included in the Day of Practice the Mountain Meditation, and discovered that for several people this proved extremely powerful. In subsequent courses I therefore added other visualisation meditations (and have taken to using them more frequently myself). One example was a Smiling Meditation which has proved particularly popular, now used twice in the programme.
As expected, feedback showed that different people preferred different meditations - all had their fans, and their detractors. This became a point of emphasis in each subsequent course - that participants should try all the meditations and activities, recognising they will have preferences, but not ignoring those they do not like. I gave as personal examples bodyscan and guided visualisations, neither of which I liked initially.
The major difficulty reported by participants in relation to content was the phrase in the Equanimity meditation "May I be free of preference and prejudice". Coupled with the issue which has appeared in every course - the role of acceptance - this raised for some the concern that the implication was that injustice is acceptable. I addressed this by introducing material from Acceptance and Commitment therapy, explaining the contrast between acceptance and acquiescence
Each session was extended by 15 minutes from the original two hours, allowing more time for discussion and reflection.
The need to emphasise that with all aspects of the course - whether it is mindfulness, compassion, forgiveness or any other quality - the facilitator is not creating these. We all have them within us, and the course provides means to enhance them.

Figure 5: The Learning Process

As I was completing the first course I discovered McCown et al.'s book 'Teaching Mindfulness' (2010), and the earlier article (McCown and Reibel 2009). These proved very helpful to practice, as well as allowing a further conceptualisation of the programme. They identified five participant learning outcomes in MBSR (McCown et al 2010, p.143), and this led me to reflect on learning outcomes for MBLE. These included their five, but expanded 'Growing Compassion' to 'Growing the Four Immeasurables', and I added two further learning outcomes, 'Cultivating Mindful Change' and 'Enhancing the Quality of Life', shown in Figure 6.

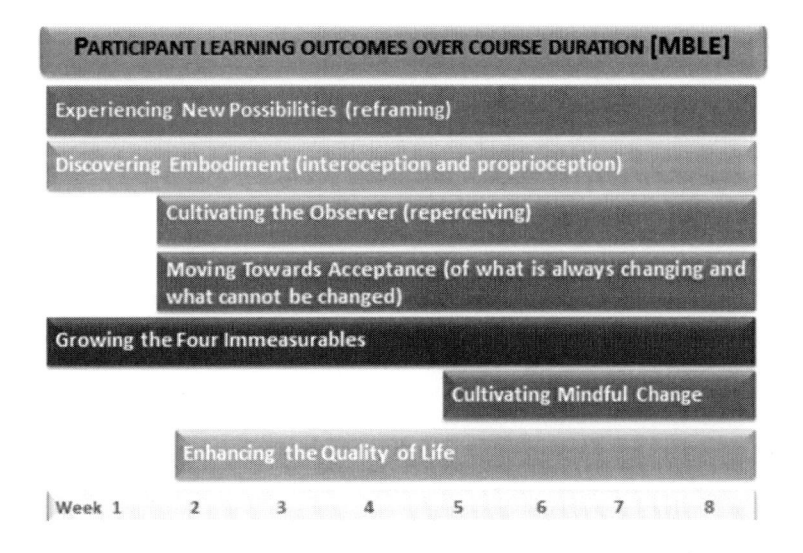

Figure 6: Participant Learning Outcomes Over Course Duration: MBLE

CHAPTER THREE: ENTER THE UNIVERSITY OF ABERDEEN

While running MBLE for the third time I came across the MSc Studies in Mindfulness at the University of Aberdeen. Given my comments in Chapter One, you will not be surprised that it immediately resonated with me. As Graeme Nixon explains in Chapter Three, it is not clinical in approach, it incorporates compassion as a central theme (and this extends in practice to all the Four Immeasurables), and it is concerned with enhancing well-being. The Insight module looked attractive, and the Research elements, including a dissertation, could be addressed by the Action Research I was already undertaking. Given all this, and the opportunity to learn in a beautiful monastic setting, which I had never visited, it was easy to decide to apply.

The programme lived up to expectations. Graeme identifies that each module involves an assignment twinning reflection on personal practice with exploration of the relevant theme in a professional context. At the time I was still doing a fair amount of lecturing at Sheffield Business School, so this worked nicely. I explored mindfulness in relation to management strategy, compassion in relation to organisational culture, and insight in relation to the theory and practice of organisational change.

The module on professional enquiry provided me with the opportunity to address a question that had become of great interest to me. I have mentioned that the Four Immeasurables are a central feature of MBLE, and I took inspiration here from several Buddhist authors, including Buddhaghosa (1956), Wallace (2004), McLeod (2001), and Nyanaponika Thera (1994). But it was important that MBLE be accessible to people from all faiths and none, and that it recognise the many ways in which these qualities have resonated over centuries. For example, Hendricks points out that "Occurring some 240 times in the Hebrew Bible, 'hesed' is one of the most important principles in Old Testament ethics. It has three basic meanings: love, strength, and steadfastness." Hesed translates as Loving Kindness, referenced in Hendricks (2006,p.111) In the Bahá'í Faith the Persian word mahabbat is translated as Loving Kindness. And the Golden Rule, which "requires kindness and care for the less fortunate" (British Humanist Association), is to be found in all faiths, and in those uncommitted to a faith.

So I used the professional enquiry assignment to explore this, by interviewing eight people drawn from different faiths or none. And while I have been researching for more than 40 years, I chose a method for this which I had never previously used, hermeneutic inquiry (Kvale and Brinkmann 2009), which involves seeking to listen to people's words within their own perspective, rather than immediately reframing them within my own. A big challenge, but it turned out be a rich learning experience for me. None of the respondents had difficulty in relating to the Four Immeasurables, though several thought one or more – particularly Empathetic Joy – were underplayed in their spiritual tradition. And all were comfortable with the approach in MBLE (six had done the course, and I explained it to the other two). There were also important lessons for the running of MBLE, some of which are given in Figure 7.

WEEK	MODIFICATION
1	Be more explicit about Buddhist background. Extend discussion of Negativity Bias to cover assumptions and beliefs.
2	Increase emphasis on self and other in relation to the Four Immeasurables and themes from Positive Psychology.
3	Extend discussion of Compassion, using Near and Far Enemies (in particular contrast with pity).
4	Expand definition of Empathetic Joy, incorporating synonyms and emphasising self and other.
5	Expand definition of Equanimity, incorporating synonyms and emphasising self and other.
6	Incorporate a practice (meditation) on self-forgiveness.
7	Incorporate a practice (reflection) on purpose and relationship to wider personal belief system and existing practices.
8	To help people continue the practice, develop a series of short (5 and 10 minutes) guided meditations.

Figure 7: Implications of Hermeneutic Inquiry for MBLE Course

My involvement in the MSc Studies in Mindfulness also provided me with a context within which to explore the teaching method I was using, Action Learning. I had incorporated in feedback questionnaires: How did you find your experience of learning about mindfulness in a group? What were the advantages and disadvantages? Some responses are given in Figure 8.

- It's useful to be part of a supportive group.
- I thought the group dynamic was good and conducive to learning about mindfulness
- I enjoyed the group and exchanging experiences with others
- It was interesting to get different views, and appreciate that we were all there for different reasons – but we were all there.
- Useful insights provided by group members and mutual support
- I like the group vibe, and group encouragement. It was good to hear that others were having similar experiences.
- Extremely helpful and supportive
- The group were all lovely and as the weeks went on, I felt more relaxed in their company
- Ideal, the perfect way for me to learn
- I am someone who can find this type of group difficult, but because of the relaxed way in which you ran the group I liked learning in this way.
- There is a sharing, a sense of everyone coming together with a common purpose (even if there are variations on that).

Figure 8: Participants' Experience of Action Learning

Some found difficulties. Once more we see the importance of addressing different learning styles, as there are those who prefer not to work this way (though there was no pressure to contribute). Several commented on the progressive opening of discussion over the weeks of the course. Overall, it was reasonable to conclude that the action learning approach adopted is fit for purpose and is an appropriate approach to take in non-clinical settings.

So, my encounter with the University of Aberdeen has proved very positive – although I should declare an interest, in that once I had completed the MSc I was invited to become a Teaching Fellow on the programme, exploring in particular the nature of mindful research in the Professional Enquiry module. And as a final bonus, David McMurtry, then Programme Director, persuaded me to publish a book on MBLE (Darwin 2015).

CHAPTER FOUR: A FAMILY IS BORN – THE CONTINUATION GROUP

During the final session of MBLE participants are invited to share their overall experience of the course. It soon became apparent to me that experiences were very varied – a further reminder of the need to address all learning styles, and not just my own preference for a theoretical approach. But although addressed in many different ways, participants picked up on the key themes of the course. They identified concerns, causal links, and practical solutions. And there was a shift from the negative to the positive, which can be summarised by returning to the link between Action Learning and the Four Noble Truths identified by Revans (Figure 4).

- The problem: our everyday state of life: anxiety, stress, negative thinking, busyness, lack of time, overcommitment, anxiety.
- The cause: the second dart, negative emotions, external factors, background, history and upbringing, mindlessness, habit, harmful emotions.
- The remedy: acceptance, compassion, mindful space, gratitude, forgiveness, cultivating mindfulness and beneficial emotions.
- The way to achieve this: Mindfulness Based Life Enhancement, with savouring and mindful movement particularly mentioned.

> **Pause and Practice**
>
> Take A Savouring Vacation! (Details at http://mindfulenhance.org/discussion-papers/)

In addition, while participants embraced the various elements of MBLE, they conceptualised it in a way I had not originally envisaged – but which made great sense. I summarised this in eight factors, which quickly became the pictogram of the course (Figure 9). At the heart of the programme, and featuring in every session, are Formal and Informal Mindfulness, together with Mindful Movement, drawn from Hatha Yoga and Qigong, and Somatic Awareness, experienced both through movement and through practices such as the Bodyscan. The other six factors embrace the Four Immeasurables, the elements of positive psychology introduced in the course, and mindful learning.

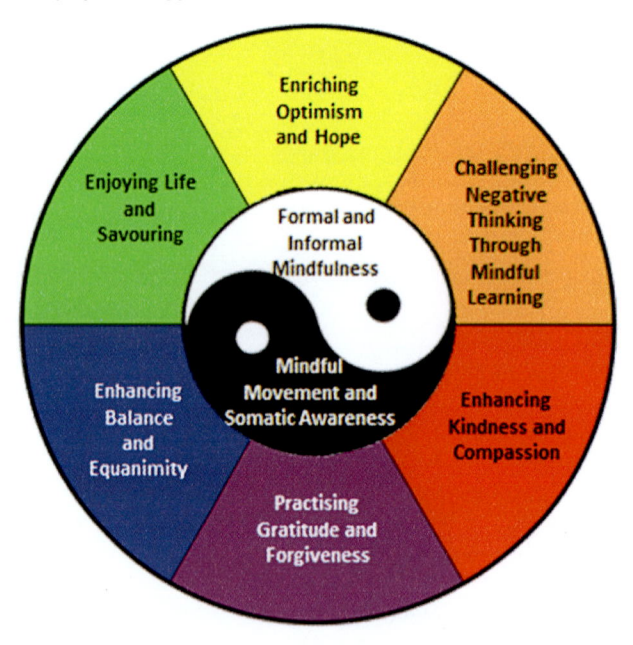

Figure 9: The MBLE Template

There was another important issue raised in the final week of the course – how do we continue our practice? While there are meditation groups in Sheffield, to which we point people, there was a strong desire not to lose the momentum of the MBLE course. And so was born the Continuation Group – a monthly open session to which all course 'alumni' were invited. As I write, this is well into its seventh year. Each session has a theme (examples are given in Figure 10), and each draws up to 30 people (and sometimes more).

Themes at the Continuation Group		
Loving kindness	Cultivating emotional balance	Savouring and Awe
Compassion	The Five Hindrances	Insight and Wisdom
Developing Self-compassion	Śamatha-Vipassanā Meditation	Forgiveness
Equanimity	Mindful Eating and Dieting	Mindful Ageing
Equanimity	The Science behind Mindfulness	Acceptance
Mindfulness and Music	Addressing Life's Transitions	Mindfulness and Art

Figure 10: Themes identified at the Continuation Group

In addition, at least twice year we have a mindful walk, sometimes taking advantage of the beauty of the Peak District National Park on our doorstep. So now we had more than a course – we had a growing community, and this was to lead to a series of important developments, summarised in Figure 11. This shows the way in which new activities have unfolded, a number of which are described in the next four Chapters.

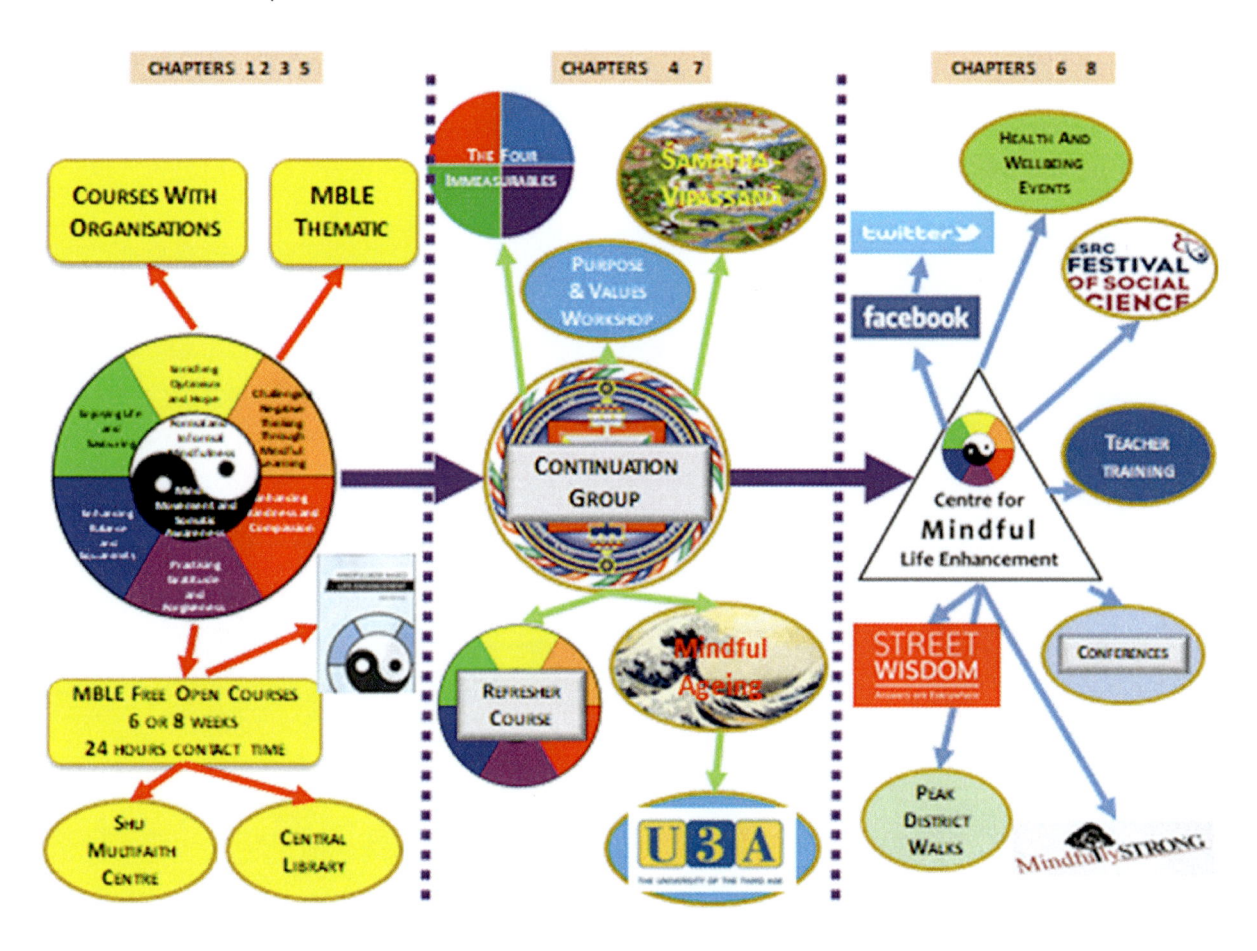

Figure 11: The Developing Mindfulness Community

CHAPTER FIVE: EXPANDING AND COLLABORATING

The next step was organisational work. Like so much of this story, it wasn't planned. A participant on one of the early courses worked for a Centre helping women who had experienced domestic violence. She asked if I would be willing to run a course specifically for the Centre's team of counsellors, both to benefit them directly and to provide them with new ideas for their counselling work. This has been followed by courses with other organisations.

And here 'I' becomes 'we' – several people who had taken the MBLE course, and had become regular participants in the Continuation Group, said that they would like to help – part of their Hero's Journey. Another unexpected development – I was being asked to teach teachers. I knew of formal mindfulness teacher training structures, but I decided on a slightly different approach, adopting an apprenticeship model, which would incorporate direct experience with formal training. This begins with participant observation – sitting in on courses and observing the teaching process, as well as having the opportunity to deepen practice through repeating the course. Then beginning to lead one or two practices, and at each iteration expanding the role until it involves also leading discussions on theme, guiding inquiry, and ultimately co-facilitating. This proved to take a minimum of two years, but to date three people have gone through the whole process, while the teaching team now numbers sixteen. With the help of one our team, Liz Biggin, we have also been able to run courses in the City Council's Central Library, which has proved more accessible for some participants.

A basic principle with the team, challenging the conventional business model, is that none of us receive remuneration. All the general courses are free, as are courses we run for charities. We charge other organisations (local authorities, police, businesses) and use this money for running costs. This has made it possible to run free courses, for example, for community groups and the local hospice.

CHAPTER SIX: THE CENTRE IS BORN

By now it was clear that MBLE was here to stay – knowledge of the course was spreading, and an increasing number of people were contacting me to say the course had been recommended by a friend or relative. This meant demand was growing, but it was still within a restricted catchment group. And an additional issue was the growing workload of organising and preparing for courses, including the need to prepare guided meditation CDs for each participant. A way of tackling these issues emerged during a journey to Samye Ling monastery with Mike Pupius, one of the first people to become involved in the teaching. By this time I was teaching on the MSc, and Mike was a student on it. We hit on the idea of creating a website which could make MBLE better known, and could at the same time be a location for the guided meditations, which participants could then download. But what to call the website? How about a Centre? And thus was born the Centre for Mindful Life Enhancement. I still get people asking me where the Centre is based and I point to the sky.

Simple in concept, the creation of a website, as well as the establishment of the Centre, have proved beneficial in many ways. The website (www.mindfulenhance.org) now contains far more than meditations, including discussion papers, weblinks, news and articles. The Centre itself has become a convenient way to reach a much wider audience and to promote activities – and this has proved important as we have extended beyond MBLE to include new courses which explore mindfulness in specific contexts.

CHAPTER SEVEN: MINDFUL AGEING

The first of these was mindful ageing. Unsurprisingly, in my seventieth year, I have a strong interest in this! How can mindfulness help address the process of ageing? There is a tendency, even in mindfulness circles, to see ageing as a 'tragedy', with all the negative connotations associated with the common stereotypes of ageing, which are sadly transferred into self-stereotyping in many people as they age, as discussed by, for example, De Hennezel (2011), Kite et al (1991), Cuddy et al (2005) and Darwin et al (1979). As Kotter-Grühn argues:

> At the societal level, negative views of aging manifest themselves in the form of age stereotypes, which result in prejudice and discrimination toward older adults. At the personal level, negative views of one's own ageing are related, among others, to poor health, lower well-being, and even shorter survival times. (2015, p.167)

I followed my initial research on this by developing with Mike Pupius a course on Mindful Ageing, specifically for people who had already done MBLE. In this course we addressed the way language distorts the image (and self-image) of elderly people and explored ways in which mindfulness practices can address this. This is part of a much wider exploration of ways in which mindful ageing can:

- Heighten and maintain mental and physical wellbeing
- Enhance life through mindfulness
- Realign toward the positive – challenging stereotypes
- Open to new possibilities and beginnings

This is a very different perspective to ageing from one which sees it as a tragedy – it is ageing as jubilation. Mindfulness practice has much to offer people as they age, and there is a need to ensure that this is adequately addressed. Conventional courses can prove very helpful, but there are also specific themes, in addition to language and stereotyping, which merit special attention; for example, the importance of attention itself, the relationship of mindful movement to the ageing process, playfulness and creativity, savouring and awe, reminiscence and reframing, and a mindful perspective on the past and future.

This relates also to wider concerns about the dominance of the market place, and its implications for the elderly. The Swedish gerontologist Tornstam (2005) argues "White, Western, middle-class, middle-life society has, since the reformation, been characterised by an overwhelmingly strong performance orientation. Productivity, effectiveness, and independence are prestige words". As a result, "we come to look down upon and hold in contempt those who are unproductive, ineffective, and dependent. We feel sorry for 'the poor, feeble, sick and lonely old people'. Moreover, our pity for old people forces us to "construct" them in such a way that the correctness of our pity is validated. We produce a negatively biased image of old people at the same time as we think their conditions ought to be improved".

These issues will be compounded in several ways by the twin developments of an ageing population and technological change. If all activity outside the monetised system is seen as unproductive, then this implies that an increasing proportion of the population will be categorised as unproductive, and, should some current predictions about the impact on the job market of technological change prove correct, elderly people will be joined in this by many younger people.

The fallacy of the argument that older people are unproductive is demonstrated in the report of the International Longevity Centre (2013) who say that "the vast majority of care (for older people) is provided by family, friends and relatives, and the care they provide is worth an estimated £119 billion per year – considerably more than total spending on the NHS". Much of this will be by older people. In addition, "the value of older people's volunteering contribution was estimated at £10.59 billion in 2010 and is expected to grow to £15.53 billion by 2030. The annual value of childcare provided by grandparents in the UK was estimated to be worth £2.73 billion in 2010 and this figure could rise to £4.47 billion per annum by 2030" (ibid). But of course a paradigm in which activity only has value if it is monetised leads inevitably to these contributions to wellbeing being discounted.

Recently we have taken this work on Mindful Ageing further, by developing programmes which we are running within the University of the Third Age. These comprise a shorter version of MBLE, lasting four weeks, with a specific orientation toward Mindful Ageing. Discussions had shown that there was strong interest, but people found it difficult to commit to eight consecutive weeks, perhaps due to health issues, or grandchild caring responsibilities. So we devised a four week course which introduces the core of MBLE, to which all participants commit, followed by a series of sessions which introduce the rest of MBLE, and which they attend when they can. Demand is proving strong.

Pause and Practice

The Celebration Tree of Life – available at
http://mindfulenhance.org/mindful-ageing/mindful-ageing-course/

CHAPTER EIGHT: NEW HORIZONS

I mentioned in Chapter Five our expansion into organisational courses, and one example has been the Facilities Directorate in Sheffield Hallam University, where we have run two, one for the senior management and one for middle management. We have been fortunate in having the Head of that Directorate, Mark Swales, as a strong supporter and advocate for our work within the University. One result of this was sponsorship for a conference we organised in 2016, the success of which led to a second in the following year. Annual conferences took a toll on our voluntary team, and we will therefore do this every other year, beginning in 2019.

As the number of people 'graduating' from our courses has increased, so has our variety of activities. We established a Facebook group – Sheffield Mindfulness Community – which at the time of writing has over 300 members. And we have also run several one-day workshops on specific themes, such as the Four Immeasurables, Values and Vision, and Self-compassion.

One of the great strengths of the team we have in the Centre is that everyone comes with their unique experience and expertise, and this has led to a series of initiatives building on this resource. The first is mine – after reading the teachings of Culadasa on Śamatha-Vipassanā Meditation: The Practice of Tranquillity and Insight, brought together in his book The Mind Illuminated (2015), I became a Teacher-in-Training with Dharma Treasure. Certain elements of this teaching have been brought into MBLE, while development courses are then offered to people who have completed the course.

The second initiative comes from Mike Pupius, whose other activities include being a volunteer park ranger in the Peak District National Park, therefore having a strong interest in mindful walking. This led him to becoming a 'Street Wizard' with the organisation Street Wisdom and we have run a number of mindful walks in the city centre and in the surrounding countryside. Mike has also found a willing audience among other park rangers, and we have been training them to run mindful walks in the Peak District.

The third initiative comes from another member of the team, Dave Hembrough, Sport Science Officer in Sheffield Hallam University and Lead Strength and Conditioning Coach. Together we have developed MindfullySTRONG, which brings mindfulness and physical training together in a programme to help people improve both physical and mental health in a friendly and social environment. This is intended to provide a nurturing and gentle guided introduction to mindfulness and physical training, designed so that it addresses the needs of those who have not trained in a gym environment before or those who are new to meditation, as well as people who work out or meditate regularly.

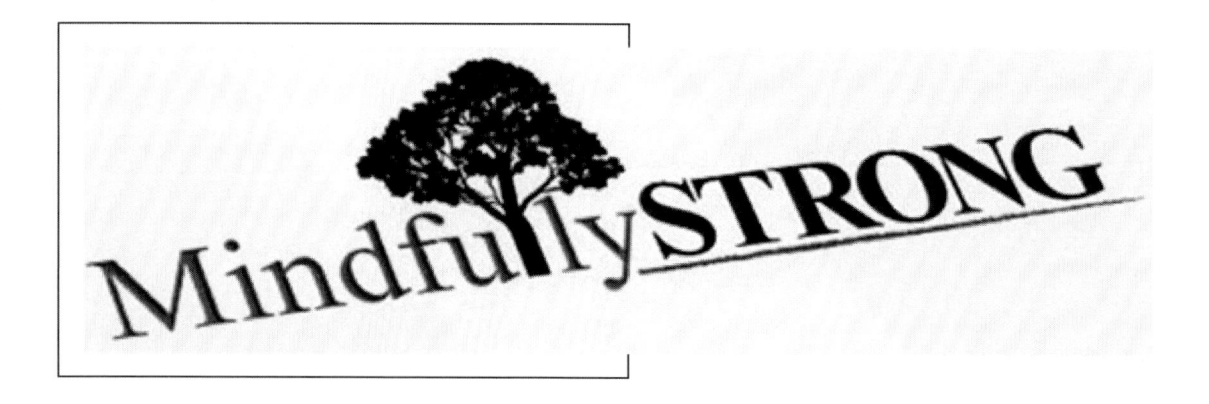

Figure 12: MindfullySTRONG logo

Each MindfullySTRONG session is split in to 3 sessions:

- Finding Focus - An initial group conversation about a mindfulness model or theory plus some mindful movement to warm up.
- Feeling Physical - A structured work out including both strength and aerobic activity, and completed mindfully to a classical music sound track.
- Finishing Flourish - A guided meditation linked to the session theme and initial discussion.

Participants on the first courses have summarised their experience:

I really found it valuable and not like any other fitness programme. At the gym, no one is going to guide you in a mindful way or take you through a meditation afterwards. To be led by someone with such expertise was fantastic too.

The combination of mindfulness and exercise worked really well. Better than I expected and I found the benefits of the both really worked for me.

A great programme delivered by experts in a novel way that's perfect for people like me who haven't been to a gym before.

Pause and Move

Try the Eight Pieces of Brocade (there are several YouTube videos showing this splendid Qigong sequence: see for example https://www.youtube.com/watch?v=DhsU1qLBF8s)

The fourth initiative, by Sue Marriott, is exploring the role of mindfulness in addressing life's transitions, which relates to our wider interest in purpose and values, both personal and organisational.

EPILOGUE

So, there you have it – an emerging community of practice. At an early stage we set one of our goals as being to make Sheffield a Mindful City. Already no less than 0.1% of the city's population have taken the course, although this does mean that we have some way to go yet! But of course, positive emotions, like negative, can be infectious, so the effect extends beyond mere numbers. For example, we ask every participant to begin committing Random Acts of Kindness every day. And we know from many comments by participants that the course's benefits have extended to their families and friends. In seven years we have come a long way – who know what else will be featured in our wild and precious life?

Pause for Reflection

What do you want to do with your one wild and precious life?

FURTHER RESOURCES

Our website, www.mindfulenhance.org, includes many additional resources. There are guided meditations which can be freely downloaded, short videos on mindfulness, and discussion papers.
The Discussion Papers, at http://mindfulenhance.org/discussion-papers/ , look at mindfulness in relation to wellbeing, emotional intelligence, creativity and innovation. There is also a detailed paper on Mindful Ageing.
For more on Samatha-Vipassanā Meditation: The Practice of Tranquillity and Insight see https://dharmatreasure.org/. This includes talks and guided meditations by Culadasa.
Ken McLeod's website, http://unfetteredmind.org/, includes valuable insights into the Four Immeasurables.
For more on Street Wisdom, visit https://www.streetwisdom.org/
A good source about ageing mindfully is Lewis Richmond's site, http://www.lewisrichmond.com/

REFERENCES

ASOKANANDA (1990) The Art of Traditional Thai Massage. Bangkok: Duang Kamol
BUDDHAGHOSA (1956) Visuddhimagga: The Path of Purification. Translated by Bhikkhu Nanamoli Singapore: Buddhist Meditation Centre
CUDDY, A., NORTON, M. & FISKE, S. (2005) This Old Stereotype: The Pervasiveness and Persistence of the Elderly Stereotype Journal of Social Issues, Vol. 61, No. 2, pp. 267--285
CULADASA, IMMERGUT, M. with GRAVES, J. (2015) The Mind Illuminated. Pearce: Dharma Treasure Press
DARWIN, J. et al (1979) Against Ageism. Newcastle-upon-Tyne: Search Project (available at http://mindfulenhance.org/mindful-ageing/john/)
DARWIN, J. (2014) Mindfulness Based Life Enhancement. Aberdeen: Inspired by Learning
De HENNEZEL, M. (2011) The Warmth of the Heart Prevents your Body from Rusting. London: Rodale
HENDRICKS, O.B. (2006) The Politics of Jesus. New York: Doubleday
INTERNATIONAL LONGEVITY CENTRE (2013) Ageing, longevity and demographic change. Available at http://www.ilcuk.org.uk/index.php/publications/publication_details/ageing_longevity_and_demographic_change_a_factpack_of_statistics_from_the_i
KABAT-ZINN, J. (1990), Full Catastrophe Living: Using the Wisdom of Your Body and Mind to Face Stress, Pain and Illness. New York: Piatkus
KITE, M., DEAUX, K. & MILE, M. (1991) Stereotypes of Young and Old: Does Age Outweigh Gender? Psychology and Aging Vol 6 No 1, 19-27
KOTTER-GRÜHN, D. (2015) Changing Negative Views of Aging Annual Review of Gerontology and Geriatrics Springer Publishing Company
KVALE, S. and BRINKMANN, S. (2009) InterViews: Learning the Craft of Qualitative Research Interviewing. London:Sage
LANGER, E. (1997) Mindfulness: The Power of mindful learning. Reading, MA: Perseus Books.
LANGER, E. (2009) Counterclockwise London: Hodder and Stoughton
MACASKILL. A (2002). Heal the hurt: How to forgive and move on. London: Sheldon Press.
MCCOWN, D. and REIBEL, D (2009) Mindfulness and Mindfulness-Based Stress Reduction Integrative Psychiatry, Weil Integrative Medicine Library, Edited by B. Beitman and D. Monti, Oxford: Oxford University Press
MCCOWN, D., REIBEL, D. and MICOZZI, M. (2010) Teaching Mindfulness. New York: Springer
MCLEOD, K. (2001) Wake Up To Your Life. New York: HarperCollins
NYANAPONIKA THERA (1994) The Four Sublime States. Buddha Dharma Education Association downloaded from http://www.accesstoinsight.org/lib/authors/nyanaponika/wheel006.html (Accessed 16 April 2018)
NYANAPONIKA THERA (2005) http://www.accesstoinsight.org/lib/authors/various/wheel170.html accessed 16 April 2018
OXFORD LIVING DICTIONARY https://en.oxforddictionaries.com/definition/compassion
REVANS, R. (1982) The Immemorial Precursor: Action Learning Past and Present in The Origins and Growth of Action Learning pp 529-545 Lund: Studentlitteratur
TORNSTAM, L. (2005) Gerotranscendence: a developmental theory of positive aging. New York: Springer Publishing Company
WALLACE, B.A. (2004) The Four Immeasurables. Ithaca: Snow Lion
WALLACE, B.A. (2008) A Mindful Balance. Tricycle Spring 2008, available at http://www.tricycle.com/a-mindful-balance?page=0,1
WU YING-HUA & MA YUEH-LIANG (1993) Wu Style. Taichichuan. Hong Kong: Shanghai Book Co.

CHAPTER 24

TURNING EMPATHIC DISTRESS INTO COMPASSION - A HERO'S JOURNEY FOR FAMILY CARERS

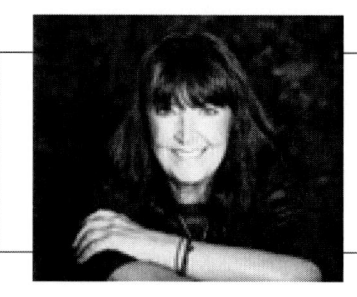

Jacqueline Seery

Jacky.seery@gmail.com

INTRODUCTION

We have learnt from other rich contributions to this book that the mind can be trained to respond more positively to stressful life events by using mindfulness techniques. After conducting a small research study into the impact of mindfulness training on the well-being of unpaid family carers, I am now convinced that showing carers how to adopt an attitude of kindness and compassion towards themselves and others plays a key role in alleviating the stress of individuals who find themselves in long-term caring roles.

This chapter not only presents the findings of my research study. It also covers my own journey over many years as I travelled from the painful depths of being an unsupported and unmindful full-time mother and carer, through learning mindfulness and self-compassion, to finding myself flourishing even when facing pretty stressful life events.

The greatest - and totally unexpected - gift I received on this exceptionally rewarding journey came about when I began to share the juicy, sweet fruits of my training in mindfulness and compassion with a small group of highly stressed family carers. The very act of opening my heart to these unsung caring heroines and then extending heartfelt compassion to them contributed so much to my own long-term healing and overall sense of wellbeing and fulfilment in life.

MY HERO'S JOURNEY

Vin Harris describes the 'departure', 'descent', 'initiation' and 'return' phases of the hero's journey in Chapter two of this book. The 'departure' indicates the moment in life when a crisis launches the hero into a journey of new realisation. The 'descent' is the next stage of the journey where the hero uncovers teachers and new skills to help him with the challenges that he will face on his journey of self-discovery and change. The 'initiation' represents the ultimate challenges to be faced and overcome on the journey, culminating in the 'return' where the hero arrives safely back having conquered his dragons and demons. He is now ready to share his story and knowledge to help others. This is my hero's journey.

Having babies didn't come easily for me. 35 years ago, it took four miscarriages before my plight was taken seriously by my doctor who put me forward for a trial treatment for recurrent miscarriage at St Marys Hospital in London. This controlled clinical trial involved identifying the presence of an antibody created during early pregnancy which immunises the mother against rejecting the foreign body of an embryo in her body. Despite my four pregnancies I had never created this antibody. The active treatment on this trial took the form of an injection of the prospective father's white blood cells. If you were in the control group however, you received just your own cells.

When I received the treatment, my arm swelled up as though someone had planted large eggs beneath my skin and so I was convinced I had received my partner's blood cells. Following the treatment, my next pregnancy was successful, and I carried the baby full term.

Following the birth, I was shocked to learn that I was in the control group. I was convinced that my strong belief that I had received the active treatment had enabled my body to create the necessary antibody. I also believed that the compassion, kindness and support I received from those running this trial in an exceptionally caring manner contributed to the positive outlook I adopted. Since then, I have firmly believed in the power of the mind, positive thought and the power of compassionate care. Looking back on my own path through life, I can now see that it was at this point that my 'departure' on my own hero's journey began. My first baby was extremely ill from birth, and so I cared for her intensely and with great stress until her death at 4 months. Years later, I became a full-time unpaid carer once again as I looked after my youngest daughter day in and day out after she developed severe anorexia as a teenager. At both these highly stressful times in my life, I didn't realise that my intense caring role went way beyond the normal demands and experience of being a mother. At neither time did I ever think of myself as a family carer in desperate need of some effective support.

Some years later a yearning for some kind of relief from my own troubled thoughts and feelings led me to train in Taoist meditation, Qigong, Tai Chi and Yoga. This is where the 'descent' into my hero's journey began. It took years for me to even understand 'letting go' and 'going with the flow of life'. But after several years of steady progress, I deepened my practice by training to teach mindfulness and compassion while completing the MSc Studies in Mindfulness with the University of Aberdeen. It was only when I began studies in mindfulness that I truly began the 'initiation' as all the pieces of the jigsaw were before me ready to be pieced together into a whole picture. Learning and practicing compassion practices in the first year of the MSc completely changed how I responded to life. I finally realised that it was time to become my own best friend so that I could keep soothing my troubled self with self-compassion and unconditional respect. This is such an important key to wellbeing as highlighted by Gilbert (2009) who states that most human beings spend too long in a destructive threat and drive system caused by the very nature of our reptilian brains.

2016 saw the spark of my 'return' ignite when I was inspired to bring mindfulness, compassion and mindful movement training to family carers. With the support of Carers in Hertfordshire, the setting up of this final research project for the MSc flowed effortlessly as I experienced the amazing phenomenon of 'wu wei'. In the Tao Te Ching, Lao Tzu (Zi, 1939) explains that 'wu wei' is a mental state in which our actions are quite effortlessly in alignment with the flow of life.

Everything had come full circle. My initial Taoist practices with meditation, Qigong and Tai Chi were now fully aligned with my mindfulness and self-compassion training. At last, I was able to pass on the fruits of my own training and practice to others with the core intention of empowering them as I had been empowered.

> **Pause and Reflect**
>
> Are there any profound moments in your life which come into your mind which you feel changed you? Are you able to see the path your life took since those times? Sit quietly and reflect on the journey. Notice how it feels.

CARING COSTS

> Mindfulness and compassion develop at the same pace. The more mindful you become, the easier you'll find it to be compassionate. And the more you open your heart to others, the more mindful you become in all your activities (Mingyur Rinpoche 2009, Location 3465)

At some point in most individuals' lives, there is a good chance that a close relative, such as spouse, child or parent, will suffer from some kind of long-term illness or disability. This not only turns life completely upside down for the family, but changes the relationship dynamic, as one member of the family takes on the role of unpaid carer – a role that over time often becomes all consuming.

At first, family carers don't usually define themselves as a 'carer'. As a mother, a woman often sees the care of their sick or disabled child as just an integral part of their parenting role. Similarly, when a spouse needs extra care due to a disabling disease or injury, a caring partner may see all their extra caring duties as just part of the normal role of a spouse who has vowed to care for the other 'in sickness and in health'.

It was only when I conducted my own research into the plight of family carers for the MSc Studies in Mindfulness that I realised that much earlier in my own life I had become a 'family carer' for two of my own daughters. At the time, I certainly did not identify myself as a caring heroine, but I do remember hoping that I could use these difficult experiences to help others someday. Miraculously, my training in mindfulness has finally provided me with that golden opportunity as part of my own hero's' journey.

As the caring demands on an inadvertent family carer increase over time, they tend to become subject to great stresses and strains that then have a seriously negative impact on their own emotional, mental and physical wellbeing. From my own experiences as a family carer and from supporting several groups of family carers with Mindfulness Courses, I now know that the impact of caring for a sick relative can be a complex cocktail of devastating emotions which can then have a devastating impact on carers' long-term health and wellbeing.

According to Carers UK (2015) 1 in 8 adults in the UK (around 6.5 million people) are carers. Furthermore:

- There are approximately 700,000 young carers aged 16-24. On average, young carers miss 48 days of school a year as a result of their caring role. It is also reported that they experience bullying at school and diminished health (Tubb, 2018).
- By 2037, it's anticipated that the number of carers will increase to 9 million.
- Carers save the economy £132 billion per year.
- People providing high levels of care are twice as likely to be permanently sick or disabled.
- 625,000 people suffer mental and physical ill health as a direct consequence of the stress and physical demands of caring.

In a study conducted by Carers UK (2012 p.6), carers reflected on their increased levels of stress, hopelessness and fatigue. One carer stated that they "did not realise how much stress caring puts on the carer and the effect it can have on your own health". 84% of respondents in this study reported increased physical and mental health problems due to their caring role. 91% reported increases in anxiety and stress and 53% reported that they were suffering from depression.

The detrimental effects of being immersed in a professional caring role have long been researched in some depth. The concept of compassion fatigue for example emerged in the 1980s when states of heightened stress, exhaustion and physical conditions were observed amongst nursing staff in a hospital emergency department (Joinson,1992). Compassion fatigue has been defined as a "deep physical emotional and spiritual exhaustion accompanied by acute emotional pain". (Pfifferling and Gilley, 2000, p.39). This can occur as a result of caring for others who are suffering, and/or through the absence of self-care and the lack of emotional support for the carer (Figley, 1995).

Lynch and Lobo (2012, p.2125) conducted one of the few existing studies into the instance of compassion fatigue amongst family carers and concluded that,

> Compassion fatigue occurs when a caregiving relationship founded on empathy potentially results in a deep psychological response to stress that progresses to physical, psychological, spiritual and social exhaustion in the family caregiver

Further distressing consequences of caring for a sick relative include isolation, becoming lost and engulfed in the caring role and feelings of grief or guilt (Wada and Park, 2009). Grief can manifest from losing a loved one to the illness or from the carer's life not unfolding as they hoped or expected. Family carers can also feel guilty every time they do something for themselves, which can prevent them finding time for self-care (Gilbert, 2009).

When family carers are continually faced with the suffering and sometimes negative moods of their sick or disabled relative, the feelings of empathy the carers experience may lead to burnout, even amongst the most devoted caregivers. Symptoms of burnout include having no energy, having disturbed sleep, depression, irritability and a decrease in quality of life (Marriott, 2003). Compassion fatigue appears to be common amongst long-term family carers. But why should a positive emotion such as compassion have such a negative effect on carers in the long run? Klimecki and Singer (2012 p.369) have proposed that,

> rather than compassion fatigue it is empathic distress that underlies the negative consequences faced by caregivers who are exposed to others' suffering

Therefore, it has been suggested that the condition of compassion fatigue should be renamed 'empathic distress fatigue' (Ricard, 2009).

Neuroscientist Tania Singer and team set up an extensive study to identify how individuals' responses to empathising with others' suffering can play a significant part in damaging their own sense of personal wellbeing. For example, 'suffering with' another can cause caring individuals to feel the other person's pain as though it were their own pain. This in turn can then lead to caring individuals suffering more stress and poorer health. Singer argued that if carers simply accept that it is the other person that is in pain not them, and if carers then cultivate feelings of compassion for the person suffering, carers can end up feeling more positive and in better overall health than if they continue to go on suffering with the person in pain or distress. See Figure 1 below.

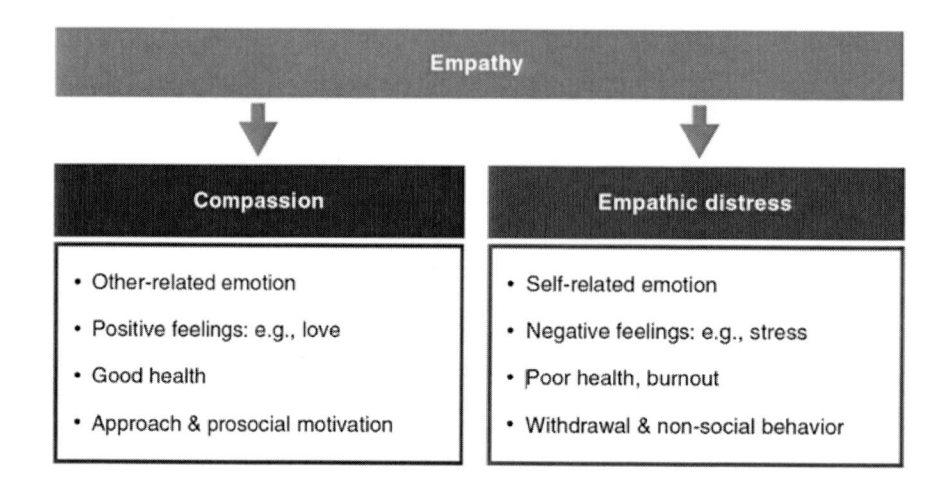

Empathy

Compassion	Empathic distress
• Other-related emotion	• Self-related emotion
• Positive feelings: e.g., love	• Negative feelings: e.g., stress
• Good health	• Poor health, burnout
• Approach & prosocial motivation	• Withdrawal & non-social behavior

Figure 1: - Compassion (Singer and Klimecki, 2014, p.875)

This concept is supported by Perry, Dalton et al., (2010, p.3) who encourage a self-care strategy for family carers by emotionally "distancing themselves from their relatives' suffering". This inspired my study in which I encouraged participants to shift from 'suffering with' their sick or disabled relative, to aiming to attain a state of compassion in which they had sympathy for, and a desire to help, their loved one, without moving into empathic distress. The results of my study indicated that this shift had occurred.

THE ALCHEMY OF MINDFULNESS, COMPASSION AND QIGONG

The benefits of mindfulness-based interventions, compassion and Qigong are well reported and include symptomatic relief to stress and depression as illustrated in Figure 2 below.

Mindfulness
- Reduces stress (Kabat-Zinn, 2013)
- Reduces depression (Segal, Williams and Teasdale, 2013)
- Increases body awareness (Kok & Singer, 2016)
- Decreases thought content (Kok & Singer, 2016)

Compassion
- Increases feelings of warmth and positive thoughts about others (Kok & Singer, 2016)
- Activates neural networks of love and positive emotions (Kok & Singer, 2016)
- Reduces negative ruminative thoughts (Kok & Singer, 2016)
- Increases sense of purpose in life (Fredrickson, Cohn et al., 2008)
- Increases the ability to cope with unpleasant emotions (Gilbert and Irons, 2010

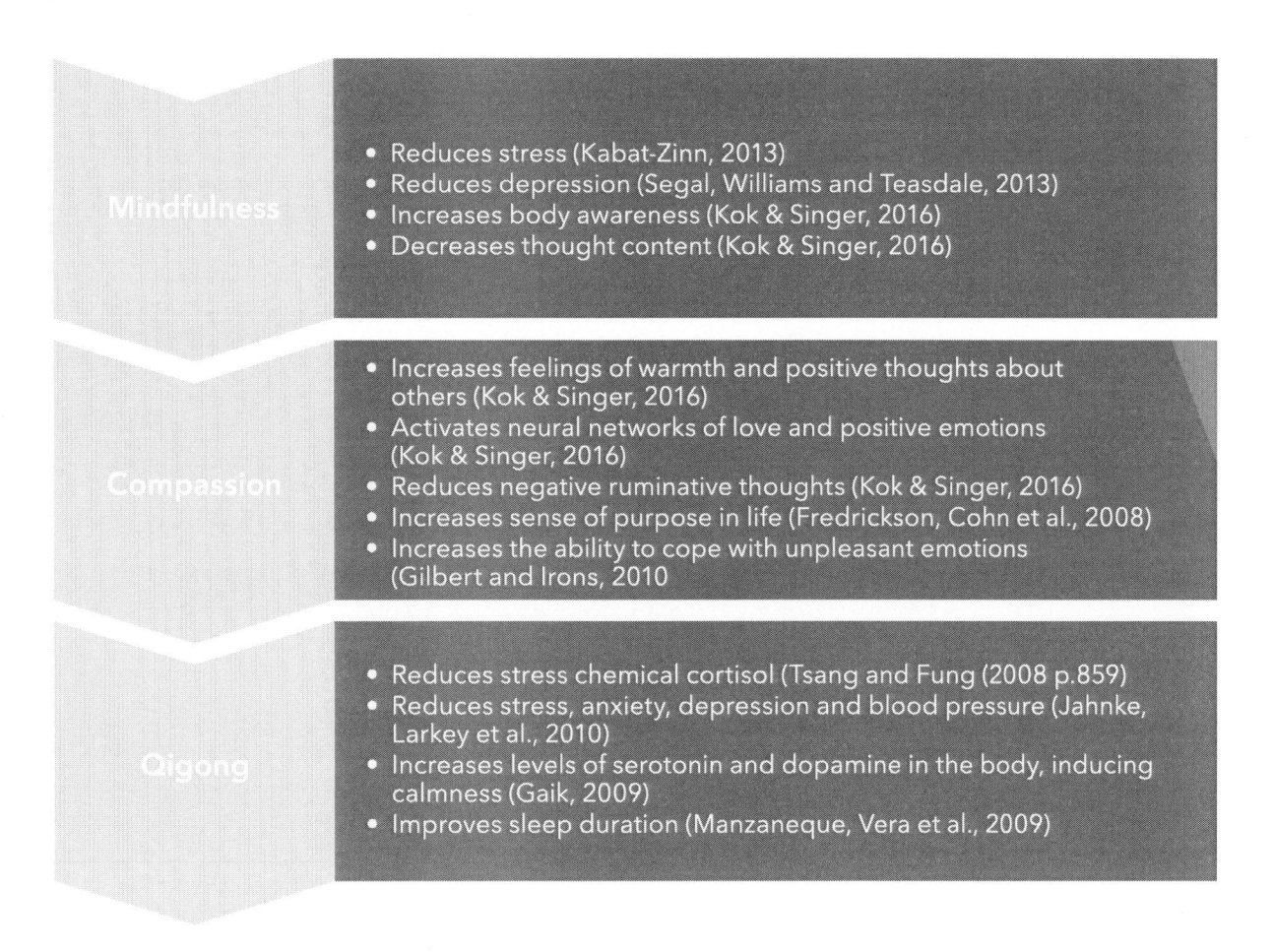

Qigong
- Reduces stress chemical cortisol (Tsang and Fung (2008 p.859)
- Reduces stress, anxiety, depression and blood pressure (Jahnke, Larkey et al., 2010)
- Increases levels of serotonin and dopamine in the body, inducing calmness (Gaik, 2009)
- Improves sleep duration (Manzaneque, Vera et al., 2009)

Figure 2: Evidence of benefits

Hoppes and Bryce et al., (2012, p148) claim that "Training in mindfulness has shown to be effective for individuals under stress and has intriguing potential for caregivers". There are many other studies which have found a positive impact of mindfulness on specific groups of family carers, for example, those who are caring for relatives suffering from specific conditions such as dementia (Waelde, Thompson et al., 2004) and parent carers of sick children (Bögels, Lehtonen et al., 2010).

The Dalai Lama was said to have asked neuroscientists to rise to the challenge of identifying the positive qualities of compassion (Jinpa, 2015, location 261). Singer rose to that challenge and investigated the impact of 'the loving kindness meditation' in comparison with the three mindfulness practices of breath awareness, observing thought and the body scan, which are typically included in an 8-week mindfulness course. In a study involving the use of psychometric tests and MRI scanners, researchers were able to analyse behaviours and activity in the brain as a direct response to specific types of mindfulness meditation practices. The results of this study are summarised and illustrated in Figure 3 below. Whilst all four practices led to increased awareness of body and decreased the tendency to become distracted by thoughts, the compassion practice of loving kindness was the only practice to increase positive thoughts in a statistically significant way.

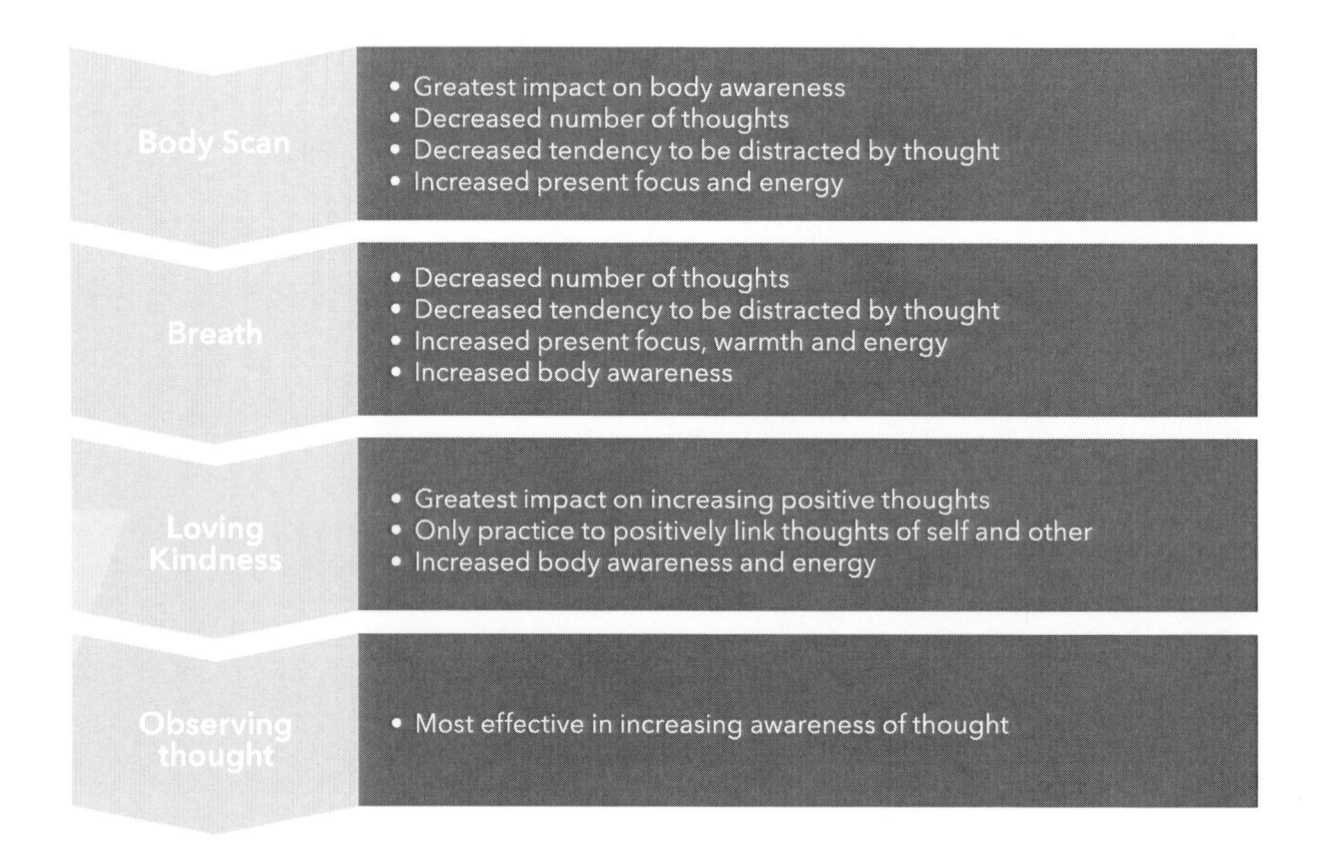

Body Scan
- Greatest impact on body awareness
- Decreased number of thoughts
- Decreased tendency to be distracted by thought
- Increased present focus and energy

Breath
- Decreased number of thoughts
- Decreased tendency to be distracted by thought
- Increased present focus, warmth and energy
- Increased body awareness

Loving Kindness
- Greatest impact on increasing positive thoughts
- Only practice to positively link thoughts of self and other
- Increased body awareness and energy

Observing thought
- Most effective in increasing awareness of thought

Figure 3: Phenomenological Fingerprints of Four Meditations (Kok, Singer, 2016, p.9).

The Loving kindness (metta) practice, derived from Buddhism some 2500 years ago, is a practice which focuses on cultivating a heartfelt wish that others may be free from suffering. Recent research has found that the loving kindness practice "activates neural networks of love and positive emotions, even in the light of distress stimuli" (Klimecki and Singer, 2012, p.370). Hutcherson, Seppala et al., (2008) found that just 7 minutes of loving kindness meditation induced positive feelings for self and others. These key findings influenced the design of my course for carers. I realised that this practice and short meditations could help transform the carers' stressful responses to their caring role and in particular the suffering of their relative to a much healthier positive response.

Whilst most research into the stress suffered by family carers has focussed on the impact this stress may have on their mental and emotional wellbeing, stress can also result in negative physical symptoms. For example, Behnke (1997) claims that suffering in the body can occur as a result of tension and emotional stress. Family carers can be said to be living in a fight or flight zone, where repeated demands from the relative they are caring for and the emotional trauma experienced from the loss of self in the caring role, may cause them pain and tension in the body. Practices which involve becoming bodily aware can help shift the experience of one's body into one of softness and ease and thus be of real benefit to stressed, tense carers.

Qigong is a system of healing medicine founded in China. The psychological and physiological health benefits of Qigong have been recognised for over five thousand years (Gaik, 2009). Qigong is known to improve mood and quality of life, whilst decreasing stress, anxiety and depression, and can thus be seen to have similar benefits to practices such as mindfulness meditation. Over a longer period of time a regular Qigong practice can strengthen the organs, nervous system and cardiovascular system as well as balancing emotions.

> **Pause and Practice**
>
> Take 10 minutes or so out of your daily life to practice this simple Qigong sequence - available at http://www.mindbodyone.co.uk/butterflysweepingqigong

RESEARCH

In my research study I came up with the following key questions designed to explore the plight of family carers and to see what types of mindfulness training would benefit them.

1. What symptoms of stress and emotional distress in response to their caring role are present in family carers that negatively affect their wellbeing and flourishing?
2. What would be the impact of a specifically designed 10-week Mindfulness, Compassion and Qigong Course (MCQC) on the overall wellbeing and flourishing of family carers?

With any desired transformational outcome there is a process that needs to be followed. The problem, solution, process and goal are highlighted in Figure 4 below.

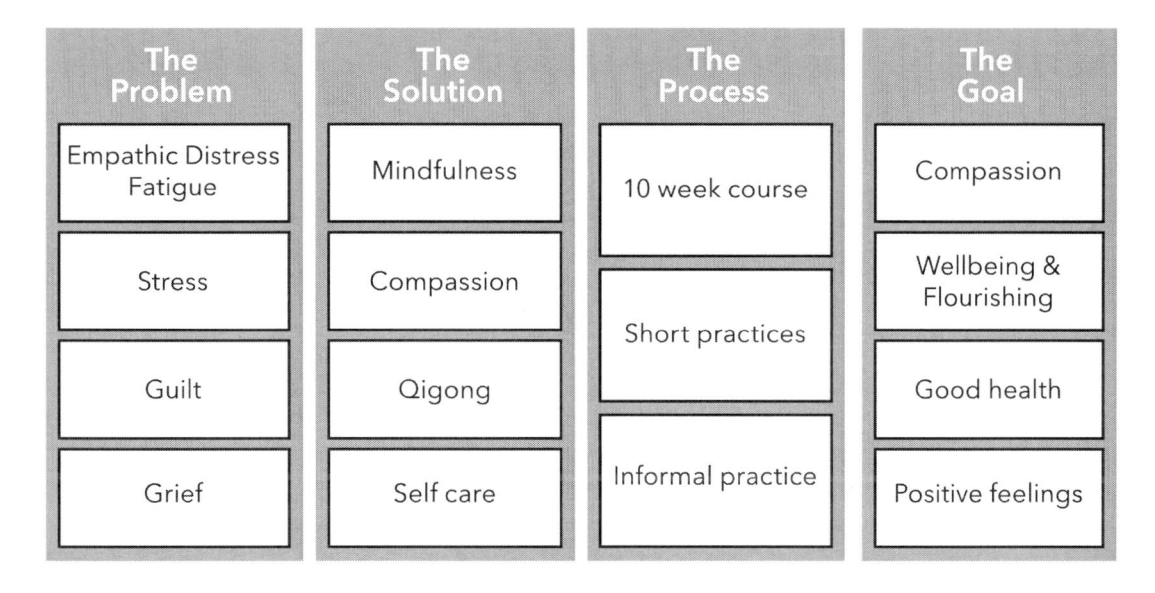

The Problem	The Solution	The Process	The Goal
Empathic Distress Fatigue	Mindfulness	10 week course	Compassion
Stress	Compassion	Short practices	Wellbeing & Flourishing
Guilt	Qigong	Short practices	Good health
Grief	Self care	Informal practice	Positive feelings

Figure 4: The process for transforming empathic distress to compassion and wellbeing

THE MINDFULNESS COMPASSION AND QIGONG COURSE

Carers in Hertfordshire kindly volunteered to support my study by recruiting twelve family carers, all women, to undertake my course. Participants had a range of caring roles including caring for sick husbands, parents and children. The course was held in a beautiful location at an old priory which provided a sense of sanctuary for the carers for their two-hour session for ten weeks.

The Mindfulness Compassion and Qigong course (MCQC) was developed using the 8-week Mindfulness Based Living Course (MBLC) as its base (Mindfulness Association, 2011). The course was extended to 10 weeks to allow for additional practices to be included from the Compassion Based Living Course (CBLC) (Mindfulness Association, 2017), Qigong movement and space for group discussion and sharing.

From my experience, family carers do not feel they have time to include a formal mindfulness practice into their lives, so in my course I emphasised informal and 'daily life' practices that would be easily achievable day by day. To encourage a regular formal practice, I recorded short 10-minute audio files of each guided practice in the MBLC course and the compassion practices for the participants to practice with at home. I taught the carers about taking comfort in small things, similar to the practice of Hygge in Denmark. Hygge (meaning wellbeing) takes its origins from Norway in the 19th Century, and means to find comfort, rest and safety whilst regaining energy and courage (Søderberg, M.T., 2016).

Pause and Reflect

Think of a pleasant event – such as the feel of sunshine, the smell of the flowers, the smile from a stranger. It could even be a simple activity you enjoy, such as drinking hot chocolate by the fire or taking a walk in a park. Notice how this activity makes you feel – the sensations in your body, your mood and your thoughts. Reflect on how you can change how you feel by changing your thoughts (energy follows focus).

One of the most important aspects of the training I provided to family carers was an emphasis on the importance of looking after themselves first and foremost. To begin with it was clear that the carers were not used to doing this. To convey this key idea, I used the analogy of the safety instructions on a flight to put your own life jacket and oxygen mask on before helping others. I also integrated Qigong into every session as a stress relieving practice. As a basis I taught them butterfly sweeping Qigong and movements from the traditional 18 move Qigong. I also taught them a further practice which involves using imagery and movements to clear out negative emotions. I showed the carers how to visualise a bubble of positive energy around themselves from which they can pour out their love and care. At the same time, I emphasised that this positive energy bubble could protect them from any negative environments and people including the negative energy of their sick loved one. I also included here the negative energy of 'the authorities' with whom most of the carers seemed to do battle on a pretty regular basis.

In order to understand how the carers were feeling and the impact of the course on their health and wellbeing I needed to collect information from them. I did this by collecting data through four questionnaires which examined the carers state of stress using the Perceived Stress Scale (Cohen, Kamarck, 1983); resilience using the Brief Resilience Scale (Smith, Dalen et al., 2008); overall wellbeing and flourishing using the Flourishing Scale (Diener, Wirtz et al., 2010) and self-compassion using Neff's (2003) Self Compassion Scale, before and after the course. Whilst the data I collected this way was revealing, the most important aspect of my research turned out to be capturing the carers' 'lived experience' through their stories, poems, paintings and heartfelt sentiments from focus groups, weekly observations and interviews. Evidence of carers' wellbeing before, during and at the end of the course came tumbling forth in a torrent of heartfelt emotion and experience. The rich narrative which emerged later formed the essence of a carer's journey from empathic stress fatigue to wellbeing, from grief to acceptance and from role engulfment to a positive self.

EMPATHIC DISTRESS TO WELLBEING

The main findings from my study confirmed that there is a big physiological and psychological 'cost of caring' for a sick relative, illustrated below in Figures 5 and 6.

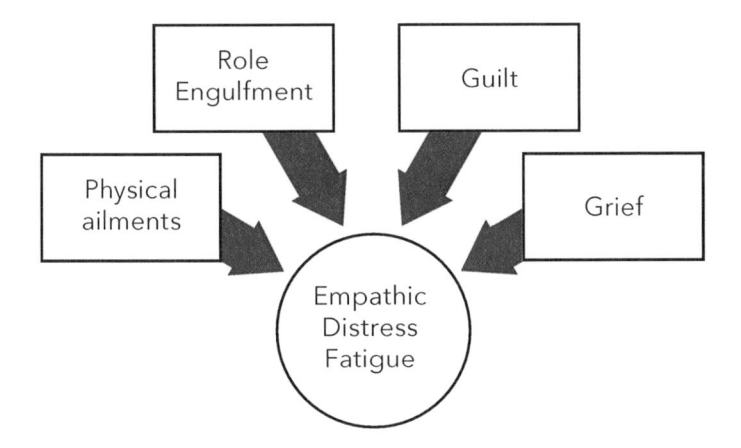

Figure 5: Symptoms of Empathic Distress Fatigue

- Physical illness
- Chronic stress
- Exhaustion
- Depression
- Chronic fatigue
- Poor sleep
- Isolation
- Anger
- Emotional exhaustion

Figure 6: Physical ailments experienced by participants pre-course

Anne shared a poem with the group, which aptly reflects the dark depths one can reach as a family carer;

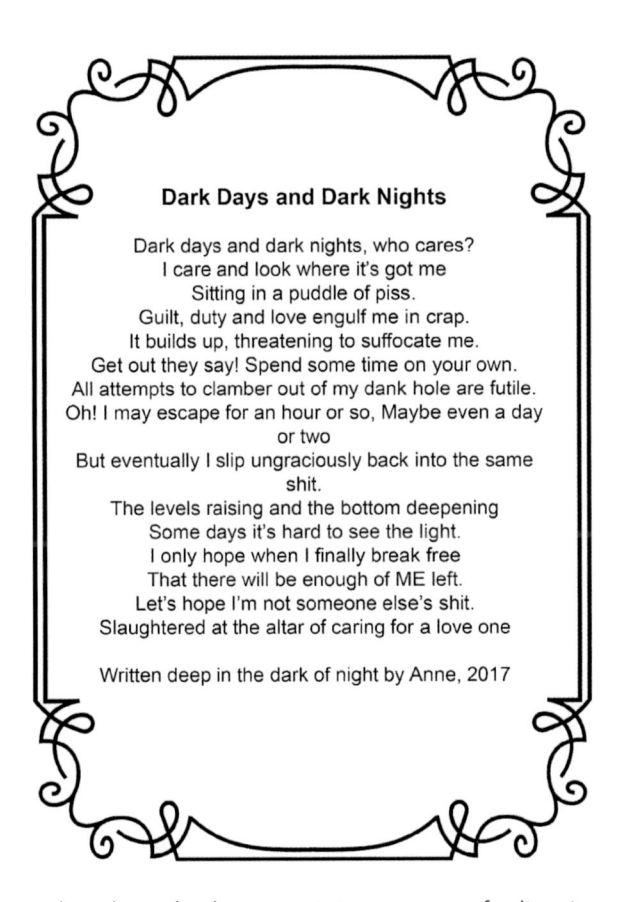

Dark Days and Dark Nights

Dark days and dark nights, who cares?
I care and look where it's got me
Sitting in a puddle of piss.
Guilt, duty and love engulf me in crap.
It builds up, threatening to suffocate me.
Get out they say! Spend some time on your own.
All attempts to clamber out of my dank hole are futile.
Oh! I may escape for an hour or so, Maybe even a day or two
But eventually I slip ungraciously back into the same shit.
The levels raising and the bottom deepening
Some days it's hard to see the light.
I only hope when I finally break free
That there will be enough of ME left.
Let's hope I'm not someone else's shit.
Slaughtered at the altar of caring for a love one

Written deep in the dark of night by Anne, 2017

By analysing the words used to describe how participants were feeling I created a word cloud below in Figure 7, which highlights emotions and ailments experienced before the course.

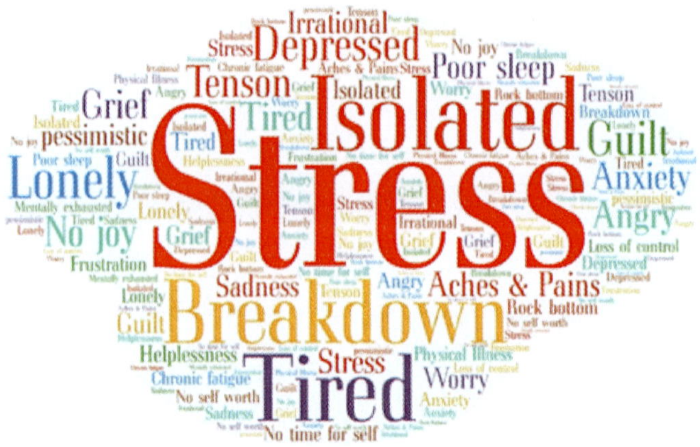

Figure 7: Pre-Course Emotions & Ailments

Pause and Practice - 3-minute breathing space

I now invite you to do a practice that the carers found very beneficial in their daily lives. Sit comfortably and close your eyes. Bring your awareness to your body sensations, thoughts and feelings. Expand your awareness to your senses to include sounds, smell and touch. Now allow your focus to rest only on the sensation of breathing. How you breathe, where you can feel it. Explore the whole sensation of breathing as if noticing it for the very first time. Do this for about a minute or so. Next allow your awareness to spread to the rest of your body and become aware of any sensations in the body, noticing contrasts of tension and warmth, tingling etc. Expand your awareness to your emotions and thoughts. Allow your senses to reengage with sounds, smells touch and sight as you open your eyes.

Check in with how you are feeling now.

TRANSFORMATION

One of the most exciting findings from my small study was that when the results from the questionnaires were analysed for the group after the course, a 32% increase in self-compassion was seen. Perceived stress levels were reduced by 32%, feelings of wellbeing and flourishing increased by 26% and resilience increased by 26%.

Six key themes became apparent which had contributed to the carer's transition from one of empathic distress to one of flourishing and improved health. I observed and recorded the unfolding process using weekly notes. The transformation represented a journey starting with mindful awareness to self-compassion and self-care, acceptance, the emergence of a more positive sense of self, improvements in carer/relative relationship and concluding with psychological and physiological wellbeing.

The word cloud in Figure 8 below, represents the positive words extracted from the carers' narrative data indicating the transformational impact of their commitment to the course and their practice.

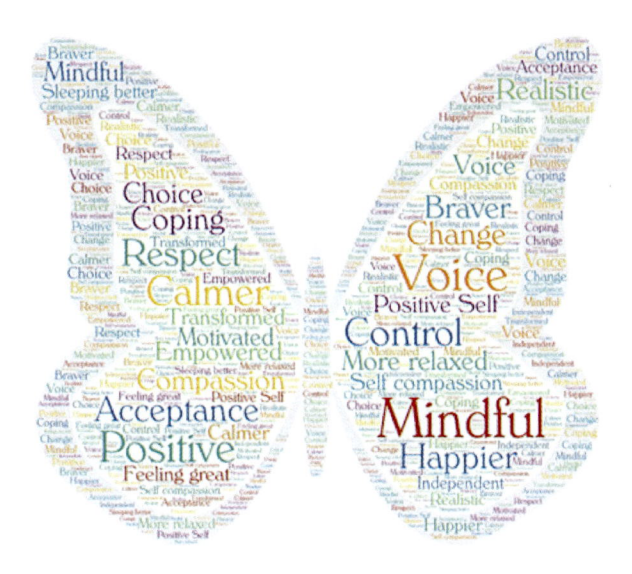

Figure 8: Post course experience

The results of my study indicated that an important shift in response to empathy had occurred as described in Figure 1. For example, one participant in my study describes:

> The turning point was when I said to him, I know you are feeling crap. I've always said – yes, I know you are in pain etc - but I have never put it to him that I am not going to take that pain on board. It's not my pain and I can't take it away for you

MINDFUL AWARENESS

The carers in my study became more mindfully aware as a result of the course. It provided them with new insights into their behaviours, thoughts and feelings and assisted them to realise that they have a choice about how they respond to stressful situations. One participant reflected;

> It's the awareness that makes the difference. I didn't realise the destructive path I was travelling down. The course has given me to the opportunity to be allowed to be aware

An awareness of how their minds worked and their usual patterns of behaviour enabled most of the participants to gain some insight into how they might be able to change their reactions to stressful triggers:

> I now realise I can change things. Whereas before I would have got annoyed by my father but this time I decided not to get annoyed. It has changed me

One participant became aware of how her mind created stories that caused her to suffer:

> I've been making up stories as I have been going along. I used to worry about what people think but now I am different. I realised I didn't need to make up a story

SELF-COMPASSION AND SELF-CARE

> Self-care is not selfish or self-indulgent. We cannot nurture others from a dry well. We need to take care of our own needs first, so that we can give from our surplus, our abundance. When we nurture others from a place of fullness, we feel renewed instead of taken advantage of (Jennifer Louden 2004, p.2)

Prior to the course, several participants described how they would forgo their own concerns and go along with the desires of others in an attempt to make them happy. But at the end of the course, they described how they had become more protective of their own wellbeing and were more self-accepting and self-compassionate. Clare stated, "I am more inclined to say I deserve a break and do something for myself". Others stated that they were doing things they wouldn't have done before, felt empowered, and that they were taking back control of their lives. Many of the participants started taking short breaks from caring and doing things for themselves like exercise and creative classes.

Joy shared her experience.

> Realising that you are only human and accepting that sometimes you are pushed to your limits and can't cope any more - that's the thing. Thinking you are a bad person because you have yelled at someone but recognising that you are only human. Recognising that it isn't an issue – it's big.

Mary stated that she was more compassionate with herself:

> I actually say to myself – you have been through an awful lot over four years and not many people I know would be able to handle that without getting to breaking point.

ACCEPTANCE

Acceptance and acknowledgment of feelings of grief were unprompted key themes which arose in the narrative from the interviews and focus groups. One participant described her grief as being paralysing:

> The course helped ground me and not allow the grief to keep taking over. Trying to let everything be, as I cannot change what has happened.

Another participant acknowledged: "Life wasn't what I expected of life. It's really a loss".

The RAIN practice is included in the MBLC course. Developed by Tara Brach (2003), the practice involves inviting a difficulty into a meditation and going through a process of 'Recognising' the difficulty, 'Allowing' it in, 'Investigating' into how this difficulty makes us feel and finally seeing if we can let it go through a process of 'Nurturing'. As a result of practicing 'RAIN' one participant shared some of her deep insights which she felt resulted from a new awareness of her thoughts and reactions:

> Looking at things from a different angle helped me to break through. I didn't realise what my undercurrent of thoughts was about. Then I realised the undercurrent was anxiety. I suppose once you know what something is, you can deal with it, realise there is no substance to it. So, let it go or at least let it pass through and go. Before I was overwhelmed, too scared to address any of it. Now it is nice to sit there and not pretend. To be authentic, true to myself, allowing it to be there

Clare reported learning how to:

> accept things as they are. The course helped me to stand back and not worry myself sick. Its major to be able to do that. I notice how I am feeling and then say – Let's cope, let's not worry if things might go wrong

---

Pause and Practice

Explore the RAIN practice for yourself by visiting Tara Brach's practice page
https://www.tarabrach.com/selfcompassion1/

FINDING POSITIVE SELF

As part of my unfolding journey, I wrote a poem in my journal during the first year of MSc Studies in Mindfulness. I realised that I had found my voice and a more positive sense of self.

One of the most remarkable findings that emerged from my research was that my small group of family carers had also begun to find their voices.

The finding of their voice was integral to the emergence of a 'positive-self' which compared favourably to carers' pre-course states of role engulfment, guilt and grief. My research has revealed that a positive-self can emerge through a combination of increases in self-compassion, self-esteem, self-confidence and social-self, as represented in Figure 12 below.

In my study, as participants' feelings of isolation were alleviated, other positive changes in their mood and emotional state followed. As the carers' self-compassion and self-confidence increased, so their self-esteem improved. Participants stated, "I started doing things for myself", and "I feel empowered. I feel I am taking back control".

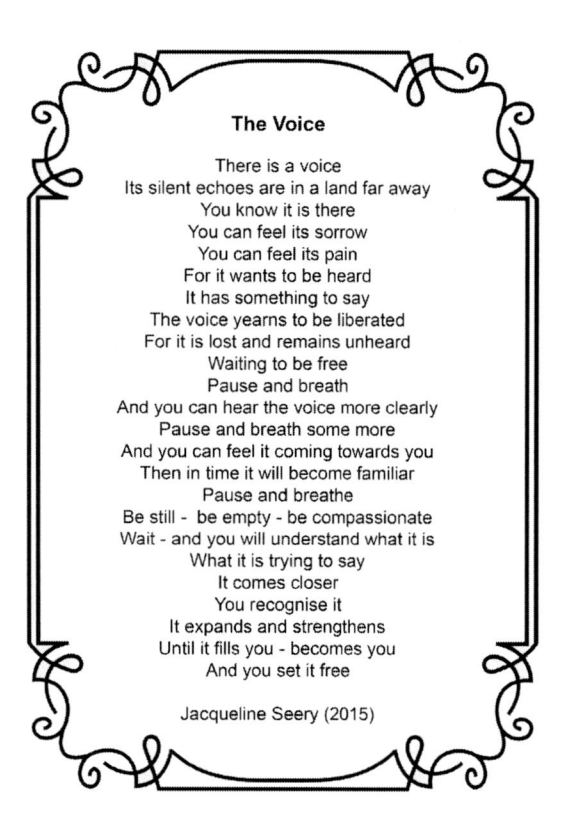

> **The Voice**
>
> There is a voice
> Its silent echoes are in a land far away
> You know it is there
> You can feel its sorrow
> You can feel its pain
> For it wants to be heard
> It has something to say
> The voice yearns to be liberated
> For it is lost and remains unheard
> Waiting to be free
> Pause and breath
> And you can hear the voice more clearly
> Pause and breath some more
> And you can feel it coming towards you
> Then in time it will become familiar
> Pause and breathe
> Be still - be empty - be compassionate
> Wait - and you will understand what it is
> What it is trying to say
> It comes closer
> You recognise it
> It expands and strengthens
> Until it fills you - becomes you
> And you set it free
>
> Jacqueline Seery (2015)

IMPROVED RELATIONSHIPS

Generally, my carers reported that their relationship with those they were caring for was more relaxed and had improved throughout the course. Some attributed this change to their own improved sense of calm and happiness. Some participants shared that they were no longer taking things so personally or feeling like a victim of their role. One participant said that,

> The relationship with my husband was as if we turned the clock back 20 years. My husband says he has seen a change in me and I have seen a change in him

Some of the participants said that they practiced mindfulness with their relative which had a positive effect on them both.

PSYCHOLOGICAL AND PHYSIOLOGICAL WELLBEING

Before the course, participants described being stressed, anxious and depressed. After the course, their levels of stress had dropped significantly. In particular one participant reflected:

> I felt really alone, really depressed and I wasn't in a very good place. The difference now is that when things happen to me, okay I am really upset about it, but I don't let it affect me as much as I did before. I think that is because I am more mindful of not letting it consume my whole being. I can feel it, live with it and know that feeling is going to pass

Participants described how they were sleeping better, feeling calmer, more relaxed and coping better. One participant described the change in how she felt thus: "I used to get angry and short tempered, but now I am more back to my philosophical self." Mary described how her body used to be in so much pain that she ended up in hospital with high levels of stress. She explained:

> My physical body, stress, anxiety and depression is better. The way I handle situations are all better. Everything is much better than it was

Another participant described how she used to feel snappy and stressed. She says, "Now I don't feel angry or stressed. The mindfulness took it to another level in how I feel about myself".

DEPARTURE

My small study revealed evidence of the symptoms of empathic stress amongst family carers. These symptoms included high levels of stress, depression, anxiety, ill health, sleep problems, grief, guilt, frustration, isolation, exhaustion and feelings of helplessness and hopelessness. My findings strongly suggested that maintaining a short daily formal practice and integrating brief moments of mindfulness and self-compassion into daily life are sufficient to bring about greater overall wellbeing in stressed family carers. All of the participants commented that the course was highly appropriate and beneficial to them and three reported that it had changed their lives.

Two of the participants described the course as 'brilliant' and that it was important that the compassion and Qigong had been a part of it. Others recognised the particular value of the compassion element within the course;

> I can see the value of the compassion element of the course. You have to have it tailored correctly for the people it's for. That's where a lot of people have a negative view of mindfulness. How you altered the course for us was brilliant

> I think this is amazing. you have given us a gift. That's how I feel about it

It had become apparent that that the carers had begun their 'departure' into hero's' journeys of their own.

THE HERO'S RETURN

Anne shared a poem she had written with the group. Her descent into her own hero's' journey had begun:

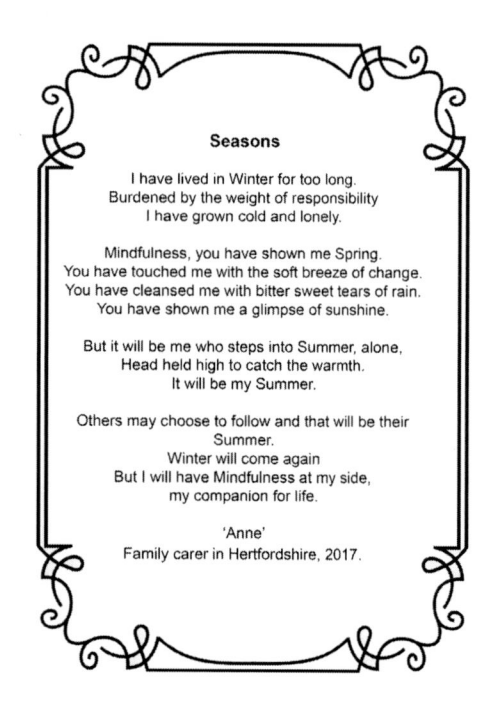

Seasons

I have lived in Winter for too long.
Burdened by the weight of responsibility
I have grown cold and lonely.

Mindfulness, you have shown me Spring.
You have touched me with the soft breeze of change.
You have cleansed me with bitter sweet tears of rain.
You have shown me a glimpse of sunshine.

But it will be me who steps into Summer, alone,
Head held high to catch the warmth.
It will be my Summer.

Others may choose to follow and that will be their Summer.
Winter will come again
But I will have Mindfulness at my side,
my companion for life.

'Anne'
Family carer in Hertfordshire, 2017.

As I conclude this story about the awful stress experienced by a small group of family carers, and their extremely positive responses to the course I ran for them, I realise the impact of my own empathic response towards their pain. Sharing their pain made me acutely aware of my own feelings as I cried along with them. I shared their journeys from suffering to glimpses of transformation, as bodies relaxed, smiles appeared, and they finally began to become much more empowered and accepting of their unavoidable caring roles.

I lived and breathed these carer's stories for twelve months. In Ricard's (2015 p.60) words I feel a "profound, heart-warming courage linked to limitless love" for the family carers in my study. I salute these unacknowledged heroines of our contemporary rather uncaring society. Spending quality time with these incredibly courageous and generous women felt to me like coming home. I had returned to a place of unconditional love and compassion for all suffering human beings, but particularly for all those amazing carers who - like my past-self - courageously keep going under the most stressful circumstances.

As I write this chapter, in June 2018, Britain is commemorating the end of WW1 and saluting all the heroes of that dark time in our history. But as well as saluting these 20th century heroes, I would like to salute here the thousands upon thousands of unsung caring heroes of the 21st Century.

I feel so privileged to have been able to hold a warm, compassionate space for these caring heroines. I feel so blessed that I was able to share with them all that I have learnt on my own heroine's journey through life. I am now so incredibly grateful that my own challenging life journey, during which I have met, and been supported by, so many incredibly wise, generous and empowering mindfulness teachers, has enabled me to offer these vulnerable, stressed carers a set of effective tools and insights to initiate them into their own heroine's' journey home to unconditional love and wholeness.

REFERENCES

BEHNKE, E.A., (1997). Ghost gestures: Phenomenological investigations of bodily micromovements and their intracorporal implications. Human Studies, 20(2), pp. 181-201.
BRACH, T., (2003). Radical Acceptance Awakening the love that heals fear and shame within us. London: Ebury Press.
BRANDEN, N., (Undated). Brainy Quote. Available: https://www.brainyquote.com/quotes/nathaniel_branden_163773?src=t_acceptance [Date Accessed: 23rd June 2018].
CARERS UK (2012). In Sickness and in Health. Available: https://www.carersuk.org/for-professionals/policy/policy-library?task=download&file=policy_file&id=208. London: Carers UK [Date Accessed 30th November 2016].
CARERS UK., (2015). Facts about carers. Available: https://www.carersuk.org/news-and-campaigns/press-releases/facts-and-figures [Date Accessed: 23rd June 2018].
COHEN, S., KAMARCK, T. and MERMELSTEIN, R., (1994). Perceived stress scale. Measuring stress: A guide for health and social scientists.
COVEY, S.R., 2006. Servant Leadership Use your moral authority to serve. Leadership Excellence, 23(12), p.5.
DIENER, E., WIRTZ, D., TOV, W., KIM-PRIETO, C., CHOI, D., OISHI, S. and BISWAS-DIENER, R., (2010). New Well-being Measures: Short Scales to Assess Flourishing and Positive and Negative Feelings. Social Indicators Research, 97(2), pp. 143-156.
FIGLEY, C.R., (1995). Compassion fatigue: Toward a new understanding of the costs of caring.
FREDRICKSON, B.L., COHN, M.A., COFFEY, K.A., PEK, J. and FINKEL, S.M., (2008). Open hearts build lives: positive emotions, induced through loving-kindness meditation, build consequential personal resources. Journal of personality and social psychology, 95(5), pp. 1045.
GAIK, F., (2009). Managing Depression with Qigong. Singing Dragon.
GILBERT, P. and IRONS, C., (2004). A pilot exploration of the use of compassionate images in a group of self‐critical people. Memory, 12(4), pp.507-516.
GILBERT, P., (2009). The compassionate mind: A new approach to life's challenges. London: Constable and Robinson Ltd (Kindle edition).
HOPPES, S., BRYCE, H., HELLMAN, C. and FINLAY, E., (2012). The effects of brief mindfulness training on caregivers' well-being. Activities, Adaptation & Aging, 36(2), pp. 147-166.

HUTCHERSON, C.A., SEPPALA, E.M. and GROSS, J.J., (2008). Loving-kindness meditation increases social connectedness. Emotion, 8(5), pp. 720.
Ivtzan, I. and Lomas, T. eds., 2016. Mindfulness in positive psychology: The science of meditation and wellbeing. Routledge.

JAHNKE, R., LARKEY, L., ROGERS, C., ETNIER, J. and LIN, F., (2010). A comprehensive review of health benefits of qigong and tai chi. American Journal of Health Promotion, 24(6), pp. e1-e25.
JINPA, T., (2015). A Fearless Heart. Why compassion is the key to greater wellbeing. London. Little, Brown Book Group (Kindle edition).
JOINSON, C., (1992). Coping with compassion fatigue. Nursing, 22(4), pp. 116, 118-9, 120.
KABAT-ZINN. J., (Undated). 76 Most Powerful Mindfulness Quotes: Your Daily Dose of Inspiration. Positive Psychology Programme. Available: https://positivepsychologyprogram.com/mindfulness-quotes/ [Date Accessed:23rd September 2018].
KABAT-ZINN, J., (2005). Coming to our senses: Healing ourselves and the world through mindfulness. Hachette UK (Kindle edition).
KABAT-ZINN, J., (2013). Full Catastrophe Living, Wherever You Go There You Are. London: Piaktus (i-book version).
KLIMECKI, O. and SINGER, T., (2012). Empathic distress fatigue rather than compassion fatigue? Integrating findings from empathy research in psychology and social neuroscience. Pathological altruism, pp. 368-383.
KOK, B.E. and SINGER, T., (2016). Phenomenological Fingerprints of Four Meditations: Differential State Changes in Affect, Mind-Wandering, Meta-Cognition, and Interoception Before and After Daily Practice Across 9 Months of Training. Mindfulness, pp. 1-14.
LOUDEN, J., (2004). The woman's comfort book: A self-nurturing guide for restoring balance in your life. HarperSanFrancisco.
LYNCH, S.H. and LOBO, M.L., (2012). Compassion fatigue in family caregivers: a Wilsonian concept analysis. Journal of advanced nursing, 68(9), pp. 2125-2134.
MANZANEQUE, J.M., VERA, F.M., RODRIGUEZ, F.M., GARCIA, G.J., LEYVA, L. and BLANCA, M.J., (2009). Serum cytokines, mood and sleep after a qigong program: is qigong an effective psychobiological tool? Journal of Health Psychology, 14(1), pp. 60-67.
MARRIOTT, H., (2003). The selfish pig's guide to caring. Polperro Heritage Press.
MINDFULNESS ASSOCIATION, Ltd., (2011). Mindfulness Based Living Course - 8-week Programme - Course Manual. Mindfulness Association Ltd.
MINDFULNESS ASSOCIATION, Ltd., (2017). Compassion Based Living Course - 8-week Programme - Course Manual. Mindfulness Association Ltd.
NEFF, K.D., (2003). The development and validation of a scale to measure self-compassion. Self and identity, 2(3), pp. 223-250.
PERRY, B., DALTON, J.E. and EDWARDS, M., (2010). Family caregivers' compassion fatigue in long-term facilities. Nursing older people, 22(4), pp. 26-31.
PFIFFERLING, J. and GILLEY, K., (2000). Overcoming compassion fatigue. Family practice management, 7(4), pp. 39-39.
RICARD, M. and SINGER, W., (2017). Neuroscience Has a Lot to Learn from Buddhism, A scientist and a monk compare notes on meditation, therapy, and their effects on the brain. The Atlantic. Available: https://www.theatlantic.com/international/archive/2017/12/buddhism-and-neuroscience/548120/ [Date Accessed 4th January 2018].
RICARD, M., (2009). Empathy and the Cultivation of Compassion. Matthieu Ricard. Available: http://www.matthieuricard.org/en/blog/posts/empathy-and-the-cultivation-of-compassion. [Date Accessed 24th July 2017].
RICARD, M., (2015). Altruism: The power of compassion to change yourself and the world. Hachette UK.
RINPOCHE, Y.M., (2009). Joyful wisdom. Random House (Kindle edition).
SEGAL, V.Z., WILLIAMS, J.M.G. and TEASDALE, J.D., (2013). Mindfulness-Based Cognitive Therapy for Depression. Second edn. New York: The Guildford Press (Kindle edition).
SINGER, T. and KLIMECKI, O.M., (2014). Empathy and compassion. Current Biology, 24(18), pp. R875-R878.
SINGER, T., KOK, B.E., BORNEMANN, B., ZURBORG, S., BOLZ, M. and BOCHOW, C., (2016). The ReSource Project: Background, design, samples, and measurements.
SMITH, B.W., DALEN, J., WIGGINS, K., TOOLEY, E., CHRISTOPHER, P. and BERNARD, J., (2008). The brief resilience scale: assessing the ability to bounce back. International Journal of Behavioral Medicine, 15(3), pp. 194-200.
SØDERBERG, M.T., (2016). Hygge: The Danish Art of Happiness. Penguin UK.
TSANG, H.W. and FUNG, K.M., (2008). A review on neurobiological and psychological mechanisms underlying the anti-depressive effect of qigong exercise. Journal of Health Psychology, 13(7), pp. 857-863.
TUBB, G., (2018). "Young carers face loneliness and isolation in summer holidays". Sky News. Available: https://news.sky.com/story/young-carers-face-loneliness-and-isolation-in-summer-holidays-11456375 [Date Accessed: 23rd June 2018].
WADA, K. and PARK, J., (2009). Integrating Buddhist psychology into grief counselling. Death studies, 33(7), pp. 657-683.
WAELDE, L.C., THOMPSON, L. and GALLAGHER-THOMPSON, D., (2004). A pilot study of a yoga and meditation intervention for dementia caregiver stress. Journal of clinical psychology, 60(6), pp. 677-687.
ZI, L., (1939). Tao te ching. Lulu. com.

CHAPTER 25

THE MINDFULNESS FOR EVERYONE PROJECT

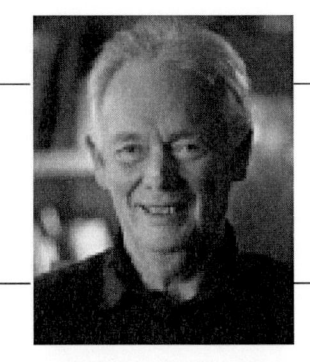

Vin Harris

trust@hartknowe.org

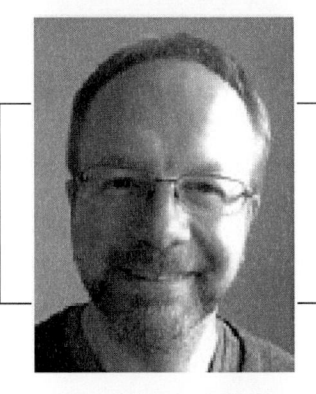

Alan Hughes

alanhughes108@gmail.com

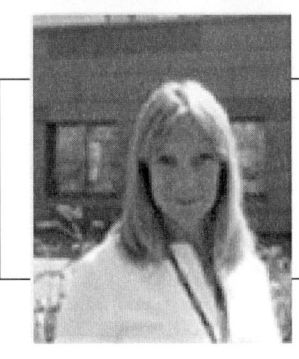

Julie McColl

juliemccoll1@gmail.com

NO HUMAN IS LIMITED

Sometimes our heroes help us to realise who we really are and why we do what we do. I recently found a new hero in an amazing man called Eliud Kipchoge, a long distance runner from Kenya who has committed himself to a quest that has long been considered impossible. He wants to run a marathon in under two hours. He is not undertaking this challenge in order to show the world how great he is, but as an affirmation of his conviction that in his own words: "no human is limited" (BBC, undated). I have no immediate plans to run a marathon but I wholeheartedly agree with him. I am inspired by his example. His story reminded me why I am involved with the Mindfulness for Everyone Project. I too believe that in reality no human is limited and I want to do whatever I can to give everyone the opportunities I sometimes take for granted.

Like all the best adventures, the Mindfulness for Everyone Project started when we noticed that something just didn't seem quite right with the world and we wanted to make it better. A series of conversations between members of the Mindfulness Association highlighted our shared concern that most people who attend mindfulness courses are able to do so because they have the freedom and resources to access the training. There's nothing wrong with that, but we began to think about all of the people who are not so lucky and might actually be expected to have an even greater need: surely they too deserve to enjoy the benefits of mindfulness practice. We asked ourselves what we could do about this.

Right from the very beginning, our mission has been just what it says on the tin: to help ourselves and others live up to our limitless potential by making mindfulness available to Everyone. This is definitely going to be a marathon and not a sprint; but at least we took the first steps instead of sitting there wondering what might have been. As we have seen in the previous chapters of this book, the wish to be free of our own limitations is universal and the wish to help others flows naturally from the heart of anyone who has had a taste of inner freedom. The Mindfulness for Everyone Project certainly has a very long way to go before we can say that we have achieved our aim and that the benefits of mindfulness really are freely available to everyone (a constant reminder that a meaningful life is more about the journey than the destination!). However, the good news is that in the past three and a half years our project has grown from the seed of an altruistic aspiration and is already helping to facilitate positive change through compassionate action.

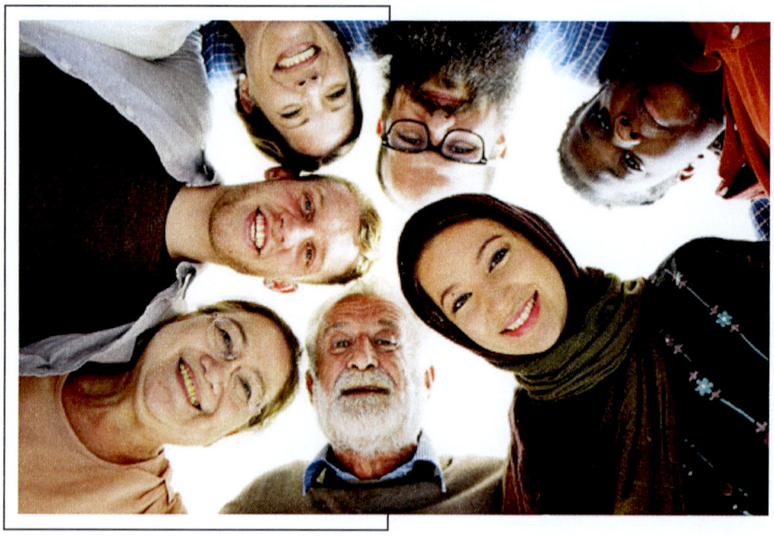

Figure 1: Mindfulness for Everyone, because no human is limited. Photo © Getty Images

COMPASSIONATE ACTION RESEARCH

A JOURNEY OF DISCOVERY IN THREE STAGES (SO FAR...)

Life can be quite messy and this being human is actually a bit of a muddle. The plots and subplots of my various endeavours feel like overlapping waves that don't quite make sense most of the time. Isn't that why we humans tend to look back and tell the story of what has happened? Stories can hold the meaning and purpose of what we have learned from experience in a form that will make sense to ourselves and others when we need it most. In this spirit I want to tell you about why we set out, what we did and what we discovered on a journey called the Mindfulness for Everyone Project. I (Vin Harris) narrate the story of the Mindfulness for Everyone Project. An important part of this story is the research to evaluate the impact of what we did and to understand what we could improve. The quantitative research was carried out by Alan Hughes and the interviews were conducted by Julie McColl. This whole initiative may well be an interconnected series of events in a tale without beginning or end. However, in order to make it easier to share what we have learnt I am going to present the account of what we did as a story of "Compassionate Acton Research", a project in three stages.

What do we mean by the term action research? The work of John Elliott whose work has been influential in the field defines it as: "the study of a social situation with a view to improving the quality of actions within it" (Elliott, 1991, p.69). This cyclical approach to research involves the researcher in a process of continuous improvement: it promotes turning curiosity into action, which results in learning, which in turn informs the next cycle.

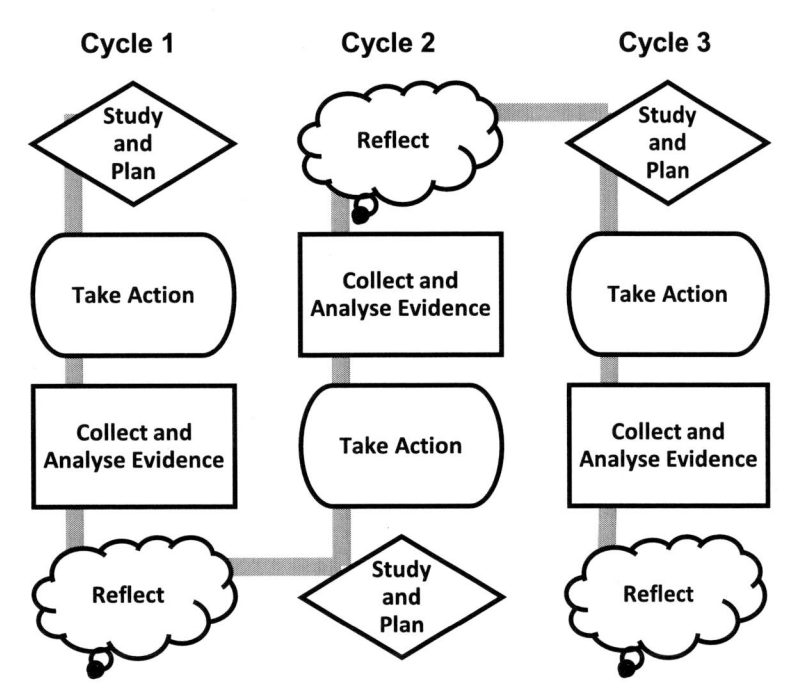

Progressive Problem Solving with Action Research

Figure 2: The flow of action research. Image by Reil, 2006

The long term aim of the Mindfulness for Everyone Project is to make mindfulness available to groups that are currently excluded and to bring about sustainable, transformational change within disadvantaged communities. The model of action research presented in Figure 2 reflects how our team has engaged with this mission: setting out together into the unknown, facing challenges, gaining insights and returning with the capacity to achieve more. It could be seen as a series of three journeys, the end of each cycle leads to the starting point for the next one. Because our underlying purpose throughout this ongoing exploration has always been to find a way to take action that will reduce suffering, it feels appropriate to describe what we have been doing as "Compassionate Action Research". I don't think it will spoil your enjoyment of the story that unfolds if you are aware of the three stages that the project has been through to bring us to where we are now.

STAGE ONE: ENLIGHTENED ENTERPRISE

We noticed that the UK demographic engaging in mindfulness training is currently overwhelmingly represented by self-funding professionals. This became apparent not only from those paying to attend the Mindfulness Association's courses, but also from the focus of the Mindful Nation UK report (MAPPG, 2015). We asked ourselves:

- "Is there anything we can do to make mindfulness accessible and inclusive?"

STAGE TWO: COMPASSION BASED MINDFULNESS TRAINING

People who engage with compassion based mindfulness practice often describe the experience as "life-changing". However, we needed to know whether training in mindfulness and compassion would be just as effective in improving the well-being of individuals from the neglected groups of people we want to help: We asked ourselves:

- "Will compassionate mindfulness be able to benefit those who might need it most?"

STAGE THREE: GROWING A GREAT IDEA

As a result of the first stage of our Compassionate Action Research project we found a way to provide access to mindfulness for groups that are generally excluded. Our evaluation of the second stage showed the difference our funded mindfulness programmes had made to people's lives. We were inspired to do more and asked ourselves:

- "Can we now reach even more people and support long term change?"

CROSSING THE THRESHOLD

Perhaps the most valuable learning from all the inspiring stories told by Mindful Heroes in our book is this: the adventure always begins with one small step which leads to another. The path is revealed by walking the path. What we discover invariably turns out to be more rewarding than could possibly have been imagined. Everything depends on having the confidence to cross the threshold into the unknown. It does get easier with practice. I like to keep in mind this quotation attributed to Goethe as a reminder that we will do well to trust the call to adventure:

> ...the moment one definitely commits oneself, then Providence moves too. All sorts of things occur to help one that would never otherwise have occurred. A whole stream of events issues from the decision, raising in one's favour all manner of unforeseen incidents, meetings and material assistance which no man could have dreamed would have come his way. Whatever you can do or dream you can, begin it. Boldness has genius, power and magic in it (Murray, 1951, p.6).

Pause and Reflect

Why not take a break, sit quietly, rest and allow your attention to be with your breathing.

Bring to mind one of your achievements that you feel good about. It doesn't matter if it is big or small, just let a few key events in the story of your project play out in your mind's eye.

Was there a particular moment when the idea came to you or did it emerge gradually over time?

At what point did you commit yourself to action and how did you feel?

Can you recall any unforeseen coincidences or people who helped you on your way?

STAGE ONE: ENLIGHTENED ENTERPRISE

AN INSIDE-OUT APPROACH

As mindfulness practitioners and tutors, returning from our own inner journeys with something of value, we set ourselves the challenge of finding a way to share what we had learnt with the world. Chloe Homewood and I have developed a mindfulness workshop called Enlightened Enterprise. The world of business may often appear to be at odds with the spirit of mindfulness and compassion but it doesn't have to be like that. You don't have to leave your values on the meditation cushion when you go out to work. Enlightened Enterprise takes an "inside-out" approach; activity in the world becomes an outer expression of inner aspirations. Our programme is influenced by The Seven Habits of Highly Effective People written by Stephen Covey (1992). He is one of my heroes. The way of working in alignment with deeper values which he promotes is far easier than wasting my energy chasing after a superficial illusion that I don't even believe in. Anyway, in developing the strategy for the Mindfulness for Everyone Project, we applied some of the timeless principles that we teach. As ever they proved to be highly effective.

WIN-WIN

Everything is interconnected. Endeavours that deliver benefits to all parties involved are more successful in the long-term than arrangements where some people gain at the expense of others. This view, expressed as "Think win-win", is the fourth of Covey's seven habits. We identified various "stakeholders", that is to say people and organisations who would have an interest in and would affect or be affected by our project:

- **Participants** could be expected to benefit from receiving mindfulness training. Their increased well-being as a result of practicing what they learnt would then have a positive impact on others.
- **Tutors** could benefit from teaching opportunities through developing their new networks. They would help participants by delivering an eight-week Mindfulness Based Living Course (MBLC).
- **The Mindfulness Association** could benefit from an opportunity carry out research to evaluate the effectiveness its MBLC training. It would benefit the project by donating funds and by using its networks to facilitate the recruitment, training and supervision of tutors.
- **The Hart Knowe Trust** could fulfil its stated charitable objective: "the advancement of education by the provision of opportunities for training and the development of human potential in order to improve the quality of individuals' own lives and to enable them to help others". It would benefit the project by donating funds and providing financial administration services.

There appeared to be a very positive balance, perhaps even a synergy, between the needs and aspirations of the main stakeholders. We decided to pursue the idea further.

BE PROACTIVE

When faced with the challenge of launching a big project (or dealing with a particularly tricky problem) it can be very easy to feel overwhelmed. This kind of thinking leads nowhere especially if you buy into the belief that there is nothing you can do. *There is always something you can do!* "Be Proactive" is the first of Covey's seven habits. The principle is simple yet profound. Waste your time worrying about what you can't influence and what you are able to achieve diminishes. Put your energy into what you can influence right now and gradually you will find yourself in a positon to achieve more than you thought possible.

OK so what resources did we have and what could we do? We had funds and administration support from the Hart Knowe Trust. The Mindfulness Association donated funds and put us in touch with tutors they had trained to teach the Mindfulness Based Living Course (MBLC) course. In spring 2016, Chloe Homewood and Heather Regan-Addis organised a weekend workshop called Compassion in Action where they shared the vision of the Mindfulness for Everyone Project. Some participants made donations and some mindfulness tutors who attended expressed their interest in being part of the new initiative. We could afford to sponsor between ten and fifteen MBLC courses. By September 2016, eleven tutors were ready to start teaching mindfulness to groups of: family carers, refugees, lone parents, volunteers, people dealing with physical and mental health and other problems arising from social inequality.

Before we knew it our first round of courses was up and running. It all came together quite easily. In my view this was because we kept it simple and didn't make it a big deal. We knew it might not be perfect but we weren't afraid to make a few mistakes: we did what we could do rather than worrying about what we couldn't do. When we started to hear back from the tutors about the positive impact the courses were having we wanted to continue.

NO FAILURE - ONLY FEEDBACK

Before taking the next step, Chloe, Heather and I took some time to reflect on what we had learnt and to consider what we might do better next time. Our application forms for the first round of funding had asked the tutors to tell us about their proposed project including information about: their own mindfulness practice; their teaching experience; the client group they would be helping; how they would recruit participants; how much it would cost to run the course. We received seventeen applications and we didn't have enough money to fund them all. We saw this as a good thing. To choose which courses to fund, we needed to clarify and prioritise our objectives. This is an example of the entrepreneurial mind-set described earlier. We were prepared to experiment and curious to learn from what happened. Isn't this what mindfulness practice is all about?

After the first round of courses, we looked back on what went well and what could have gone better. Some key themes came into focus: it was important that the tutors had a personal or professional affinity with the proposed client group; the most satisfactory way to recruit participants was through an organisation or charity already involved in supporting that group; projects with active support from a partnering organisation were more likely to go well; we had limited funds so it was important to get good value for money. The grant application form for subsequent rounds of funding was amended to include this statement:

Please remember that priority will be given to applications that meet the following criteria:

- *A clearly defined client group with significant needs that is likely to be helped by Mindfulness Training.*
- *Support from a partnering organisation with shared values that will be able to help you recruit participants.*
- *Offer good value for money, keeping costs low by working locally so as to minimize travel expenses and working with an organisation that is contributing its own resources to the project.*

As a result of what we had learnt we reduced the number of unsuitable grant applications and we were able to improve the assessment process. Subsequent projects ran more smoothly for the benefit of all concerned. We may be motivated by compassionate aspirations but we can still follow the tried and tested principles of effective action.

RESULTS OF STAGE ONE – ENLIGHTENED ENTERPRISE

Until now we have funded four rounds of projects, delivered in autumn 2016, spring 2017, spring 2018 and spring 2019. The courses have reached a total of sixty seven groups in locations throughout the UK. Around seven hundred participants have learnt how to practice mindfulness and what happens when they become more compassionate towards themselves and others.

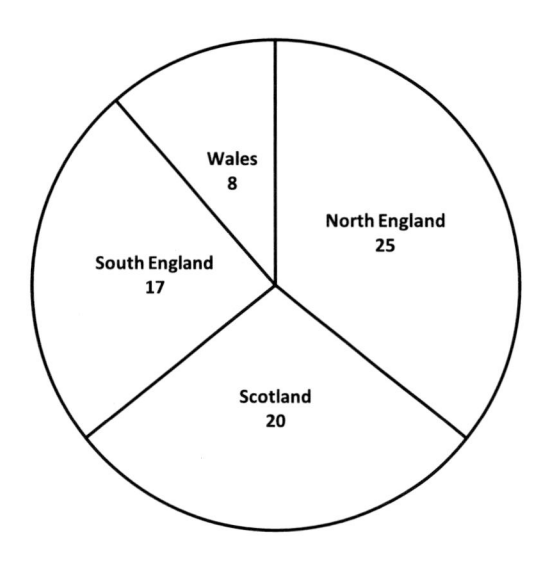

Figure 3: Numbers of courses delivered across four regions of the UK

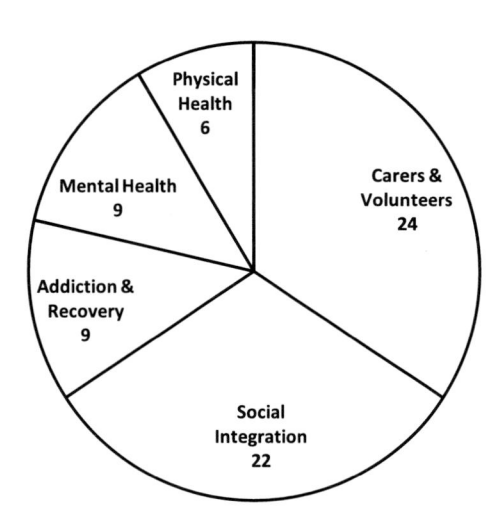

Figure 4: Numbers of courses delivered to five categories of client groups

There is not much point in pursuing activity that is efficient unless it is effective. So this brings us to Stage Two of our Compassionate Action Research which evaluated the impact of mindfulness training on the lives of participants in our courses

> **Pause and Plan**
>
> Do you have a project you would like to pursue if only you could but you can't see how it is possible?
>
> Maybe you could try this experiment. Sit quietly for a while and allow your mind to rest. Without worrying about what you can't do, ask yourself this question:
>
> Is there something simple and easy that I can do right now to get started?

STAGE TWO: COMPASSION BASED MINDFULNESS TRAINING

TRAINING IN MINDFULNESS AND COMPASSION

There are a number of recognised mindfulness courses available but the Mindfulness Based Living Course (MBLC) is distinctive in its focus on both mindfulness and compassion as a means of improving well-being. The key to compassion is the desire to prevent and help alleviate the suffering of others and the cultivation of well-being for oneself (Gilbert and Choden, 2013; Goetzz, et al., 2010; Van Dam, et al., 2011; Neff, 2011). It is difficult, although not impossible, for someone who is in the midst of significant suffering to extend compassion to others. Maybe compassion needs to begin at home. Self-Compassion is defined as having three basic components:

> 1) extending kindness and understanding to oneself rather than harsh self-criticism and judgement; 2) seeing one's experiences as part of the larger human experience rather than as separate and isolating; 3) holding one's painful thoughts and feelings in balanced awareness rather than over identifying with them (Neff, 2003, p.224).

In our modern society it is common to be excessively self-critical, even though this does not serve oneself or others well. I find that the more I am aware of my own suffering and truly mindful of the habitual processes that create it, the more genuine kindness and compassion I feel for others who share this human condition. The MBLC course is a compassion based mindfulness training; it teaches practices to awaken compassion for self and others and it is taught with compassionate motivation. The Mindfulness Association (MA) developed the MBLC course is based on their Level 1 Mindfulness Training (to find out more about the MA and the MBLC see Further Resources). It is an 8-week course consisting of eight classes, which are typically two hours long, preceded by an introductory class before the eight week course begins and concluded by a follow up class after the eight week course ends. A day of mindfulness practice is often included between weeks 6 and 7.

The weekly themes are:

- Introductory Session – What is Mindfulness and Why Practice It?
- Week 1 – Start Where We Are
- Week 2 – The Body as a Place to Stay Present
- Week 3 – Introducing Mindfulness Support
- Week 4 – Working with Distraction
- Week 5 – Exploring the Undercurrent
- Week 6 – Attitude of the Observer
- A day of Mindfulness Practice
- Week 7 – Self-acceptance
- Week 8 – A Mindfulness Based Life
- Follow Up – The Rest of Your Life

The Mindfulness for Everyone Project works with tutors who have been evaluated by the MA as ready to teach the MBLC course. They are committed to following the Good Practice Guidelines of the UK Network of Mindfulness Teacher Training Organisations. We wanted to ensure that people in disadvantaged communities would have access to the highest quality training available. As practitioners ourselves we recognised the value of including a compassionate attitude in our own practice and we felt it was particularly appropriate to offer mindfulness training that includes compassion to the vulnerable groups who we were hoping to benefit.

Pause and Learn

Go to the Mindfulness Association website where you can learn more about their compassionate approach to mindfulness and the MBLC training provided through the Everyone Project.

You could just follow your curiosity and have a look around the site or maybe you could watch some of the short videos by tutors and course participants. If you have time why not do one of the guided practices that are available in the free audio resources section.

www.mindfulnessassociation.net

QUANTITATIVE AND QUALITATIVE RESEARCH

The groups involved in our research came from various backgrounds. They all met our criteria for awarding grant funding; a clear indication that their lives were full of challenges most of us can only imagine. Participants and the organisations who hosted the projects were asked to help with research to evaluate the extent to which the MBLC training might contribute to improving well-being. Our tutors who collected information for the research assured participants that procedures were in place to ensure that all responses would be anonymous.

The **quantitative** research summarised here was carried out by Alan Hughes (to access the full version of Alan's research see Further Resources). Course participants were asked to complete three questionnaires at the beginning and end of their MBLC course:

- The WHO-5, Well-Being Index questionnaire: measures current mental well-being.
- The PSS-10, Perceived Stress Scale: measures the degree to which situations in a person's life are appraised as stressful.
- The MAAS, Mindfulness Attention Awareness Scale: measures the core characteristic of dispositional mindfulness

The **qualitative** research was carried out by Julie McColl. It provides a rich source of information and insight into participants' thoughts and feelings so as to gain a deeper understanding of the results from the questionnaires:

- Tutors conducted interviews with selected participants who had completed the course to inquire into how the MBLC course had affected their lives.

THE WHO-5 QUESTIONNAIRE

The World Health Organisation's Five Wellbeing Index Questionnaire is a widely used measure of psychological well-being. Participants are asked to assess their feelings over the past two weeks. In previous research studies, mindfulness has been found to be effective in improving psychological well-being. The participants attending our courses were from groups in society that do not normally have access to mindfulness training and so we wanted to know if mindfulness would be able to help with potentially more difficult issues.

Participants were asked to measure their own well-being according to a 6 point scale ranging from 5 (all of the time) to 0 (at no time) in response to the following five statements:

- I have felt cheerful and in good spirits
- I have felt calm and relaxed
- I have felt active and vigorous
- I woke up feeling fresh and refreshed
- My daily life has been filled with things that interest me

There was an overall increase in psychological well-being as measured by WHO-5 between the beginning and the end of the course, indicating that the course participants felt that their lives had improved in terms of their mental and physical well-being. This was a positive result for the participants.

PERCEIVED STRESS SCALE (PSS)

It has been well established in previous studies that there is an improvement in perceived stress as a result of mindfulness interventions. The Perceived Stress Scale asks people to look back over the past month and consider the degree to which situations in their own lives have been stressful. Participants were asked to say how the felt at the beginning and at the end of the courses using a scale of 0 (never) to 4 (very often) when answering the following ten questions:

- In the last month have you been upset because of something that happened unexpectedly
- In the last month, how often have you felt that you were unable to control the important things in your life
- In the last month have you felt nervous and stressed
- In the last month, how often have you felt confident about your ability to handle your personal problems
- In the last month how often have you felt that things were going your way
- In the last month, how often have you found that you could not cope with all the things that you had to do
- In the last month, how often have you been able to control irritations in your life
- In the last month, how often have you felt you were on top of things
- In the last month, how often have you been angered because of things that were outside of your control
- In the last month, how often have you felt difficulties were piling up so high that you could not overcome them

The overall result was a decrease in stress levels across the groups of participants although this was not the case for all individuals. Nevertheless, it was encouraging to observe this measurable overall improvement, given that many lived in highly stressful social situations.

MINDFUL ATTENTION AWARENESS SCALE (MAAS)

The Mindfulness Awareness Scale measures open or receptive awareness of and attention to what is taking place in the present. Responses are indicated on a 6 point scale ranging from 1 (almost always) to 6 (almost never). Participants are asked to assess the following fifteen statements:

- I could be experiencing some emotion and not be conscious of it until some time later on
- I break or spill things because of carelessness, not paying attention, or thinking of something else

- I find it difficult to stay focused on what is happening in the present
- I tend to walk quickly to get to where I'm going without paying attention to what I experience along the way
- I tend not to notice feelings of physical tension or discomfort until they really grab my attention
- I forget a person's name almost as soon as I've been told it for the first time
- It seems I am "running on automatic" without much awareness of what I am doing
- I rush through activities without being really attentive to them
- I get so focused on the goal I want to achieve that I lose touch with what I am doing right now to get there
- I do jobs automatically without being aware of what I'm doing
- I find myself listening to someone with one ear, doing something else at the same time
- I drive places on "automatic pilot" and then wonder why I went there
- I find myself preoccupied with the future and the past
- I find myself doing things without paying attention
- I snack without being aware of what I'm eating

There was a significant increase in the scores for all questions meaning that participants felt that they were living more in the present moment and were paying more attention to what was happening at any given time. These themes were also apparent in the participant interviews with featured in the following section.

PARTICIPANT INTERVIEWS

Five in depth interviews were carried out with participants by the mindfulness tutors leading the individual courses. The participants who had volunteered to take part in these interviews were promised anonymity. The interviews lasted approximately one hour and were recorded and transcribed. The participants were asked a series of open questions designed to explore their thoughts and feelings about how the course had affected their lives. They were asked to explain in their own words:

- Why they had chosen to enroll on a mindfulness course.
- What their feelings were towards themselves at the beginning of the course, if and how these feelings may have changed.
- Whether their stress levels had changed and if they dealt with stress differently at the end of the course.
- Were there any feelings of compassion towards themselves and others they wanted to talk about?
- If anything had changes in the way they relate to problems that arise and if they noticed any difference in the flow of their thoughts.
- Any difficulties they may have experienced: what had been the positive aspects of their ongoing mindfulness practice and the journey over the past eight weeks.

INTERVIEW RESULTS

Why they started

Most participants chose to attend a mindfulness course because they, or someone close to them, had experienced anxiety or/and they wished to support colleagues and clients at work. A few felt that they wanted to try using mindfulness to deal with anxiety rather than use medication. One person in particular was trying to help someone close to them who suffered from clinical depression. A recurring issue for this participant was the need to "rescue" people and mindfulness had made her more aware of this "rescuer tendency". Two participants, who had some prior experience of mindfulness, found it useful and wanted to explore it further:

> I think I really needed to be part of a group to get that motivation going and also there was a purpose to it if I could use it and understand it in my role as a counsellor.

Another participant from an asylum seekers group wanted to feel more positive about herself and had come to the course as recommended by her counsellor. This person had experienced particularly traumatic events in her life which had manifested in nightmares associated with the trauma, feelings of depression, fear and lack of confidence.

Feelings towards themselves

At the beginning of the course, participants admitted feeling worried about past and future, feeling as if they never had enough time, experiencing feelings of numbness. One participant said:

> I couldn't concentrate or think about things in detail. I started to question my confidence....this affected my work life.

Participants reported that as the course progressed, they became conscious of the changes in themselves even if they had not fully understood or grasped the practices when they were taught. One participant mentioned they had noticed the impact each session had on them. This had motivated them to continue with the course. Another felt less irritated by people, more able to accept what was happening without trying to control situations. Another noticed she was able to place more value on her own needs:

> I'm important. My mental health is important. There is still a sense of guilt....but now I know I'm not sitting doing nothing. I'm doing something

One person felt at the beginning of the course that mindfulness was for "hippies", however, by the end of the course he felt more relaxed and chilled, more able to deal with situations as they arose at work, "enjoying the journey!"

Stress levels and dealing with stress

Participants started the course with different feelings about how stressed they were. All felt some level of stress in their lives and all felt that their stress levels had reduced. Three participants felt stress was directly related to work or home life, the inability to say no or to worry about their work when they were there and at home. Two spoke about not being able to "leave work behind". One had now moved to a less stressful job. All felt able to cope better with stress and able to use the practices when stressful situations arose. One mentioned that the breathing space exercise had been very useful, another shouted less at people when driving. A participant, who had experienced a very traumatic situation in their past, reported at the beginning of the course suffering from flashbacks, feeling numb and having nightmares on a regular basis. She said she still felt stressed but now she was able to take some action to help to reduce her stress levels. She felt mindfulness had decreased her stress levels and helped to calm her down:

> It can help me when I feel that life is not worth living. I am still struggling with finance and accommodation so my situation hasn't changed....If I feel stressed I can remember how to relax. If I feel pain the breathing in and out helps. My stress has improved.

Compassion for self and others

Only one participant admitted not feeling more compassionate towards themselves at the end of the course. The other participants felt they were kinder towards themselves and felt less guilty about having time to themselves. One said this was an area of her life she was working on:

> I have worked on being kind to myself. That has been part of my recovery, developing kindness to myself and not thinking so horribly about myself.

The participant who had suffered trauma felt she was responsible for her situation and found it difficult to be compassionate towards herself because of what she had been through. She reported feeling that the compassionate practices had been hard, particularly the compassion practices for herself. However, she was coping with her life better and said she felt much better at the end of each session:

> I used to cut myself off for two to three years. I fragment my body….the course makes me feel I can put my body together.

All participants felt more able to deal with or communicate with people around them. One reported feeling more confident and less threatened by their boss and dealt with situations that arose in a more effective manner. Others said they felt they were more compassionate and more caring to the people close to them. Participants reported feeling less overwhelmed:

> Before mindfulness…I would drink or I would shout. Things like that…now my response is more balanced. I feel more in control and I respond in a more controlled way.

One person, who feared travelling on public transport because they felt discomfort at having people in their personal space, used mindfulness and compassion to help her when travelling and had been able to make journeys she had not been able to make previously. She also felt very strongly that she now wanted to help people who were in pain.

Problems and the flow of thoughts

Participants were asked if they related to or dealt differently in any way with problems that might arise in their lives. Most reported feeling a greater level of acceptance of things that happened and having a greater sense of perspective about what did and did not matter. One felt this was the result of her mindfulness training and practice. Most participants had used their mindfulness practices to help them through difficult situations. For example, one used the body scan regularly and another found it useful to bring her attention to her breath:

> I concentrate on one thing at once now. I recognise when I am becoming distracted and my mind is getting busy overthinking things. When this happens I talk really fast and get much louder. It's as if I have to say everything as quickly as I can. Sometimes it isn't even relevant stuff I'm blurting out. This has significantly reduced. My mind is calmer now. When I spot the racing mind I can bring my attention onto my breath and slow down.

Participants generally felt their flow of thoughts during the day was now calmer; one felt it was helping her to help herself feel in control. Another felt calmer and more considered in what she said whereas previously she might "offload a stream of thoughts". She felt this was beneficial to the people who worked closely with her and she now had a better relationship with her children. Others reported feeling more focused, able to deal with one thing at a time, feeling more positive and more able to enjoy work and home life:

> I am doing the three minute breathing space at night and during the day, remembering to be positive…..and what a difference.

Positives and negatives

All participants had enjoyed the course and felt it had been beneficial to them. They understood now that they were not alone in how they felt. They had enjoyed hearing of other people's experiences and sharing their own. All now wished for mindfulness to continue to be part of their lives, a few had sought to find people to practice with on an ongoing basis:

> It's a journey that I want to continue. I want it to be part of my life. I might not do it every day but it's made a difference.

The only negative aspects of mindfulness for the participants was finding time and space for their practice. All realised they were on a journey and that they would feel more confident of their practice in time:

> I am not alone. I feel connected to people. I feel their pain and problems. I felt it was just me but I am not alone. I will try to keep in contact with my peers. We can text each other to remind us to do mindfulness. I came up with that idea last week. I am just trying to take baby steps.

Finally, participants would have liked follow up mindfulness courses provided so that they could continue their practice with a group of like-minded people.

RESULTS OF STAGE TWO: COMPASSION BASED MINDFULNESS TRAINING

The data from the questionnaires gives an overview of the impact of the MBLC training provided by the Mindfulness for Everyone Project. The courses were successful in improving overall well-being, decreasing perceived stress levels and improving perceived mindful awareness of the participants. The interviews allowed the participants to tell their own moving stories of how compassion based mindfulness training changed their lives and affected the lives of those around them. In Stage One we found a way to share mindfulness with parts of our society that had previously been missing out. Stage Two of our Compassionate Action Research confirmed our supposition that mindfulness can indeed be effective in helping Everyone. So what's next?

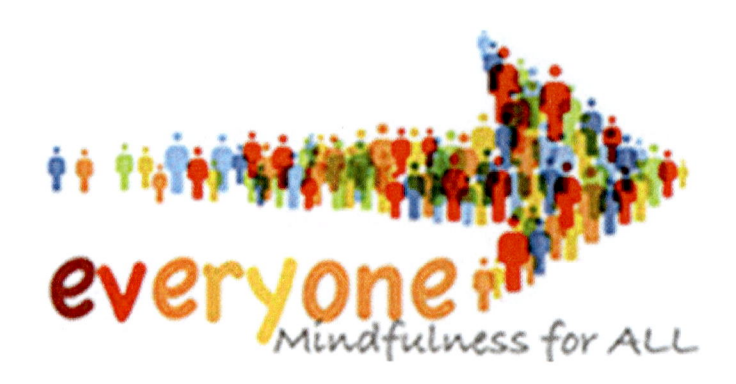

Figure 5: Logo © Everyone Project (2019)

STAGE THREE: GROWING A GREAT IDEA

As we move into Stage Three we have asked ourselves: What can we do better and how can the Mindfulness for Everyone Project operate on a bigger scale? I don't know who first said it, but I do like the saying: "It is difficult to make predictions, especially about the future!" There's not much to be gained by talking about plans that may well change, but I am happy to tell you a little about our grand aspirations: Who knows, maybe there is something you can do to help us to grow this great idea?

LEARNING ACTION

The Mindfulness for Everyone Project cannot exist without the tutors. They are skilled in delivering the MBLC course, but they also have a special personal or professional affinity with the client groups they work with which helps them understand the particular needs of the participants. The genuine kindness of the tutors is evident in the way they have been so committed in helping others. They are true mindful heroes. The tutors have also been responsible for making connections with local community organisations throughout the UK. These organisations are generally charities or non-profit organisations working with disadvantaged communities and they facilitate access to the courses by recruiting participants and providing community-based premises and other support.

We have always done our best to support the tutors through holding online meetings where members of the team can share with each other the challenges they face as well as the creative solutions they have found. Much of what we have learnt and many of the ideas for improvement we hope to implement in this stage have come from dialogue with the tutors and from their written feedback.

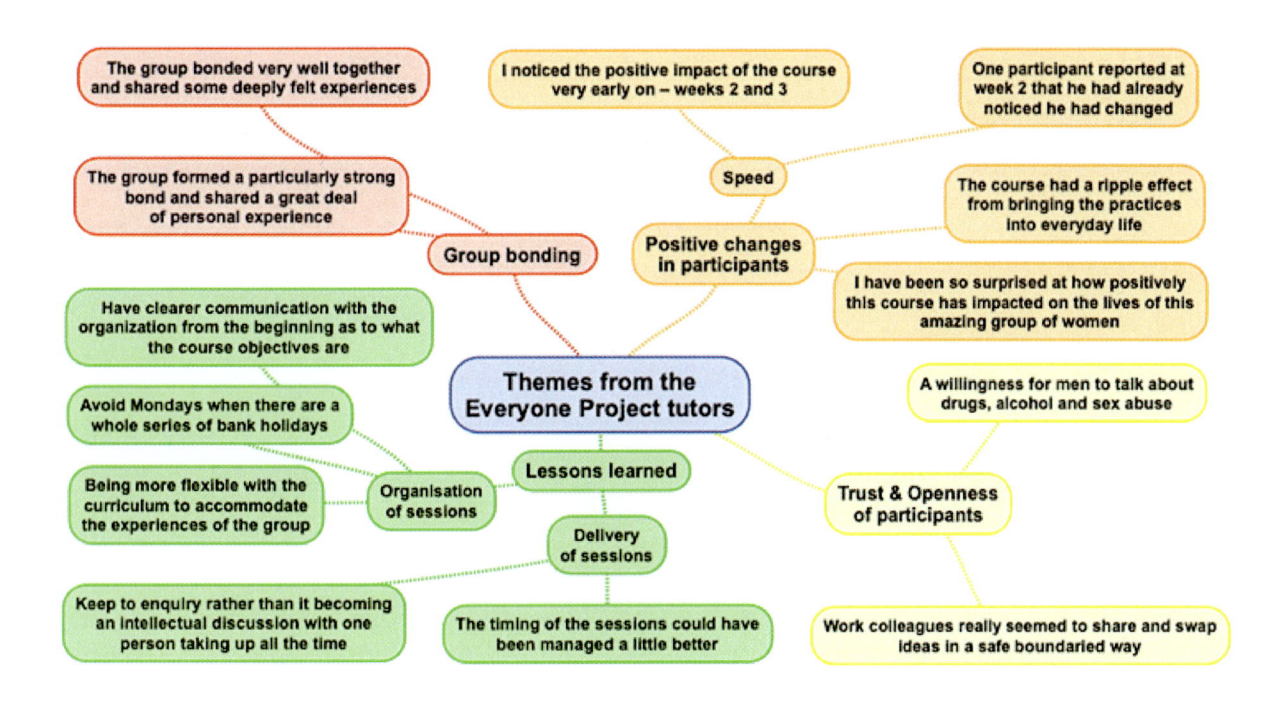

Figure 6: Example of tutor feedback report highlighting some common themes (McPhail, 2018)

Here are some examples of issues that have surfaced and a few ideas we are considering:

Importance of Support
Learning and practicing in a group of friends creates its own magic. It is not easy for anyone to establish a regular practice without some support, even when they have witnessed the benefits of mindfulness for themselves. We would like to be able to offer tutor led practice groups so that mindfulness becomes embedded in the communities we work with.

Need for Flexibility
The Everyone Project tutors have adapted the way they deliver the MBLC, improvising in order to meet the particular needs of the participants without compromising the integrity of the training. This challenge requires kindness, skill and balance. The tutors have also had to accept that the chaos of people's lives does not always conform to the timetable we set. We hope to create a forum for communication and learning from their experience.

Language and Learning
For some Everyone Project participants, English is not their first language. Others found the questionnaires difficult to understand. We can't assume that everyone is able to read the course manuals we provide. We plan to make audio recordings of the course materials. If we want to make a difference we must be willing to meet people where they are.

Time Constraints
Many participants found the recordings of guided practices too long. It was not easy to take so much time out to practice between course sessions. We want to create a library of shorter recorded practices to help people fit mindfulness into their busy unpredictable lives.

Organisations
Staff and volunteers working in organisations that look after others also need support. Many of them lead busy and stressful lives. Our courses are particularly effective when they are championed by someone within the host organisation. We want to explore initiatives for co-operation based on shared values to achieve a lasting positive impact.

THE EVERYONE PROJECT:
A SCOTTISH CHARITABLE INCORPORATED ORGANISATION

This section might sound a bit official but don't worry; we won't mistake the necessary means for the compassionate ends we keep in our hearts and minds. The Mindfulness for Everyone Project began as an informal collaboration between the Hart Knowe Trust and the Mindfulness Association. Representatives of these two organisations along with other helpers who joined the team discussed how best to grow the project to the next level. We wanted to create a vehicle suitable for this next stage of the adventure and so we founded a charitable organisation called The Everyone Project with the following mission and purposes:

To give the gift of mindfulness to help everyone in society to flourish through:

> The advancement of education and health primarily by making the benefits of mindfulness and related skills available in accordance with the Mindfulness Association Approach

> The advancement of science by researching the impact of mindfulness interventions to inform future developments (Everyone Project, 2019).

We intend to follow our successful strategy of encouraging tutors to establish links with local community organisations that can host courses as well as helping to recruit and support participants. Commitment to building mutually beneficial relationships remains at the heart of our plans for increased activity. Since the Mindfulness Association continues to train tutors who can deliver Mindfulness Based Living Courses (MBLC), the Everyone Project will be able to rely on the availability of qualified tutors. The Mindfulness Association is also providing funding for research into the effectiveness of future rounds of MBLC courses. Details of the proposed research can be found on the Everyone Project website (see Further Resources).

The Everyone Project continues to receive on-going financial support from Hart Knowe Trust in line with its stated charitable objectives. The Everyone Project SCIO is the asset lock for the Mindfulness Association which is a Community Interest Company and so profits that are not reinvested in the business are donated to the Everyone Project. However, it seems unlikely that our ambitious aspirations to grow the project to meet the needs we have identified can be funded solely by the Hart Knowe Trust and the Mindfulness Association. It is time to explore other sources of funding.

FINDING THE FUNDING

A friend of mine once asked his spiritual teacher who was about to embark on a large project; "Where is the money we need for this going to come from?" His teacher replied: "Wherever it is now!" Throughout the development of the Mindfulness for Everyone Project we have made the occasional leap of faith backed up by sound business principles and common sense. It has worked well so far. We have finished the Hobbit and we are about to start Lord of the Rings. I know it may be a lot bigger but it is more or less a continuation of the same story and the same principles will apply.

Members of our team have been preparing detailed proposals so that the Everyone Project can make applications for grant funding: and why not? We know we can take mindfulness to places it has not been before and we know how beneficial it is to the people mindfulness has not yet been able to reach. We also want to activate connections with the mindfulness community, people like you and me whose lives have been transformed by our practice of mindfulness and compassion. As we learn to accept who we are and discover who we could be, I trust we will all continue to look out for fresh opportunities to share our good fortune with others.

Don't Pause - Take Action!

I hope you are feeling inspired by this journey of Compassionate Action Research. I will be very happy if you now feel ready and able to do more than you thought possible.

Do you want to be part of the Everyone Project? Go to our website to find how you can help.

www.everyoneproject.org

ACKNOWLEDGEMENTS

The Mindfulness for Everyone Project is the journey of an ever growing team of mindful heroes who have each done their best to help others. It has fallen to me to tell the story and I want to honour: the vision and commitment of the project team; the kindness and skills of the tutors; the courage of course participants who have been willing to face the situations in which they find themselves; the generosity of so many organisations and individuals who have given their time and resources to make this altruistic aspiration a reality.

FURTHER RESOURCES

Keep up to date with the activities of the Everyone Project (SC048133)
www.everyoneproject.org

Find out more about the Mindfulness Association
www.mindfulnessassociation.net

CHODEN & REGAN-ADDIS, H., (2018).The Mindfulness Based Living Course. Alresford, UK: O-Books.

Mindfulness Association Research (including the research by Alan Hughes summarised in this chapter)
https://www.mindfulnessassociation.net/resources-and-research/research/

REFERENCES

BBC. (undated). https://www.bbc.co.uk/sport/athletics/48055305 [Date Accessed: 07/05/2019]
COVEY, S.R., (1992). The Seven Habits of Highly Effective People. Great Britain: Simon & Schuster.
ELLIOTT, J., (1991) Action Research for Educational Change. Milton Keynes and Philadelphia: Open University Press.
EVERYONE PROJECT, (2019). www.everyoneproject.org
GETTY IMAGES. https://www.istockphoto.com/gb/photo/people-of-different-ages-and-nationalities-having-fun-together-gm871518740-243462210 (purchased 20/05/2019)
GILBERT, P., & CHODEN., (2013). Mindful Compassion: Using the Power of Mindfulness and Compassion to Transform Lives. London: Robinson.
GOETZ J.L., KELTNER, D., & SIMON-THOMAS, E., (2010). Compassion: an evolutionary analysis and empirical review. American Psychological Association, 136, (3), pp 351-374.
https://commons.wikimedia.org/wiki/File:Riel-action_research.jpg
MAPPG, (2015) Report by the Mindfulness All-Party Parliamentary Group. Available: https://www.themindfulnessinitiative.org.uk/publications/mindful-nation-uk-report
MCPHAIL, D., (2019). Figure 6: Tutor Feedback Report for Everyone Project.
MURRAY, W.H., (1951) The Scottish Himalayan Expedition. London: J.M. Dent & Sons.
NEFF, K. (2003). The development and validation of a scale to measure self compassion. Self and Identity, 2, pp 223-250.
NEFF, K. (2011). Self Compassion: Stop Beating Yourself Up and Leave Insecurity Behind. London: Hodder and Stoughton.
REIL, M.(2006). Action research Spiral of change. Wikimedia Commons.Creative Commons 3.0 license. https://commons.wikimedia.org/wiki/File:Riel-action_research.jpg
VAN DAM, N.T., SHEPPARD, S. C., FOTSYTH, J. P., & EARLYEWINE, M., (2011). Self compassion is a better predictor than mindfulness of symptom severity and quality of life in mixed anxiety and depression. Journal of Anxiety Disorders, 25, pp 123-130.

THE EDITORS

TERRY BARRETT

I am an Assistant Professor in Educational Development at University College Dublin. I am currently the Programme Director of the postgraduate programmes in University Teaching and Learning at UCD. I have over twenty years of experience of working with problem-based learning (PBL). I have presented keynote papers on problem-based learning in Ireland, England, Finland and Australia. I co-edited (with Sarah Moore) New Approaches to Problem-based Learning: Revitalising Your Practice in Higher Education. New York: Routledge. My other research and teaching interests include curriculum design, creativity in higher education, peer observation of teaching, collaborative academic writing and mindfulness and compassion in education. I have published peer-reviewed papers in each of these areas. See https://scholar.google.com/citations?user=wUg_ZRYAAAAJ&hl=en for research publications. I have had a meditation practice for over 30 years. I facilitate workshops on mindful learning in higher education and coordinate a weekly guided mindfulness practice session for staff at UCD.

VIN HARRIS

I have studied and practiced meditation for more than 40 years under the guidance of many great Tibetan Buddhist masters. I have always aspired to follow the example of my main teacher Akong Rinpoche who taught me that it is possible to express spiritual values through practical action. It never seemed necessary to escape from the world. As well as establishing a very successful business, I have found the time to be a project manager for the construction of the Temple and College at Samye Ling the Executive Producer of an award-winning film. I founded the Hart Knowe Trust and I am a Trustee of the Everyone Project. I teach and develop mindfulness training programmes for individuals and organisations in the UK and Europe who appreciate my ability to communicate the subtle meaning and purpose of meditation practice in everyday language.

GRAEME NIXON

I am a senior lecturer at the University of Aberdeen. For the last nine years I have been the programme director of the University's MSc Studies in Mindfulness programme. I practice, publish on and supervise research projects on mindfulness. In this field I am particularly interested in debates about the possibility of secular mindfulness, Buddhist origins and criticisms of mindfulness. Formerly a secondary teacher of Religious, Moral and Philosophical Studies, I retain an interest in the manifestations of meditation across multiple wisdom traditions (religious or otherwise). As a teacher educator I am particularly interested in the development of thinking skills in schools and I have written on this as well as delivered training for professionals on how to weave a suite of thinking skills approaches (including mindfulness) into their life and work.

THE CONTRIBUTORS

JOHN ARNOLD

Mountain outdoor life and nature have always held an attraction for me and I now share my passion through leading mindfulness mountain retreats in the Italian Alps. You can find out about this on my website: In summer I am a keen hiker and yogi; during the winter I am a skier. I have qualifications and experience in life coaching and mentoring as well as coaching snow sports. I graduated in 2014 from Aberdeen University with an MSc in Mindfulness Studies and have qualified through the Mindfulness Association to teach mindfulness. You can find out more about me and my work at http://www.mindfulmountains.com/about/people/john-arnold/

HEATHER GRACE BOND

I am a mindfulness and compassion teacher (children and adults) and author of self-help book, 'Awakening Child: A journey of inner transformation through teaching your child mindfulness and compassion'. I have taught mindfulness to children of all ages and stages in both school and family settings and I am currently studying for a PhD in Education with the University of Aberdeen, researching the role (if any) of self-compassion in Scottish secondary schools.

MISHA BOTTING

I was born in Moscow (Russia) and trained in Moscow Bolshoi Ballet Academy. My professional classical ballet career started in Moscow and finished in Glasgow. I am very keen to bring my experiences and knowledge to future generations of performers in arts and sport. I now lead a team of sport psychologists in Sportscotland Institute of Sport and have the highest qualification for professional sport psychology: High Performance Sport Accreditation (BASES). I was a part of Team GB during Winter Olympic Games in Sochi 2014 and PyongChang 2018. My particular area of interest is developing mindfulness and compassion in team sports.

GAVIN CULLEN

I am a lecturer in mental health practice in the School of Health and Social Care at Edinburgh Napier University, having previously worked as a nurse, mainly in an NHS child and adolescent mental health service. I completed the Mindfulness Association and University of Aberdeen's wonderful MSc Studies in Mindfulness in 2014. I practice and teach mindfulness whenever I can and have recently begun PhD research exploring mindful compassion training for student nurses. I am particularly interested in how nurses and their colleagues can sustain resilience, and in how we could build a community of mindful practitioners to benefit everyone.

PAUL D'ALTON

Over the course of my career I have been blessed to find environments where this radical act of turning up to suffering is encouraged and supported. I have taught the 8-week Mindfulness Based Cognitive Therapy (MBCT) programme to close to 500 patients in acute care at the hospital where I am Principal Clinical Psychologist and Head of Department. I am also an Associate Professor at University College Dublin where I founded and co-direct the MSc in Mindfulness Based Interventions. I am the external examiner at the Centre for Mindfulness at the University of Bangor, Wales.

JOHN DARWIN

Following community work in north east England, I joined Newcastle City Council, later moving to Sheffield City Council, where I became a Chief Officer. My third career was academic. I have master's degrees in Mathematical Logic and Business Administration, and a Doctorate on "Complexity Theory and Fuzzy Logic in Strategic Management". My books include The Enterprise Society and Developing Strategies for Change. I have practised meditation and yoga for more than 25 years, and my fourth 'career' is teaching mindfulness. I completed the MSc [with distinction] in Studies in Mindfulness at University of Aberdeen. I am a Teaching Fellow there and Visiting Fellow at Sheffield Business School. I am also an authorised teacher of Śamatha-Vipassanā with Dharma Treasure Sangha.

TARJA GORDIENKO

I work as a journalist and as a communications professional in Finland. I am Finnish, and I hold a master's degree in communications and social sciences from the Helsinki University. My true passion is writing, and I firmly believe that you can shape your life by writing about it. This has led me to use an auto ethnographic approach in writing to explore my personal experience of work addiction in my dissertation which I completed in 2018 for the MSc Studies in Mindfulness at the School of Education, University of Aberdeen.

DONALD GORDON

I completed my MSc in Studies in Mindfulness in 2014. This included a work-based dissertation on the effects of mindfulness on children with autistic spectrum condition. Along with my background in mindfulness, I have broad experiences working in education within secondary, tertiary and the special needs sectors, as well as working in the area of biodiversity conservation as an employee and environmental consultant. I currently teach science at the college level and I am becoming increasingly interested in combining aspects of nature, environmental education and mindfulness in supporting the wellbeing of young people as well as helping to address current environmental challenges.

SUSAN GRANDFIELD

I have a passion for enabling people to become more conscious and purposeful in their personal and professional lives. For over 20 years I have worked with individuals, teams and leaders in the UK and globally to help them become more self-aware, more effective and more resilient. My approach combines psychology and neuroscience with my business experience and is underpinned by my long-standing mindfulness practice. I have a particular interest in conscious leadership and frequently write blogs and receive invitations to speak at events on the topic. I completed the Aberdeen University Studies in Mindfulness MSc in 2018.

ALAN HUGHES

I became interested in Buddhism, and started meditating, in my late teens. In the 1990s, I started practicing within the Tibetan tradition, and eventually started attending courses and retreats with Rob Nairn, whenever he was in the UK. This naturally led me to become involved with the Mindfulness Association, and to do the MSc Studies in Mindfulness course at Aberdeen University. In 2011, I gave up my job as a marine biologist to deepen my interest in Buddhism and meditation and worked as a full-time volunteer at Kagyu Samye Dzong London for five years. I now focus on teaching mindfulness and helping out with administration for the Mindfulness Association.

TERRY HYLAND

I have taught in schools, colleges and universities throughout the UK and retired as Professor of Education at the University of Bolton in 2009. I am currently a Director and Trustee at the Free University of Ireland in Dublin where I teach philosophy and mindfulness to 'second chance' mature students. I have over 200 publications - including 8 books, 24 book chapters and over 180 articles - on a diverse range of philosophy of education topics. A book very relevant to this publication is: Hyland, T. (2011) Mindfulness and Learning: Celebrating the Affective Dimension of Education. (Dordrecht, The Netherlands: Springer Press).

NAOMI McAREAVEY

I have been trying to practice mindfulness for five years and have experienced its positive effects on my life and work. I have brought some contemplative practices into the classroom in University College Dublin where I teach Shakespeare and Renaissance literature. I research and write on the literature and culture of early modern Ireland and I am co-editor, with Julie A. Eckerle, of Women's Life Writing and Early Modern Ireland (University of Nebraska Press, 2019) and, with Fionnuala Dillane and Emilie Pine, of The Body in Pain in Irish Literature and Culture (Palgrave, 2016).

JULIE McCOLL

I am Professor of Marketing at York St John University. With a background in business education, I joined the MSc Studies in Mindfulness at Aberdeen University in 2014 having explored the subject through popular psychology over many years. I completed the MBLC teacher training in 2016, have taught on the Everyone Project and have been involved in running mindfulness courses for students in the UK and abroad with very positive results. As an academic, I have also been research active, publishing in the area of mindfulness in education and, with colleagues from the Mindfulness Association, mindfulness for healthcare staff. I continue to maintain a personal practice in mindfulness.

LARRY McNUTT

I am currently the Registrar and a member of the senior management at the Technological University Dublin - Blanchardstown Campus. I have over 35 years' experience in the Higher Education both in Ireland and Australia. I am a Fellow of the Irish Computer Society and am a member of the board of AHEAD (https://ahead.ie/) and my research interests and publications include distance education, educational technology, instructional design, computer science education and universal design for learning. I studied computer science in University College Dublin (UCD) and hold a master's degree in Education (Multimedia) from the University of New England, Australia and a Doctorate in Education from NUI Maynooth.

SARAH MOORE (FITZGERALD)

I am an award-winning professor, teacher and novelist. Based at the University of Limerick my academic career has focused on enhancing teaching and learning through creative practice. As well as a researcher and teacher, I am the author of four published novels, with a further one now complete and due for publication in July 2019. My fiction has been translated into seventeen languages and also adapted for the stage. I have presented at many festivals and conferences throughout the world. I am currently part of the Creative Writing team at the University of Limerick, part of the UL Frank McCourt summer school teaching team and founder of UL's Creative Writing Winter School for professional writers.

KARL MORRIS

I am author of the recently released book The Lost Art of Putting as well as Attention –the secret to YOU playing great golf and Golf –The Mind Factor with Ryder Cup captain Darren Clarke. I have personally trained over 1000 certified Mind Factor coaches (www.themindfactor.com). From other sports my clients include Ashes winning England captain Michael Vaughan, premiership footballers including recently England capped Tom Heaton. My passion is to provide golfers of all levels with simple and effective tools to get the very best from their game. My Mind Factor seminars have been presented all over the world.

JANE NEGRYCH

I am the Programme Manager at the Sanctuary in Dublin Ireland, where I develop and teach mindfulness and compassion courses. Previously, I have worked as the Communications Manager for the Mindfulness Association, where I am still part of their tutor team. I have taught for the University of Winnipeg, as well as the University of Aberdeen. I also teach mindfulness and compassion in a number of different contexts for DCU's (Dublin City University) Recovery College.

JANA NEUMANNOVA

Although I initially trained as a physiotherapist in the Czech Republic, after moving to Scotland in 2002 I started working with homeless, disabled clients, people experiencing mental health issues and people in substance recovery. I also completed the MSc in Mindfulness programme at the University of Aberdeen in 2017. I believe that working directly in local community is the best way to improve people's wellbeing and I like sharing with others what I have learnt from mindfulness practice.

SUSANNE OLBRICH

I am a musician and music educator. I am a qualified teacher of Mindfulness-based Stress Reduction (MBSR) and Mindfulness-based Living (MBLC), and I was authorised by Thich Nhat Hanh to teach the Plum Village approach to mindfulness. I have led many workshops and retreats in the UK and Germany, and I especially enjoy combining mindfulness with creative expression. As a pianist and composer, my work embraces classical, jazz and folk. Recordings include my album 'Continuations'. I am currently completing an MSc Studies in Mindfulness with the University of Aberdeen, researching the links between mindfulness meditation and creativity.

JOANNE O'MALLEY

I am a passionate and committed mindfulness and compassion practitioner, teacher and speaker. My mission is to help people strengthen their connection to their inner voice and wisdom, so they can be more aware, present and wholehearted at work and live more deeply and fully. I set up Mindfulness at Work https://mindfulnessatwork.ie/ in 2012 to offer Corporate Mindfulness Programmes that improve both individual and organisational leadership, wellbeing, resilience and relationships. I am privileged to have spoken at conferences and taught a range of Corporate Mindfulness Programmes in many of Ireland's top organisations and abroad. I share positive, practical tools and practices that move people to work more cohesively with vitality, resilience and compassion.

IAN RIGG

I have been studying and practicing mindfulness since 2004 under the guidance of Rob Nairn and have participated in a number of week long and month long retreats with a variety of teachers in the U.K., South Africa and India. In 2010, I enrolled on the first cohort of the Studies in Mindfulness MSc and graduated from this programme with an MSc in 2013. I have been teaching mindfulness since 2012 and I am currently employed by the NHS to design, deliver and research mindfulness-based interventions for staff as well as being a lead tutor for the Mindfulness Association. I have a particular interest in mindful movement and also teach martial arts and yoga.

JACKY SEERY

I work as Communications Manager for the Mindfulness Association. I graduated with the MSc Studies in Mindfulness with the University of Aberdeen in 2018 and I am a fully trained mindfulness and compassion teacher. Having held a lifelong fascination with the benefits of Eastern health practices, I completed 10 years of training courses in Tai Chi, Qigong and Chi Yoga and I am a dedicated practitioner and teacher. I combine compassion-based mindfulness and mindful movement and run courses, workshops and retreats in the UK, Sweden and Spain.

DAVID WARING

I graduated from The Laban Centre for Movement and Dance in 1987 and I am currently Artistic Director of Transitions Dance Company at Trinity Laban Conservatoire for Music and Dance. I have performed, choreographed and taught both in the UK and internationally with a range of companies and as an independent dance artist. Recently, I have been making and performing my guerrilla style 'hustler' series. In 2017 I completed my University of Aberdeen MSc Studies in Mindfulness. I have studied Zero Balancing and I want to train as a Breath Coach.